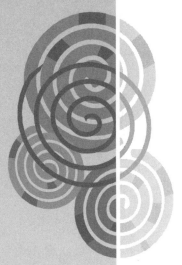

The Auditory System
Anatomy, Physiology, and Clinical Correlates

Frank E. Musiek
University of Connecticut

Jane A. Baran
University of Massachusetts Amherst

PEARSON

Boston • New York • San Francisco
Mexico City • Montreal • Toronto • London • Madrid • Munich • Paris
Hong Kong • Singapore • Tokyo • Cape Town • Sydney

Executive Editor and Publisher: Stephen D. Dragin
Editorial Assistant: Meaghan Minnick
Production Managing Editor: Joe Sweeney
Editorial–Production Service: nSight, Inc.
Composition and Prepress Buyer: Linda Cox
Manufacturing Buyer: Megan Cochran
Cover Administrator: Kristina Mose-Libon
Electronic Composition: Laserwords

For related titles and support materials, visit our online catalog at www.ablongman.com.

ISBN: 0-205-33553-5

Printed in the United States of America

10 9 8 7 6 5 4 3 2 1   VHP-IA   10 09 08 07 06

Contents

2 THE EXTERNAL EAR: ITS STRUCTURE AND FUNCTION   38

3 ANATOMY AND PHYSIOLOGY OF THE MIDDLE EAR   48

4 FUNCTIONAL ANATOMY OF THE COCHLEA   71

5 COCHLEAR PHYSIOLOGY I: MOSTLY MECHANICS   97

6 COCHLEAR PHYSIOLOGY II: MOSTLY ELECTROPHYSIOLOGY 112

7 STRUCTURE AND FUNCTION OF THE AUDITORY NERVE 150

8 THE FIRST CENTRAL AUDITORY STRUCTURE: THE COCHLEAR NUCLEUS 172

11 THE MEDIAL GENICULATE BODY AND AUDITORY THALAMUS   222

12 THE AUDITORY CORTEX AND SUBCORTEX   235

13   THE CORPUS CALLOSUM AND AUDITORY INTERHEMISPHERIC FUNCTION   264

14   VASCULAR ANATOMY OF THE AUDITORY SYSTEM   284

15 THE EFFERENT SYSTEM   299

Preface

The Auditory System: Anatomy, Physiology, and Clinical Correlates was written to provide a comprehensive text on the anatomy and physiology of the peripheral as well as the central auditory systems. The approach to this book is slightly different than what is generally planned for books on the structure and function of the auditory system. This book is written primarily for clinicians, with the hope of drawing more practitioners into the important process of reading and learning more about the anatomy and physiology of the auditory system. After conducting surveys as well as extensive discussions with clinicians, we have learned several concepts and approaches that may make a book on anatomy and physiology more appealing to clinicians. These concepts and approaches follow and provide the impetus for this book.

1. As noted by the title of this book, we will highlight clinical correlates to the basic science principles that are being presented. Whenever possible, a case study, a brief review, or a clinical comment will be connected to the basic science principle being discussed. This added clinical information will be highlighted in the text as *clinical or pathologic correlates*. The purpose of this feature is to help establish the link between science and practice in a brief but relevant way. We believe this will make this text more interesting and useful for the clinically oriented student and professional.

2. This book makes generous use of secondary references because many review chapters and articles are often easier to follow and are more relevant to the clinician. Our interaction with clinicians has taught us that basic science articles are not usually read—even when recommended. Instead, review articles are sought for a better grasp on the subject. Hence, we have tried to provide some key basic science readings (original or key articles) for each of the topics covered, and whenever possible, we have also included review articles or chapters as supplementary references. Finally, we have tried to select basic science articles that have a clinical slant or clinical implications for inclusion in this text.

3. In the past decade or so, considerable interest and research has been focused on neuroscience and the central auditory system. However, prior to this time, there was far more attention devoted to the peripheral system. In this text, we have tried to balance the coverage of both peripheral and central systems so that the reader can be exposed to both portions of the auditory system in sufficient depth to be able to appreciate the nature of the processing that occurs at the two levels. The text will present information regarding the similarities in the auditory processes conducted at the two levels, as well as the unique types of processing that occur not only between the two levels, but also among some of the structures within each level of the auditory system.

4. Although it has been difficult to do, we have tried to use the human model as much as possible in our discussion of the anatomy and physiology of the auditory system. So much work has been completed on animals and so little on humans that it often was a challenge to limit the discussion to the human model—but a serious effort has been made to do this in this book.

5. This book is aimed not only at the clinician, but also at the student—especially those enrolled in doctor of audiology (Au.D.) programs who need to understand the anatomy and physiology of the human hearing mechanism as it is relevant to clinical audiology. A number of Au.D. programs have split their hearing science course into two courses: one on anatomy and physiology and one on psychoacoustics. We feel this is an appropriate approach and one for which this book is well suited.

6. The fields of anatomy and physiology have exploded, with large quantities of new research information appearing in the literature on a regular basis. Most of this is important indeed, but it is not always relevant to the clinician. We therefore have tried to sort out what is most salient to the audiologist (perhaps our most difficult task) and keep the book a reasonable length.

Importance to the Clinician

An understanding of the biological aspects of the auditory system is essential to the knowledgeable clinician. At first glance many clinicians perhaps wonder how knowledge of anatomy and physiology of the auditory system will help them in their everyday activities. However, if one closely reflects upon what a clinician in hearing and hearing disorders does in any given day, the role of biology becomes obvious. A number of clinical activities come to mind that are dependent on the provider being familiar with the structure and function of the auditory system.

Communication with other clinicians in the same as well as different disciplines can be enhanced greatly by understanding anatomy and physiology. Long-lasting opinions are formed in the clinical arena by brief discussions of difficult patients, diagnoses, and treatments. One who is well grounded in anatomy and physiology can better understand and contribute to these types of discussions.

Clinicians are responsible, to varying degrees, for test selection and interpretation. These are the evaluation tools that are critical to the proper diagnosis of the patient. Tests are a measure of function and function is intimately related to structure. Knowing how to administer a test but not understanding the underlying functions that it is assessing is doing only half the job. For example, an absent acoustic reflex is of little value if one does not know the anatomy of the acoustic reflex circuit. Clinicians well oriented toward anatomy and physiology are in a much better position to optimally utilize tests and test results than those who are not.

Radiological information is becoming more available and more sophisticated. Diagnostic clinicians can be helped by radiological information on a patient. However, radiology is a specialty that is based on anatomy. Without anatomical knowledge, radiological information cannot be utilized efficiently. Correlations of test results to radiological findings is the backbone of diagnostic audiology, and these correlations (or lack of them) cannot be accomplished without a solid anatomical grounding.

Clinicians work with people who have a variety of auditory disorders. In order to understand a given disorder, the locus and function of the structure(s) affected must be known. At times the anatomy and physiology related to a given disorder may provide insight as to the nature of the problem and what is to be expected. For example, we know that kernicterus primarily compromises the cochlear nucleus in the brainstem even though it often manifests as a high-frequency sensorineural hearing loss, which could be interpreted as a peripheral problem. Utilizing only a peripheral audiologic evaluation would miss the key aspects of this disorder.

Finally, patient counseling is dependent on knowledge of the anatomy and physiology of the auditory system. Better explanations of the patient's problems come from clinicians who understand the basics of structure and function. Anatomical models and illustrations can help enhance understanding for the patient. With common use of the Internet, patients are more knowledgeable and can ask demanding questions about the underlying anatomy and physiology of their disorders. Many of them know and appreciate what has been known in science for many years: that anatomy along with its physiology is the common denominator for understanding how we hear or do not hear. It therefore is critical for hearing healthcare professionals to have a solid grounding in anatomy and physiology in order to be able to effectively counsel patients with auditory disorders and to be able to answer their patients' questions with knowledge and confidence.

Closing Comments

We trust that this book has helped make explicit the link between the structures and functions of the auditory system and the specific clinical correlates that are tied to the underlying basic science principles and concepts that have been presented. It was with much deliberation and careful consideration of this intent that we decided on the title for our text: *The Auditory System: Anatomy, Physiology, and Clinical Correlates*. Finally, we hope, the reader of this book will become a better, more informed provider of care to individuals with hearing loss and hearing deficits, having gained these insights.

Acknowledgments

I am grateful to many people who have helped me in a variety of ways with this book. For many years Jane Baran, my coauthor, has been a close friend and colleague. Her many contributions to the completion of this work have been immeasurable, and I thank her for these and her continued support. A special thanks is in order for doctoral student Jeff Weihing, whose fine computer skills and great work ethic were critical to the completion of this book. Recent graduate Jennifer Shinn and doctoral student Jennifer Paulovicks were of great assistance to me in many aspects of this effort and deserve mention here.

Kent Morest's ongoing support and sage advice as well as his insightful comments on this book are deeply appreciated. I thank Tony Sahley, Bill Loftus, Jim Kaltenbach, Jacek Smurzynski, East Tennessee State University, Dennis Phillips, Albert R. De Chicchis, The University of Georgia, John A. Ferraro, University of Kansas Medical Center, Laura Ann Wilber, Northwestern University, Craig A. Champlin, University of Texas at Austin, and Deborah Moncrieff, University of Florida for their useful comments and reviews on various segments of this book. Richard Salvi, Ann Clock Eddins, and Jian Wang are acknowledged for the fine chapter they contributed.

Two special people have positively influenced me and my career and I would like to mention them. The late Marilyn Pinheiro and the late Dudley Weider were colleagues and friends who helped me in many ways and they will always be remembered.

Finally I wish to thank my gracious and lovely wife, Sheila, and my two wonderful sons, Erik and Justin, for their constant support and interest in everything I do. — FM

I also am grateful to the many fine individuals who have contributed in many important ways to this book. I first and foremost want to thank my colleague and coauthor, Frank Musiek. I have had the privilege and honor of working with him for a number of years, and this book is but one of the fruits of this collaboration. Without his diligence, persistence, and insights, this book would not have become a reality. He is one of those rare individuals who is not only a good colleague but also a valued and trusted friend.

I also would like to recognize the individuals that Frank Musiek has mentioned in his acknowledgments. I will not mention all of these individuals again here, but I would like to add my sincere thanks and expression of appreciation to all of these individuals, as each of them has made an important contribution to the success of this book. I would also like to recognize Beth Ann Jacques, who is a graduate student at the University of Massachusetts Amherst. Beth Ann provided invaluable technical assistance with the generation of the reference list for this book.

Finally, I especially want to thank my husband, David Hoffman, and my daughter, Sarah Jane, who continually offered their encouragement, assistance, and support throughout this endeavor. —JAB

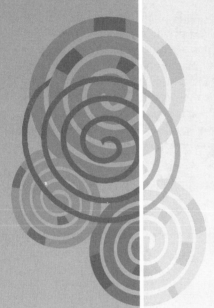

1

Overview of the Anatomy and Physiology of the Auditory System

Introduction to the Auditory System

The auditory system is often divided into peripheral and central components (Figure 1.1). The peripheral system includes the outer ear, the middle ear, the cochlea, and the auditory nerve (AN). The central auditory system includes the cochlear nucleus (CN), the superior olivary complex (SOC), the lateral lemniscus (LL) (both nuclei and pathways), the inferior colliculus (IC), the medial geniculate body (MGB), the auditory subcortex (subcortical white matter and basal ganglia region), the cortex, and the interhemispheric pathways (including the corpus callosum).

The peripheral auditory system is located for the most part in the temporal bone, part of the cranium, and the central auditory system is located in the brain. Specifically, the CN, SOC, and LL are situated in the pons, the IC is in the midbrain, and the MGB is in the caudal thalamus. The auditory subcortex and cortex involve structures such as the internal capsule, the insula, Heschl's gyrus, the planum temporale, and other parts of the superior temporal gyrus. Auditory responsive areas also include segments of the frontal lobe, the parietal lobe, the angular gyrus, the supramarginal gyrus, and the corpus callosum. This entire system is often referred to as the auditory afferent system, meaning it courses from the ear up to and including the brain. There is also an efferent system, which is almost the reverse of the afferent system in that it runs a similar route but from the cortex down to the cochlea.

CLINICAL CORRELATE

In diagnostic audiology, considerable effort is expended in differentiating conductive hearing loss from sensorineural hearing loss. Conductive hearing loss involves dysfunction or compromise of the conductive apparatus (i.e., the outer and/or middle ear). Most conductive hearing losses can be medically or surgically corrected, whereas the majority of sensorineural losses are not typically amenable to medical intervention, which means that they tend to be permanent. The hearing deficits associated with conductive and sensorineural losses are quite different in their nature; therefore, it is important for the clinician to differentiate these two types of losses so that the best management approaches can be implemented.

Although much of the early diagnostic work in audiology was directed toward differentiating conductive versus sensorineural hearing

(continued)

losses, the focus for many years was centered on differentially diagnosing conductive versus "sensory" hearing losses (i.e., hearing losses originating within the inner ear or cochlea). More recently, however, because of advances in both basic science and diagnostic methods, it has become important for the audiologist to identify cochlear versus retrocochlear (all structures past the cochlea) dysfunction. This need to differentially diagnose cochlear versus retrocochlear losses was initially driven by the fact that most lesions of the AN were acoustic tumors or serious lesions of the brain. Hence, the accurate identification of the site of lesion had important implications for the medical management for many patients with retrocochlear lesions. Even more recently, it has become important for audiological management purposes that cochlear sites of lesion be differentiated from retrocochlear sites even if the lesions are benign.

Again, this is because a different set of hearing problems arise from compromise of the retrocochlear system compared to those seen with involvement of the cochlea. Most recently, audiologists have begun to diagnose and manage central auditory disorders or central auditory processing disorders (CAPDs). These disorders are caused by dysfunction or compromise of the auditory system in the brain. Central auditory disorders are retrocochlear disorders that exclude the AN.

It has become important in the clinical domain to know and define the different areas of the auditory system because various regions are responsible for various auditory functions. Each area contributes its own special aspect of processing acoustic signals. It is also important to realize the auditory system is well orchestrated and works as a whole. The different parts of the auditory system are interdependent. •

● Figure 1.1

Highly schematized drawing of the peripheral and central auditory systems.

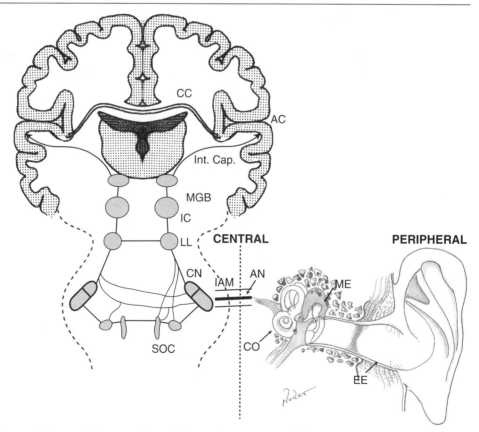

EE = external ear and canal, ME = middle ear, CO = cochlea, AN = auditory nerve, IAM = internal auditory meatus, CN = cochlear nucleus, SOC = superior olivary complex, LL = lateral lemniscus, IC = inferior colliculus, MGB = medial geniculate body, Int. cap. = internal capsule, AC = auditory cortex, CC = corpus callosum.

In general, the auditory system performs two kinds of processing of acoustic stimuli—sequential and parallel. Sequential processing is the transferring of information from one area or level to the next. Sequential processing lends itself to a hierarchical organization as one ascends the auditory afferent system. Parallel processing involves overlapping functions that occur at about the same time along different channels. Both of these major types of processing are needed for optimal function of the auditory system. Sequential processing takes place in the entire auditory system, but parallel processing takes place, for the most part, in the neural system. Examples of parallel processing are noted throughout the auditory neural system. The AN has type I and type II fibers that proceed in parallel to the brainstem. Likewise, the left and right sides of the brainstem pathways proceed in parallel to the cortex. The cortex is highly sequential but also has separate groups of fibers coursing in parallel between the primary and secondary auditory cortex as well as to other areas of the brain (Rouiller, 1997).

Another principle that applies to the entire auditory system, although it is manifested primarily at the cochlear, AN, and brain levels, is the influence of inhibition and excitation. More evidence is emerging to indicate that a balance between excitation and inhibition processes in the auditory system (as well as other systems) is critical for normal function. It is speculated that such maladies as tinnitus and hypersensitivity to sound may have as their bases an imbalance between inhibition and excitation in the auditory system.

THE PERIPHERAL AUDITORY SYSTEM

External and Middle Ear

• *Anatomy and Physiology*

Sounds entering the auditory system do so by initially traveling through the outer ear to the middle ear and then they are passed on to the inner ear and the neural pathways of the peripheral and central auditory nervous systems (Figure 1.2). As part of this process of sound transmission within the auditory system, the sounds detected by the ear are converted from acoustic energy at the outer ear to vibratory (or mechanical) energy in the middle and inner ears to a neural representation of the acoustic signal at the cochlea and beyond. Anatomically, the outer ear consists of the pinna and the external auditory meatus (EAM), also known as the ear canal. The pinna protrudes from the side of the head and has a foundation of ligaments and cartilage that is covered by skin. This outer ear structure has a number of ridges and depressions and probably serves as collector of sound energy. Because of the unique configuration of ridges and depressions or grooves in this structure, it tends to respond maximally to some sounds within the high-frequency range (around 5000 Hz). The result of this preferential response is that acoustic signals in this frequency range are differentially enhanced or amplified before they are directed to the ear canal. The differential sound-collection properties of the pinna are believed to assist in sound localization (Yost, 2000).

The EAM accepts the sounds arriving at the ear and directs these acoustic signals to the tympanic membrane (TM). Because of its configuration, which is much like a pipe or tube that is closed at one end and open at the other, the EAM generates an ear canal resonance that is determined, at least in part, by the dimensions of the ear canal. In adults, this resonance (the enhancement of an acoustic signal) typically occurs at a frequency in the vicinity of 3000 to 4000 Hz. The presence of this

● **Figure 1.2**

Main structures of the peripheral auditory system and cross section of the cochlea.

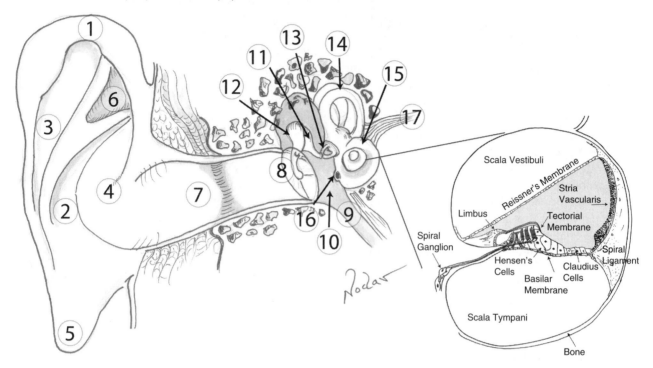

1 = helix, 2 = anti-helix, 3 = caphoid fossa, 4 = concha, 5 = lobe, 6 = triangular fossa, 7 = external auditory meatus, 8 = tympanic membrane, 9 = Eustachian tube, 10 = middle ear space (tympanum), 11 = incus, 12 = malleus, 13 = stapes, 14 = superior semicircular canal, 15 = bony cochlea shell (otic capsule), 16 = round window, 17 = eighth nerve.

ear canal resonance is important for the natural perception of sound. The loss or compromise of the normal ear canal response can result in the perception of speech and other acoustic signals as being "unnatural" or "tinny." Such perceptions are often noted by patients who have their ears occluded by earmolds or hearing aids.

The middle ear is an air-filled space within the temporal bone, sometimes referred to as the tympanum. The TM (or eardrum) forms the lateral wall of this structure, while the medial wall is formed by the dense portion of the temporal bone that houses the inner ear. Two openings within the part of the temporal bone that forms the medial wall of the middle ear allow for communication between the middle ear and inner ear (i.e., the oval and round windows). The other borders of the middle ear space are formed by portions of the temporal bone. Important structures within the middle ear include the three smallest bones in the human body (i.e., malleus, incus, and stapes), which collectively form the ossicular chain, and the Eustachian tube, which provides fresh air to the middle ear space and equalizes middle ear pressure when necessary. Other structures within the middle ear include the tendons from two middle ear muscles (i.e., tensor tympani and stapedius) and a branch of the facial nerve, which transverses the middle ear space. The two muscle tendons help support the ossicular chain within the middle ear space and they contract in response to loud stimuli, resulting in a stiffening of the ossicular chain known as the acoustic reflex.

The middle ear's main function is to increase the energy that is imparted to the cochlea. This is accomplished by two mechanisms: an area differential between the TM and the footplate of the stapes and the lever action afforded by the configuration of the ossicular chain. Since the TM is considerably larger in area than the stapes' footplate, energy from vibrations arriving at the eardrum is concentrated on the smaller stapes with an increase in applied force. An additional increase in force is realized because the ossicular chain works as a lever in conducting sounds to the cochlea. This overall increase in energy is needed because of an impedance mismatch between the outer ear (low impedance) and the cochlea (high impedance). This mismatch is primarily created by transfer of energy from an air to fluid medium (Yost, 2000).

The Cochlea

● *Anatomy*

TEMPORAL BONE   The cochlea as well as the middle and external ear, vestibular apparatus, and seventh and eighth cranial nerves are all housed in the temporal bone. The **temporal bone,** which is part of the skull base, is a hard bone that has myriad cavities, channels, and canals that subserve the organs of hearing and balance; hence, the term *labyrinth* is often applied to several of the structures housed within the temporal bone. The temporal bone has four main segments: the squamous (superior to the ear canal), the mastoid (posterior to the pinna), the petrous (deep in the cranium housing the inner ear), and the tympanic (ear canal). The petrous segment is where the middle ear apparatus, cochlea, vestibular structures, and the internal auditory meatus (IAM) are located. The triangle-shaped petrous segment divides the cranial skull base into the posterior and middle fossa. The IAM houses the facial, auditory, and vestibular nerves and opens into the lateral aspect of the brainstem (see Anson and Donaldson, 1967).

THE BONY COCHLEA   The bony cochlea is imbedded in the petrous portion of the temporal bone and is a totally enclosed structure resembling the shell of a snail. It has two openings covered by membranes: the oval window and round window, which interface with the middle ear cavity (Figure 1.3). The bony cochlea has about $2\frac{1}{2}$ turns, with the basal turn (closest to the middle ear) being larger than the apical turn. A perforated bony central core called the modiolus runs through the cochlea. The **osseous spiral lamina** is a shelf-like structure that winds around the modiolus from base to apex (Figure 1.4a,b). This lamina looks like a fir tree, with the cochlear base correlating with the wider branches and the apex of the cochlea correlating with the narrower branches at the top. Small perforations in the lateral-most aspect

● Figure 1.3

Photograph of the bony cochlea exposed in the temporal bone. The top layers of bone have been drilled away so the coils of the cochlea can be observed. (Courtesy of Marilyn Pinheiro.)

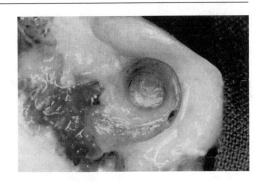

● **Figure 1.4**

(a) The osseous spiral lamina. The bony shelf spirals around the modiolus (within the dotted lines) from base to apex of the structure. (b) An exposed (chinchilla) osseous spiral lamina from base (bottom) to apex (top) with the stapes footplate in the oval window (arrow). (Courtesy of Richard Mount, Hospital for Sick Children, Toronto.)

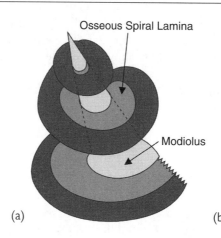

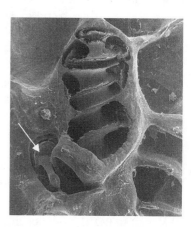

(a)   (b)

of these shelf-type structures are referred to as the habenula perforata. These perforations allow the AN fibers (from the hair cells) to pass through the openings and form the modiolus and (eventually) the AN trunk. The spiral lamina shelf is wider at the base than at the apex and it helps form the beginnings of the anatomical divisions of the cochlea by serving as an anchor to the medial aspect of the basilar membrane (Gulya, 1997).

THE MEMBRANOUS COCHLEA   The osseous cochlea is lined with elastic, membranous structures that follow the shape of the bony cochlea. The membranous cochlea has three ducts: the scala vestibuli (superior), the scala media (middle), and the scala tympani (inferior). The three divisions of the cochlea (ducts) are created by two important membranes. The **basilar membrane** (BM) separates the scala tympani from the inferior portion of the scala media and **Reissner's membrane** divides the superior aspect of the scala media from the scala vestibuli. At the apex of the cochlea, the scala vestibuli and scala tympani communicate, and this point of communication is termed the **helicotrema.**

The membranous cochlea is a fluid-filled system. The scala tympani and scala vestibuli are filled with perilymph, and the scala media contains endolymph and cortilymph (see Yost, 2000 for review). Perilymph has essentially the same chemical composition as cerebral spinal fluid (CSF). It is low in potassium and high in sodium and has a 0-mv electrical charge. Endolymph is high in potassium and low in sodium and has a +80-mv electrical charge. **Cortilymph** (0-mv electrical charge) is similar in chemical composition to perilymph. Endolymph is most likely produced by the stria vascularis, which is a highly vascular structure located on the lateral wall of the cochlear duct next to the spiral ligament (Figure 1.5).

Playing an important role in the hydrodynamics of the cochlear fluid system are the vestibular (endolymphatic) and cochlear aqueducts. Within the **vestibular**

● **Figure 1.5**

Cross-section of the cochlea (the scala media; inner hair cells and outer hair cells are shaded in light to dark shades, respectively).

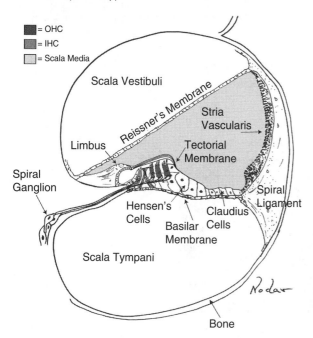

aqueduct are the **endolymphatic sac** and the **endolymphatic duct**. The vestibular aqueduct connects the posterior aspect of the vestibule to the posterior side of the petrous bone. This channel is thought to be a type of overflow valve for excess endolymph. The **cochlear aqueduct** courses from the basal turn of the cochlea to the posterior aspect of the temporal bone. It permits the transfer of cerebral spinal fluid to the scalae tympani and vestibuli (Gulya, 1997).

CLINICAL CORRELATE

The fluid dynamics in the membranous cochlear labyrinth are critical for appropriate function of the cochlea. If the fluid system doesn't function adequately, inner ear disorders can result, such as meniere's disease (endolymphatic hydrops) and related disorders such as perilymph fistulas (see Schwaber, 1997; Thai-van, Bounaix and Fraysse, 2001). Meniere's disease symptoms include episodic vertigo, hearing loss, and tinnitus. The exact etiology of meniere's disease is not known, but its basis is believed to be an overproduction of endolymph possibly related to dysfunction of the stria vascularis. There could also be excess endolymph in the scala media because the fluid is under-absorbed related to dysfunction of the endolymphatic sac and/or duct. In the pathological state, meniere's disease is characterized by an expanded cochlear duct and sometimes even ruptures of Reissner's membrane, usually in the apical end of the cochlea. This is thought to be related to the low-frequency hearing sensorineural loss typically seen in meniere's disease. A perilymphatic fistula is a tear in the oval or round window membrane through which perilymph leaks. This leakage causes a condition similar to meniere's disease because there is unequal pressure between the scala media and the other scalae. The administration of diuretics often alleviates the symptoms of meniere's disease. These drugs increase osmotic action in the cochlea and may rid the cochlea of excess endolymph—at least temporarily (see Chapter 4 for more on meniere's disease and cochlear fistulas).

The hearing loss, tinnitus, and vertigo associated with meniere's disease fluctuate with the episodic nature of the disease. Early on, symptoms completely clear after a so-called meniere's attack. This is best demonstrated by changes in the pure-tone audiogram, which after an episode returns from a low-frequency sensorineural loss back to normal hearing sensitivity. Long-term meniere's disease often results in permanent hearing loss, although fluctuations in hearing often continue to occur. A type of auditory evoked potential procedure, electrocochleography (Ecog), is used in the diagnosis of meniere's disease (see Chapters 5 and 6). Ecog recordings often show a large summating potential (SP) relative to the AN action potential (AP); this is known as an abnormal SP/AP ratio (Schwaber, 1997). ●

The BM runs the length of the cochlea (25–35 mm) and is wider at the apex than at the base. It is composed of fibers that are stiffer at the base than at the apex. This allows better high-frequency tuning at the base and better low-frequency tuning at the apex. Reissner's membrane is a thin, elastic membrane that is responsible for keeping separate the perilymph of the scala vestibuli from the endolymph in the scala media (Figures 1.5, 1.6). This membrane and the BM define the upper and lower boundaries of the scala media (see Gelfand, 1998).

THE ORGAN OF CORTI   Resting on the BM is the **organ of Corti**, that is, the end organ of hearing. The organ of Corti is composed of sensory cells, supporting cells, and a variety of membranes. It runs the entire length of the cochlear duct. The top of the organ of Corti is defined by the **tectorial membrane**, which on its underside touches the taller cilia of the **outer hair cells** (OHCs). The **inner hair cells'** (IHCs) cilia do not touch the tectorial membrane. At the base of the stereocilia is the **reticular lamina,** which forms a tight juncture around the cilia. The reticular lamina prevents the endolymph from entering the area of the hair cells and is formed by a flattened top surface of supporting **(Deiters' cells)** and the **cuticular plate** at the top of the hair cells.

Figure 1.6

A drawing looking down on the basilar membrane from above showing changes in the width of the membrane from the apical to basal end and corresponding frequency representation along the length of the basilar membrane.

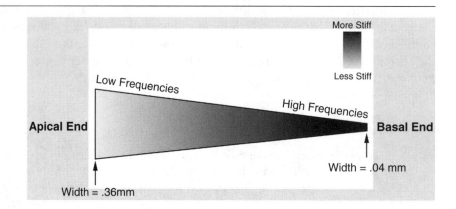

The sensory cells in the organ of Corti are the IHCs and the OHCs. The OHCs have three to five rows and the IHCs have only one row.

Arranged on both sides of the **pillar cells** (which define the tunnel of Corti) are the OHCs and the IHCs (Figure 1.7a). In the human, there is a single row of about 3,500 IHCs that run the length of the cochlea and multiple rows of about 12,000 OHCs that also run the length of the cochlea (Figure 1.7b). The IHCs are flask-shaped and robust in their appearance. The OHCs are cylinder-shaped and are thinner and longer than the IHCs. The electrical charge in the hair cells is −40 to −70 mv. At the top of the hair cells are stereocilia (also called cilia), and at the bottom are AN fiber connections (often called terminal buttons). The cilia on the hair cells are graded in length. The OHCs' cilia form a "W" shape, while the IHCs' cilia form a flattened "U" shape (Figure 1.7a). Located on the cilia, probably on the top, are pores that open when the cilia are bent toward the lateral wall of the cochlea duct. **Tip-links** are small filaments that are connected to other cilia on the hair cells

Figure 1.7

(a) Photograph looking down on the top of inner (one row) and outer (three rows) hair cells and the reticular lamina (area in between cells) after removal of the tectorial membrane. The region between the row of inner hair cells and first row of outer hair cells is the pillar cell region. Note that the cilia of the outer hair cells form a "W," while the inner hair cells look like a flattened "U." (Courtesy of Richard Mount, Hospital for Sick Children, Toronto.) (b) Hair cells and related structures. (Modified from Sahley et al., 1997 and the Cleveland Clinic Foundation, with permission.)

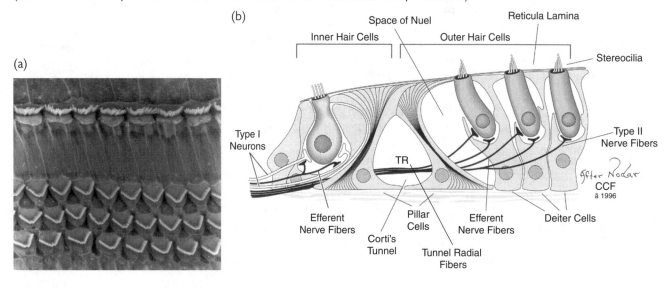

and help with the opening and closing of the pores (which allows K+ ions to flow into the cell and start the transduction process). **Cross-links** are similar to tip-links; however, they are located at the sides of the cilia (Figure 1.8). The cross-links help the cilia move in concert when the cilia are stimulated. Hair cells are present along the entire length of the cochlea. The hair cells at the basal end respond best to high frequencies, and those at the apical end respond to low frequencies (see Raphael and Altschuler, 2003).

CLINICAL CORRELATE

High-intensity noise exposure typically results in damage, primarily to the OHCs. If sound is of high enough intensity and/or there is a sufficiently long duration of exposure, then the IHCs and supporting cells can also be damaged. The basal portion of the cochlea is most susceptible to damage from high-intensity sound. Most people with noise exposure incur the greatest amount of hearing loss at 4 kHz, with the adjacent frequencies of 3 and 6 kHz also often affected. Susceptibility to hearing loss from high-intensity sound is highly variable, with some people being highly vulnerable while others are affected minimally.

Ototoxic drugs also damage hair cells, with the OHCs being the most susceptible. Audiologically, the high frequencies are affected first, with subsequent progression to the mid and low frequencies. Because of this trend for high-frequency compromise to occur prior to mid- and low-frequency compromise, two specialized audiometric procedures (high-frequency audiometry and otoacoustic emissions) have been used to define early ototoxic effects on hearing. Probably the two most known categories of ototoxic drugs are the aminoglycosides (the myacins, for example, gentamyacin) and the salicylates (aspirin). While most ototoxic drugs result in permanent hearing loss, the hearing loss associated with salicylates is often reversible. Ototoxic drugs can also damage the vestibular system and, in at least some cases, the balance system is affected before the auditory system.

Autoimmune disorders, head trauma, viral and bacterial infections, and vascular disorders are other maladies that can damage the hair cells. In most instances the OHCs at the basal end are more susceptible to damage. Therefore, in most of these disorders high-frequency hearing loss is more common than low- or mid-frequency hearing loss. ●

The organ of Corti is highly dependent on not only hair cells, which are sensory transducers, but also supporting cells. The **phalangeal cells** support the IHCs, and Deiters' cells support the OHCs. The hair cells rest on the bases of the supporting cells, with the stalks of these supporting cells angularly, projecting upward across the cells to form the reticular lamina. Pillar supporting cells are at angles facing each other to form a triangular structure known as the **tunnel of Corti.** More supporting cells (Hensen and Claudian) are seen as one views the more lateral aspect of the organ of Corti as it progresses to the lateral wall (Figures 1.7, 1.8) (see Slepecky, 1996; Geisler, 1998).

The lateral wall of the cochlea marks the end of the organ of Corti and it encompasses two key structures. Progressing laterally, one first encounters the stria vascularis and then the spiral ligament, which rests against the osseous, cochlear wall.

● Figure 1.8

An outer hair cell (OHC) and its supporting structure.

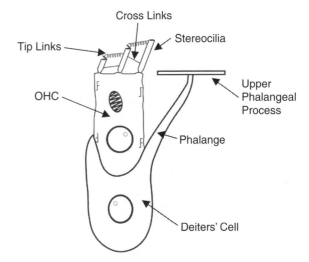

● Cochlear Physiology

How does the cochlea work to help provide the hearing experience? From a general perspective, the cochlea performs some key functions. It changes vibratory energy (sound) into electrical impulses so the brain can utilize these signals. The cochlea also provides fundamental coding of the intensity, frequency, and temporal aspects of sound.

COCHLEAR MECHANICS   Cochlear physiology begins with the mechanical input from the stapes via the oval window, which is accommodated by expansion of the round window membrane. When a compression sound wave is introduced, the stapes is pushed in and the oval window bulges; the opposite happens when the acoustic input is a rarefaction wave.

The vibratory input from the stapes to the cochlea sets up a traveling wave (TW) in the cochlear fluids that moves down the length of the BM. This TW moves faster at the basal end (nearly 100 m/second) and slower at the apical end (3 m/second) (Zwislocki, 2002 and interpolated from Tonndorf, 1960). This velocity difference is related to the physical characteristics of the BM (short stiff fibers at the basal end equal fast velocity; longer, looser fibers apically equal slow velocity). A compression wave results in the initial movement of the BM being downward, and a rarefaction wave results in an initial upward movement of the BM. The BM movement is influenced by where it is attached. The inner part of the BM is attached to the osseous spiral lamina, which serves as a fulcrum for the BM and the organ of Corti. The lateral edge of the osseous spiral lamina is almost directly below the inner pillar, which provides support for BM movement. The outer part of the lateral aspect of the BM is attached to the spiral ligament. The lateral aspect of the BM, as one would expect, is more elastic than the inner aspect; hence, it moves more easily (Raphael and Altschuler, 2003).

FREQUENCY AND INTENSITY   Frequency representation at the cochlea is accomplished by the place principle and/or temporally by the rate of neuron firing. Different frequencies produce TWs that reach their maximum deflection at different places along the cochlear partition (Figure 1.9). Simply stated, the point of maximum deflection on the BM is the result of the resonance characteristic of the BM that matches the frequency of the stimulating sound. The BM is tuned from high (basal end) to low (apical end) frequencies. Hence, the point of maximum deflection along the cochlear duct relates the frequency of the sound (the higher the frequency, the more basal the location of maximum deflection; the lower the frequency, the more apical the point of maximum deflection). A long-standing problem that surrounded this view was that the frequency tuning of the BM was too broad to explain the psychoacoustic measurement of frequency discrimination (behaviorally, frequency discrimination was much sharper than could be predicted by the frequency tuning of the BM alone). Hence, the temporal theory of frequency analysis was entertained.

At low and mid frequencies the BM vibrates in a whip-like motion at the rate of the frequency of the stimulating sound (if the sound has a frequency of 700 Hz, the BM vibrates 700 times per second and stimulates the AN at this rate) (Figures 1.9, 1.10). This BM vibration happens within

● **Figure 1.9**

The traveling waves and their envelopes (dotted lines) for (a) low (500 Hz), (b) mid (1500 Hz), and (c) high (3500 Hz) frequency tones.

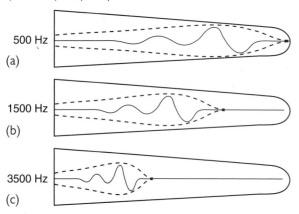

● **Figure 1.10**

Close-up sketch of the whip-like fine motion of the basilar membrane and the envelope of its displacement. The peak of maximum displacement is the place on the basilar membrane that corresponds to the frequency of the acoustic stimulus.

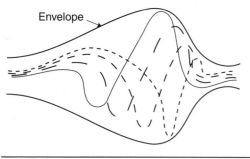

the envelope of the TW (often termed the fine movement or structure of the envelope). This also may be how frequency is temporally coded at low to mid frequencies either in addition to or perhaps in place of the place principle. At higher frequencies the temporal theory runs into problems, and it becomes more difficult to support this concept (for more discussion of this topic, see Chapter 6). Many agree that both place and temporal theories contribute to frequency coding (see von Bekesy; 1970; Hudspeth, 2000a,b).

Intensity representation in the cochlea is related to the amplitude of the TW envelope. That is, the more intense the stimulus, the greater the magnitude of the maximum deflection of the BM. Because of its physical characteristics, the BM has greater deflections at its apical end than at its basal end (for the same intensity stimulus). As the stimulus intensity increases, the TW envelope becomes not only greater in amplitude but also broader in shape. The broadness of the TW envelope at high intensities decreases the frequency selectivity of the BM. Hence, BM frequency tuning is sharper for low-intensity than for high-intensity stimuli. The greater the amplitude and broadness of the BM deflection, the greater the number of hair cells that are stimulated. This in turn creates a greater neural response and eventually greater loudness perception.

A critical concept in intensity representation in the cochlea is its nonlinearity. Basilar membrane deflection is certainly greater for high-intensity stimuli than for low-intensity stimuli, but there is progressively less change in BM deflection amplitude as the intensity of a sound increases. Stated another way, there is compression in the cochlea for intensity representation at high levels (Ruggero, 1992).

HAIR CELL MECHANICS   Hair cells change vibratory energy to electrical energy. A key aspect of this transduction process is the mechanics of the hair cells, which begins at the level of the cilia. The OHCs' cilia articulate with the tectorial membrane in an interesting manner. The TW of an acoustic compression wave depresses the BM downward. When this happens the organ of Corti also moves downward, and this results in a shearing motion of the tectorial membrane that pushes the cilia toward the limbus, which causes the tip-links to close the pores in the cilia. This in turn causes a hyperpolarization of the hair cells (inhibition). When the BM moves upward, the cilia are pushed in the opposite direction (away from the limbus), causing the tip-links to open the pores in the cilia and K+ to enter the cell and the cells to fire (depolarization) (Figure 1.11).

The IHC cilia do not touch the tectorial membrane; hence, there must be another means of moving these cilia so that these cells can fire. The leading hypothesis explaining how this happens is that fluid flow between the reticular lamina and the tectorial membrane caused by OHC cilia movement results in the IHC cilia rotating in the same direction as the cilia from the OHCs (Geisler, 1998).

Both IHCs and OHCs are responsible for the transduction process; however, the OHC's responsibility primarily is one of expansion and contraction. That is, it has been shown that when the OHCs are stimulated, contractile proteins in the cells allow them to expand and contract. This motility works in such a manner that when the BM is moved upward the OCHs contract and when the BM is pushed downward the OHCs expand. Since these cells are firmly connected to the tectorial membrane superiorly and to the Deiters' cells inferiorly (which are connected to the BM), contraction lifts the BM, creating a greater displacement of it. When the BM is pushed downward, the cells expand and again cause greater displacement of the BM. This hair cell motility works like an amplifier by increasing BM movement and causing greater stimulation—hence, the term *cochlear amplifier*. The OHC

CLINICAL CORRELATE

At high intensities there is less frequency selectivity—especially if there is hair cell damage. Amplification increases input to the cochlea and thus creates greater broadness of the TW envelope. This broadness creates greater intensity representation at lower sensation levels in individuals with hearing impairment when compared to individuals with normal hearing. In addition, frequency discrimination is compromised. For these reasons, it becomes important when fitting hearing aids to determine the lowest level of amplification that results in sufficient audibility. This is because the lower the intensity level, the better the chance for proper intensity and frequency representation. This physiologic concept relates to essentially all audiologic suprathreshold procedures. ●

● **Figure 1.11**

Sketch showing the deflection of the outer hair cells by the tectorial membrane for movement upward and downward from the basilar membrane. Upward movement results in depolarization of the hair cells, while downward movement results in hyperpolarization. Note the pivot points at the limbus and near the (inner) pillar cells. Although the inner hair cells' cilia do not touch the tectorial membrane, it is theorized that the endolymph flow (shown by arrows) and its related forces deflect the inner hair cells' cilia. (Modified from Perkins and Kent, 1986, with permission.)

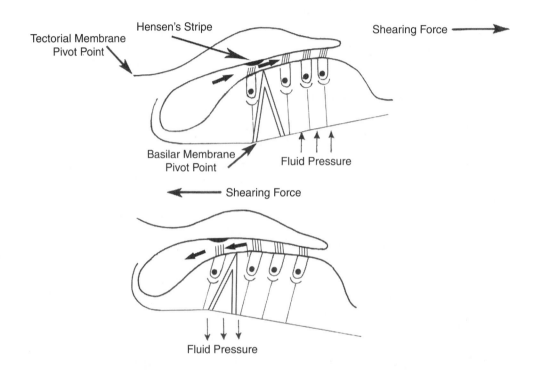

motility that operates at the peak of BM displacement also sharpens the membrane's tuning by reducing the broadness of the membrane's peak. This cochlear amplifier action takes place only for low intensities and is lost for high-intensity stimuli. This is one of the reasons high intensities result in poorer frequency selectivity (see Geisler, 1998).

The expansion and contraction of the OHCs is believed to be the basis for the generation of the small acoustic signals that are referred to as otoacoustic emissions (OAEs). OAEs are not typically present when there is hearing loss or when there is damage to the OHCs. The intensity range over which OAEs are operational is similar to the operating intensity range of the cochlear amplifier. Damage to the IHCs, AN, or central auditory nervous system (CANS) do not generally affect OAEs. Salicilate ototoxicity, which appears to compromise OHC function, arrests OAE activity as well as creates reversible sensorineural hearing loss. By stopping salicilate intake, hearing sensitivity will typically return, as will the patient's OAEs. These research findings, as well as other similar data, have strongly associated OHC motility to the generation of OAEs (Brownell, Bader, Bertrand, and de Ribaupierre, 1985; Geisler, 1998).

CLINICAL CORRELATE

OAEs, first discovered by Kemp (1978), have become a highly used clinical tool. Three main types of OAEs have emerged. These include transient (or click) evoked OAEs (TEOAEs, CEOAEs), distortion product OAEs (DPOAEs), and spontaneous OAEs (SOAEs). Briefly, TEOAEs result from click stimuli presented to the ear at mid to moderately high intensities. A microphone placed in the ear canal picks up the sound oscillations generated by the cochlea (OHCs) that are conducted back through the middle ear apparatus into the ear canal. These sound emissions (oscillations) are subaudible and represent most of the frequencies in the range of hearing tested clinically. The subaudible sounds in the ear canal are represented by oscillations similar to sound waves and represent a wide frequency spectrum. The oscillations, like sound waves, have amplitude and frequency information (Figure 1.12). The high frequencies have a shorter latency and appear first in the recording that is made, and these are then followed by mid and low frequencies. The high frequencies are depicted by tight (narrow) and the low frequencies by broad oscillations. The amplitudes of these oscillations can be correlated to norms that indicate normal or near normal hearing. TEOAEs are seldom present if hearing loss is greater than 30 dB HL. The TEOAEs can be quite frequency specific in that if hearing loss is present at a given frequency, then TEOAEs are absent at (or near) that frequency.

DPOAEs evolve from the presentation of two tones at slightly different frequencies. The frequency ratio of the two tones should hover around 1.2. These two tones result in a distortion production in the cochlea that is manifested by a lower intensity and lower frequency third tone in the cochlea that can also be measured in the ear canal. The frequency of the third tone follows the formula 2f1-f2, with f1 and f2 being the frequencies of the stimulating tones. DPOAEs are generated by tone pairs presented at discrete frequencies across the frequency range being assessed. Hence, this method of OAEs is highly frequency specific. DPOAES are recorded similarly to TEOAEs. They have been recorded in individuals who have 40 to 45 dB HL hearing loss; hence, their intensity range is greater than TEOAEs. DPOAEs are frequency specific and can mimic the contour of the audiogram.

SOAEs are present without acoustic stimulation. They are essentially only present in people with normal hearing, but not all people who have normal hearing have SOAEs.

Most research indicates that 90% or more of people with normal hearing have normal TEOAEs or DPOAEs; this is far more than people with normal hearing who have SOAEs. Hence, most clinical applications involve TEOAEs or DPOAEs. Presently, OAEs are primarily used for screening newborns for hearing loss, but they can also be used for detection of psuedohypacusis and assistance in differential diagnosis of neural versus sensory involvement (see Robinette and Glattke, 2002). ●

● Figure 1.12

An otoacoustic emission from a click stimulus. The arrow at the left indicates the amplitude of the oscillations, and the latency is noted along the bottom. The higher frequencies of the waveform are at the left. The oscillations here are closer together and are of a shorter latency. The low-frequency responses are on the right. Note that the oscillations are wider apart.

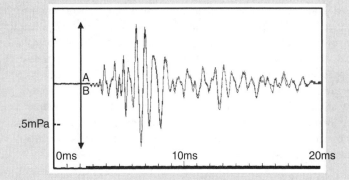

● Cochlear Electrophysiology

Cochlear mechanics begins the transduction process. The BM, moving in an upward direction (rarefaction sound wave), results in a shearing action at the TM, which pushes the cilia away from the limbus, and the hair cell depolarizes. When the BM moves downward (compression sound wave) the hair cell is in hyperpolarization and doesn't fire. Associated with the hair cell depolarization are three cochlear electrical potentials: the endocochlear or resting potential, the cochlear microphonic (CM), and the SP. The AP is generated by the AN and follows the SP in time.

The endocochlear potential is observed by passing an electrode through the different fluid compartments of the cochlea and noting how voltages increase to +80 mV when it enters the scala media. This positive voltage creates a large differential with the −40-mV to −70-mV charge in the hair cells. The endocochlear potential is probably generated and maintained by the stria vascularis and is responsible for moving positively charged K+ ions through the channels of the hair cell stereocilia (Wangemann, 2002).

The CM is generated mostly by the OHCs, with a minor contribution from the IHCs, and is regarded as mirroring receptor currents as they flow through the hair cells; that is, the CM mimics the incoming stimulus. As the intensity of the sound increases, the CM increases in amplitude up to relatively high levels where it will saturate and then decrease in its output. Reversing the polarity of the sound signal reverses the polarity of the CM (Dallos, 1973). Therefore, an alternating polarity signal, when averaged, will cancel the CM (Figure 1.13). The CM is almost instantaneous in its response to the stimulus and it is essentially unaffected by the rate of presentation (Dallos, 1973).

The SP is an extracellular direct current (DC) response that follows the envelope of the stimulus. It is most likely generated by the IHCs but with some contribution from the OHCs. The SP accommodates high intensities quite well and doesn't saturate at high intensity levels. To record the SP most efficiently, high-intensity stimuli work best (see Geisler, 1998).

The AP (also called the compound action potential) is not a cochlear potential but is closely associated with cochlear potentials. The AP is generated by the AN and can be a good estimate of behavioral hearing threshold. The AP is the same as wave I of the auditory brainstem response (ABR) (Figure 1.13).

The OHCs are motile and can better tune the response of the BM. Damage to the OHCs broadens their tuning curves and can shift hearing sensitivity significantly (40–60 dB). The OHCs are more susceptible to damage than are the IHCs. The OHCs help with tuning and sensitivity while the IHCs transmit information to the AN (see Geisler, 1998; Moller, 2000).

The neurotransmitter in the IHCs is an amino acid called glutamate. The neurotransmitter of the OHCs is not known. Depolarization of the hair cells results in the release of the neurotransmitter and activation of the AN across the synaptic cleft (Geisler, 1998).

CLINICAL CORRELATE

The CM, SP, and AP can be recorded in humans by using standard evoked-potential recording techniques. The clinical recording of these potentials is termed electrocochleography (Ecog). For the best recording of these potentials, special electrodes are placed in the ear canal (canal or extratympanic electrode), on the TM itself (tympanic electrode), or onto the promontory of the cochlea after a needle electrode has been inserted through the TM. The closer the electrode is placed to the cochlea, the larger are the CM, SP, and AP responses. Although Ecog can be used to estimate threshold hearing sensitivity, to measure the integrity of the cochlea, and/or to detect malingering, its most common use is in the diagnosis of meniere's disease or as a procedure to enhance wave I amplitude for the ABR. In meniere's disease, a key finding involves an amplitude comparison of the SP to the AP. In normal individuals the amplitude of the SP is usually less than .4 that of the AP. In patients with meniere's disease, however, the AP/SP ratio is typically greater than .4. Usually the Ecog is conducted with an alternating polarity stimulus. This allows the CM to be cancelled out and permits a clearer reading of the SP and AP waves. Ecogs are conducted at high intensities when they are used to assist in the diagnosis of meniere's disease (see Schwaber, 1997). •

● Figure 1.13

An adaptation of an electrocochleographic recording from a human subject showing the cochlear microphonic (CM), summating potential (SP), and action potential (AP) of the auditory nerve. This Ecog was done with a transtympanic needle electrode. The sound (click) was delivered through an ER-3A insert phone (hence a delay of 0.9 msec). The top tracing was derived from an alternating click stimulus that cancelled out the CM. The bottom tracing depicts a tracing from a rarefaction stimulus that allows the CM to be present. The AP is approximately 4 microvolts in amplitude.

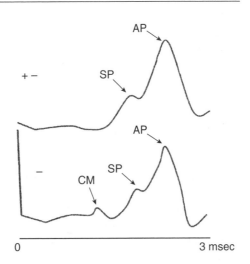

The Auditory Nerve

The AN carries electrical impulses from the cochlea to the brainstem. All the information that has been coded by the cochlea passes through the AN before it reaches the brain. The AN is one component of the eighth cranial nerve. Much of what is known about the anatomy of the human AN has come from surgeons who operate on or in the vicinity of this nerve. Disorders such as acoustic tumors and the application of rehabilitation devices such as cochlear implants have caused many investigators to focus on the structure and function of the AN.

● Anatomy

The AN in the adult human ranges from approximately 22–26 mm and has about 30,000 fibers. The AN runs from the terminal buttons on the hair cells to the habenula perforata, which are small openings in the bony shelf of the osseous spiral lamina. The AN fibers next proceed to Rosenthal's canal, which is an enlarged area that accommodates the spiral ganglion cells. The AN fibers then form a trunk, the modiolus, and extend into the IAM before entering the cerebellopontine angle (CPA) and connecting to the CN. The AN courses through the IAM along with the facial and vestibular nerves. The AN fibers (type I) are unmyelinated before they reach the habenula perforata and become myelinated thereafter. Type II AN fibers are generally unmyelinated in both portions of the fibers.

The two types of AN fibers are termed type I and II. Type I fibers are larger and more myelinated than type II fibers. Approximately 90% (or more) of AN fibers are type I fibers, which connect to the IHCs. The other 10% (or less) of the AN fibers are type II fibers, which connect to the OHCs. Therefore, many AN fibers may innervate one IHC, whereas a single AN fiber may innervate many OHCs (Figure 1.14). The AN has a definite tonotopic organization. In general, high-frequency fibers are located on the outside (of the nerve trunk) and low-frequency fibers are in the core (Spoendlin, 1972; Moller, 2000).

● Figure 1.14

An example of the auditory nerve fiber afferent connections to the outer hair cells (OHCs) (type II fibers) and to the inner hair cells (IHCs) (type I fibers). The type I fibers are myelinated, type II fibers are not.

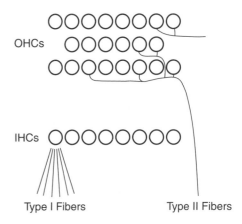

CLINICAL CORRELATE

A serious disorder to which audiologists have contributed many advances is the acoustic neuroma. The acoustic tumor is (at least 90% of the time) a vestibular schwannoma; that is, these tumors most often arise from the vestibular nerve(s) in the IAM and encroach upon the AN. Since the outside of the AN is typically the first region to become involved, a gradually progressive, high-frequency hearing loss is often the first symptom of this pathology. Balance problems (although seldom vertigo) and unilateral tinnitus are common symptoms associated with acoustic neuromas. In advanced stages the facial nerve may become involved, but early on, facial nerve symptoms are rare (Johnson, 1977; House and Luetje, 1979).

Besides high-frequency sensorineural hearing loss, patients with acoustic neuromas can suffer from poor speech recognition, elevated or absent acoustic reflexes, and reduced or absent caloric responses on electronystagmography testing. OAEs may be normal or abnormal, depending on whether the cochlea is compromised or not. Clearly, the best audiologic test for acoustic tumor detection is the ABR (about a 90% hit rate). The ABR waves may be absent or the inter-wave intervals may be extended in patients with acoustic tumors (Musiek, McCormick, and Hurley, 1996). In addition, wave IV-V of the ABR is often delayed for the involved ear when compared to the uninvolved ear. This comparison is known as the interaural latency difference (ILD) (Figure 1.15).

Auditory neuropathy is a dysfunction of the AN that may have a number of different etiologies. It can be present in newborns, children, or adults. There are differences of opinion as to the diagnostic criteria for auditory neuropathy. It seems clear, however, that the ABR should be absent to make this diagnosis. Acoustic reflexes are often abnormal and OAEs are usually, but not always, normal. Hearing sensitivity may be affected. However, when it is affected, it is likely related to neural compromise; hence, normal OAEs are expected. The diagnosis of auditory neuropathy is typically made on an audiologic basis because MRIs or CTs are often normal (Starr, Sininger, Nguyen, Michalewski, Oba, and Abdala, 2001). ●

● Figure 1.15

An ABR from a middle-aged patient with a medium-sized acoustic neuroma. The top tracing is from the noninvolved ear and the bottom tracing is from the ear with the lesion. Note on the bottom tracing the delay of the IV-V wave and the absence of wave III relative to the results depicted in the upper tracing.

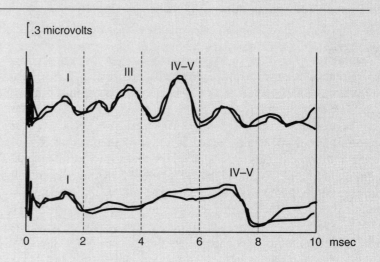

● *Physiology*

The frequency to which an AN fiber best responds (lowest intensity) is considered its characteristic frequency (CF). Generally, the further away in frequency from the CF a stimulating tone is, the greater is the intensity required for the fiber to fire or respond. If these intensity levels are plotted as a function of stimulus frequency, a tuning curve (TC) results (Figure 1.16). The sharper the TC, the better the frequency selectivity of the fiber. The frequency representation (as mentioned earlier) for the AN is high frequency on the periphery and low toward the middle of the nerve trunk. Tuning curves are generally sharper for high frequencies and are broader for low frequencies. Damage to the cochlea's OHCs results in a decrease in TC sensitivity and sharpness (Harrison, 2001).

Frequency is coded by place and temporal (or firing rate) characteristics. AN fibers that are connected to hair cells running from the apical and basal end of the cochlea by their spatial (place) location are graded from low to high in frequency. The temporal coding is related to phase-locking (generally this involves a particular place on the waveform such as the compression or rarefaction phase of the signal where the nerve fiber fires each time). The waveform and firing rate of the fiber are related to the frequency of the stimulus (i.e., low frequency equates to a low firing rate, high frequency to a higher firing rate). A key question concerning how phase-locking relates to frequency coding is whether the AN fiber can fire rapidly enough to represent each stimulus waveform— even at high frequencies. Because the best responding AN fibers can only fire at a rate of 1000 per second, the answer is probably "no." This is where the **volley principle** comes in. For high-frequency sounds, the AN fibers may fire on every second, third, or fourth cycle of the sound stimulus. It is important to realize that even though a nerve fiber (NF) may not phase-lock on every cycle (but rather every second or third cycle, etc.), it is still considered a phase-locking neuron. Other AN fibers are recruited to lock onto the cycles not locked onto by the initial fiber(s). In this manner, frequency coding is maintained at high frequencies (Johnson, 1978).

Intensity is coded at the AN by the number of fibers involved (more for high intensities) and the firing rate (greater rates for high intensities). Many nerve fibers with similar CFs will reach their response threshold at moderate to high intensities, but a reduced number will reach this threshold for a low-intensity stimulus. Interestingly, some AN fibers respond better to low intensities, while others respond better to high intensities. It seems the AN fibers with low spontaneous rates are better high intensity coders, whereas fibers with high spontaneous rates are better suited for low-intensities (Kim and Parham, 1997).

When recordings are made from the AN that reflect large numbers of fibers firing synchronously, an **evoked potential** (EP) can be recorded. Evoked potentials can be recorded from near-field (electrode on or near the AN) or far-field (usually electrodes on the head) approaches. Waves I and II of the auditory brainstem response (ABR) are generated by the AN.

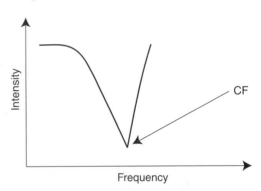

● **Figure 1.16**

The typical type of tuning curve obtained from an auditory nerve fiber. The characteristic frequency (CF) is the frequency to which the fiber is most sensitive. The nerve fiber will respond to other frequencies, but only at higher intensities.

THE CENTRAL AUDITORY SYSTEM

The Cochlear Nucleus

● *Anatomy*

The AN is the final structure of the auditory periphery. The CN is the first structure of the central auditory nervous system (CANS) (Figure 1.17a). The CN is located on the latero-posterior aspect of the caudal pons. The CN has three major divisions: the dorsal (DCN), the posterior ventral (PVCN), and the anterior ventral

• Figure 1.17

(a) Posterior view of the brainstem and thalamus. (From Waddington, 1984, with permission.) (b) Template of a coronal section of the brain schematized to show the key auditory ascending tracts and nuclei.

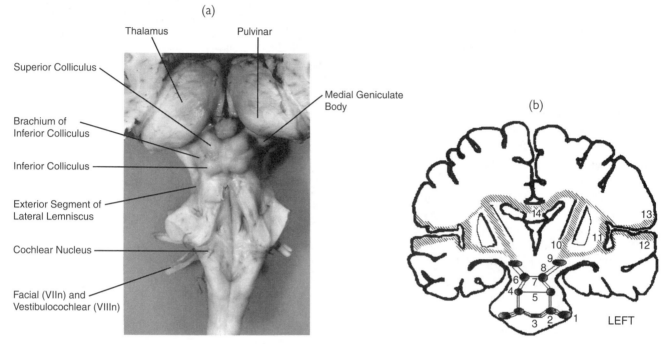

1 = cochlear nucleus, 2 = superior olivary complex, 3 = trapezoid body, 4 = nuclei of the lateral lemniscus, 5 = commissure of Probst, 6 = inferior colliculus, 7 = commissure of inferior colliculus, 8 = brachium of the inferior colliculus, 9 = medial geniculate body, 10 = internal capsule, 11 = insula, 12 = Heschl's gyrus, 13 = inferior central gyri of the parietal lobe, 14 = corpus callosum.

(AVCN). The AN fibers project to the CN and enter between the AVCN and PVCN, sending major branches to each of the three areas of the CN.

In the CN complex there are a number of cell types. Most notable among these cells are pyramidal, octopus, globular, multipolar, and spherical types. These cell types are generally located in specific areas of the CN (Pfeiffer, 1966; Osen, 1969).

The neural outputs from the CN take three primary routes—the ventral, dorsal and intermediate stria (Helfert, Sneed, and Altschuler, 1991). The ventral stria is also referred to as the trapezoid body tract. The DCN output fibers course along the dorsal stria, the AVCN fibers leave along the ventral stria and the PVCN exit via the intermediate stria. The ventral and intermediate stria are primarily contralateral pathways leading to the SOC although ipsilateral routes are also present. The dorsal stria leads mostly to the contralateral LL. Besides the stria, the CN has fibers that project directly to the SOC and IC via ipsilateral and contralateral routes (Moller, 2000).

In cats, it has been shown that sectioning the dorsal and intermediate stria has little or no effect on the threshold of hearing for tonal or noise stimuli presented monaurally. However, sectioning the ventral stria resulted in major decreases in sound detection ability (Masterton and Granger, 1988). A follow-up study demonstrated that sectioning the dorsal and intermediate stria did not change the ability to detect relevant sounds in noise, but that sectioning the ventral stria did compromise the cat's ability to hear in noise. Given these findings, it is possible that it could be either the afferent fibers, the efferent fibers, or both operating in concert that contribute to enhancement of hearing in noise (Masterton, Granger, and Glendenning, 1994).

● *Physiology*

Each of the cell types in the CN either modifies or preserves the AN firing pattern (Pffeifer, 1966). These firing patterns are called post-stimulatory time histograms (PSTHs) and they represent the firing rate of the fiber over time. PSTHs take different forms depending on the cell type that produces them. For example, some neurons may respond vigorously (high firing rate) at the beginning of a stimulus and then not respond to the remaining part of the sound. Other nerve fibers may respond to the entire stimulus but in a graded manner. The spherical and globular bushy cells in the AVCN can yield "primary-like," "primary-like with notch," and "on" types of responses. The octopus cells from the PVCN have only an "on" response, while the pyramidal (fusiform) cells in the DCN can provide pauser and "build up" responses (specifics about these patterns are provided in Chapter 7). The AN provides one type of firing pattern to the CN. The different cell types of the CN modify this pattern into a variety of other patterns, hence, better defining the input it receives from the AN. Some of the cell responses are quick and simple, such as the "on" type PSTH, while others are complex and slower, like the "chopper" PSTH. These responses are representative of the complex processing of various sounds that occurs at the CN.

The frequency representation at the CN follows that of the AN in each of its segments. Low-frequency AN fibers project to the lateral regions and the high frequencies to the medial-dorsal regions in the AVCN, PVCN, and DCN (Sando, 1965; Romand and Avan, 1997). This means that each segment of the CN has its own tonotopic arrangement. The TCs at the CN are similar to those noted at the AN. Sharper tuning is noted for low-intensity sounds than for high-intensity sounds.

In the CN, as intensity of the acoustic stimulus increases, the firing rate of neurons increases monotonically. More neurons fire at higher intensities. The intensity range for most fibers is 30–40 dB, but some fibers, although these are in the minority, have a much greater intensity range (Rhode and Smith, 1986). The CN fibers respond well to amplitude modulated tones. Many CN neurons have larger dynamic ranges for amplitude-modulated tones than they do for steady state tonal stimuli (Moller, 2000).

Temporal coding integrity is usually measured and judged by the ability of neurons to phase-lock onto a periodic stimulus. In small animals, some CN fibers can phase-lock for tones in the 3–4 kHz range (Moller, 2000). Hence, the CN has precise timing ability and neurons that can fire at high rates.

In regard to EPs and the CN, this structure contributes to wave III of the ABR. This wave occurs about 2 msec after wave I and is of relatively large amplitude in normal hearers (Moller, Jannetta, and Jho, 1994).

CLINICAL CORRELATE

Hyperbilirubinemia and jaundice have been associated with auditory neuropathy (Starr et al., 2001). This association has been made primarily because many of the cases of hyperbilirubinemia and jaundice provide an audiologic profile that is similar to that noted in auditory neuropathy and dysynchrony. Perhaps there could be some secondary involvement of the AN in cases of high bilirubin, but it is important to realize that high bilirubin, based on pathological evidence, is primarily a disorder that affects brain tissue and not the AN. Specifically, in hyperbilirubinemia, the CN appears to be involved—perhaps more frequently than any other central auditory structure (Dublin, 1986; Moller, 2000).

Damage to the CN will show up on central auditory tests such as the ABR. The ABR generally shows a normal wave I (if hearing sensitivity is good) and a delayed or absent wave III (if the CN is compromised). Behavioral central auditory tests such as dichotic listening show ipsilateral deficits for disorders of the CN (Musiek, Gollegly, Kibbe, and Verkest, 1988). ●

The Superior Olivary Complex

• Anatomy

The SOC is the next major auditory structure in the pons after the CN. The SOC has a number of individual nuclei groups that are located in the medial to lateral, ventral, and caudal pons in the human. From a caudal to rostral perspective, the SOC is at about the same level as the CN but it is located deep in the pons. In the cat the main nuclei of the SOC (which are located in the rostral medulla) include the **lateral superior olive** (LSO), which is the largest, the **middle superior olive** (MSO), and the medial nucleus of the trapezoid body (MNTB). There are also periolivary nuclei in the regions of the LSO and MSO that are considered part of the SOC. The ventral acoustic stria, along with the intermediate and dorsal acoustic stria, cross the midline of the caudal pons to connect the CN and the SOC and other parts of the brainstem pathway (see Moore, 2000).

In regard to cell types found within the main SOC structures, the MSO has primarily multipolar and bipolar cells and the LSO is primarily made up of one cell type: the principal or fusiform cell (Helfert et al., 1991).

As is the case for the CN, a tonotopic arrangement is noted in the SOC. In the LSO, higher frequencies are located medially and low frequencies are found laterally within this structure. The MSO has high frequencies represented toward the ventral end and low frequencies at the dorsal end (at least in cats) (Moore, 2000). In comparing the relative tuning of the LSO and MSO, the LSO (especially in small animals) seems to be tuned higher than the MSO.

The output connections from the LSO and MSO have been viewed structurally as an acoustic chiasm (after the optic chiasm) (Glendenning, Hutson, Nudo, and Masterton, 1985). The acoustic chiasm involves primarily the crossed connections between the LSO, the MSO, and the IC. The SOC, in general, also has ipsilateral connections to the IC as well as connections to the dorsal nucleus of the lateral lemniscus (DNLL) (Adams, 1979). These connections, however, are not as large or dense as the nerve tracts in the acoustic chiasm. The SOC, along with its neural input and output connections, makes for a very dense auditory region in the caudal pons.

• Physiology

The SOC is essentially the first place in the auditory system where there is bilateral representation of monaural acoustic input. This binaural representation allows a precise comparison of ipsilateral and contralateral inputs to the SOC. These complex comparisons, especially along temporal and intensity domains, are the basis for key functions of the SOC such as fusion, lateralization, and localization. Fusion is the combining and integration of information arriving from the two ears. Lateralization has to do with where (on a lateral plane) in an individual's head a sound image is perceived. Localization is where in auditory space a sound is perceived.

The SOC is highly sensitive to interaural time and intensity differences. The perception of these differences is the basis for localization and lateralization. The SOC has a wide array of neurons that are sensitive to interaural time and intensity differences, as well as neurons that help define left and right inputs and associated auditory fields. These kinds of functions are associated with neurons in the SOC that are excitatory (neuronal firing rate that increases above the spontaneous rate), inhibitory (neuronal firing rate that decreases below the spontaneous rate), or are unaffected by certain inputs (Rouiller, 1997). There are complex interactions between excitatory and inhibitory neurons in the SOC that contribute to localization. For example, generally inputs from the contralateral auditory field are more

CLINICAL CORRELATE

Conductive or sensorineural hearing loss in one ear will compromise accurate sound localization or lateralization. This is a good example of the role that interaural timing and intensity differences play in a clinical situation. Because of reduced input to the SOC on one side caused by hearing loss, stronger inputs (reduced latency and greater intensity) will result in a tendency to localize to the side without hearing loss. Damage to the CN and/or the SOC will also "scramble" timing and intensity cues at the SOC and result in poor localization. •

excitatory than inputs from the ipsilateral fields. This could be the result of inhibition of neurons responding to ipsilateral sounds and the enhancement of contralateral inputs via excitatory neurons (Boudreau and Tsuchitani, 1968). Localization on the horizontal plane is toward the side for which the sound first arrives or for which the sound is most intense. This action has a physiological correlate to interaural timing and intensity differences.

Tuning curves generated by neurons in the SOC are usually quite sharp and are sensitive to a change in frequency. The number of cell types and related PSTHs in the SOC are fewer than at the CN. In the MSO, PSTHs take the forms of primary and primary-like with a notch. The LSO has chopper type and primary-like PSTHs. The neurons in the SOC have good phase-locking ability with some neurons in small animals phase-locking to tones up to the to 2–3 kHz range.

Intensity coding at the SOC is similar to that of the neurons in the CN. The intensity function curves are nonlinear, with little increase in firing rate at low and high intensities. Some neurons have a dynamic (intensity) range of nearly 80 dB (Boudreau and Tsuchitani, 1968).

The SOC plays a key role in the generation of the ABR waveform. A study by Moller and colleagues (Moller, Jho, Yokota, and Jannetta, 1994) suggested a strong response near the SOC that correlated with wave IV of the ABR. More specifically, these investigators noted that the wave IV was probably generated from SOC structures at or close to midline in the brainstem.

● The Acoustic Reflex

The acoustic reflex (AR) is mediated at the SOC, although it is dependent on appropriate functioning along the entire auditory system up to and including the SOC. It is therefore accurate to refer to this response as the acoustic reflex arc in which the SOC is a key player. The AR pathway begins in the external ear where sound enters the auditory system. The middle ear directs the sound into the cochlea, and from the cochlea the electrical impulses are imparted to the AN. The AR pathway involves primarily the ventral nucleus of the lateral lemniscus (VNLL) and from there one set of fibers courses directly to the facial nerve motor nucleus ipsilaterally and another set of fibers travels through the trapezoid body and on to the LSO and MSO on the other side. From the SOC there are connections to the facial nerve motor nucleus. Hence, there are both ipsilateral and contralateral inputs to the facial nerve motor nuclei. The efferent pathway leads from the facial nerve nuclei to the facial nerve that courses through the IAM (medial to lateral) and out to the middle ear where a branch of the facial nerve (stapedius nerve) is sent to the stapedius muscle (Borg, 1973; Moller, 2000).

CLINICAL CORRELATE

Interaural timing has much to do with a clinical test in audiology called masking level differences (MLDs). Briefly, MLDs are a product of changing the phase of a tonal or speech signal imbedded in noise. When the signals are out-of-phase at the two ears (or when the noise is out-of-phase with the signal), there is better hearing in noise than when the signal or the signal and noise are at the same phase. This improvement in hearing ability when the signal or the signal and noise are out-of-phase is known as a release from masking effect. The acoustic basis for this phenomenon is that when one reverses the phase of a low-frequency signal, it creates a time disparity at the two ears or with the noise. This time disparity is recognized at the SOC, which uses it to discriminate the two inputs from each other and gain an advantage toward identification of the sounds. This results in better hearing of the signal in noise. The MLDs are greater for the low frequencies because the time disparities related to the phase changes are greater. Of great interest is that damage to the SOC region drastically reduces the MLD, and therefore MLDs have become an attractive clinical tool. The MLD, however, as a clinical tool, is grossly underutilized by clinicians (see Noffsinger, Martinez, and Schaefer, 1985). ●

CLINICAL CORRELATE

It has been shown that a specific lesion of the midline in the caudal pons (region of the SOC) has resulted in an extension of the III–V interval on the ABR (Musiek et al., 1988). There was no effect noted on wave I or III. Lesions in this region often create bilateral deficits on the ABR because there are a considerable number of crossing fibers and a heavy auditory neural network that can be compromised by lesions in this area. ●

The function of the AR is likely related to protection of the ear from high intensity sounds. At relatively high intensities the AR is initiated and results in the contraction of the stapedius muscle in the middle ear in individuals with normal hearing and AR function. This contraction attenuates the amount of energy reaching the inner ear. Hence, it is logical to reason that the AR is, at least to some degree, a protection system. Stimulating one ear (at a sufficient intensity level) will result in contraction of the stapedius muscle bilaterally. This is based on the presence of both crossed and uncrossed tracts that are activated when an intense signal is presented to one or both ears.

Intensity is a key factor in the generation of the AR. Most studies indicate that normal acoustic reflex thresholds for humans are in the 80–90 dB HL range with little effect of frequency over a 250–4000 Hz range. The degree of stapedius contraction increases with increases in intensity level above the AR threshold (Wilson and McBride, 1978).

The latency of the AR is dependent on a number of factors such as the intensity and type of sound used in stimulation. Moller (2000) reports that AR latencies can range from 25 to over 100 msec.

The Lateral Lemniscus

● *Anatomy*

Preceding up the auditory pathway in the brainstem, the next major group of nuclei includes the dorsal nuclei of the lateral lemniscus (DNLL) and the VNLL. These nuclei are located in the upper pons. The main pathway coursing from the SOC up to the IC is termed the lateral lemniscus (LL). The LL tract courses rostrally and dorsally along the lateral-most aspect of the pons before reaching the IC. The nuclei of the LL on each side of the pons are connected by the commissure of Probst (Parent, 1996).

The VNLL receives mostly contralateral inputs from the AVCN and the trapezoid body. The DNLL is connected on each side by the commisure of Probst and also receives inputs bilaterally from the AVCN and LSO and ipsilateral inputs from the MSO and VNLL (Glendenning, Brunso-Bechtold, Thompson, and Masterton, 1981; Schwartz, 1992).

Cell types found in the VNLL and DNLL include stellate, multipolar, globular, elongated, and ovid cells (Covey and Casseday, 1986).

The main outputs from the nuclei of the LL are to the IC on both sides (mostly ipsilaterally) via the commisure of the IC (Helfert and Aschoff, 1997).

● *Physiology*

The PSTHs of the nuclei of the LL are primarily onset, sustained, and chopper types (Aitkin, Anderson, and Brugge, 1970). The tonotopic arrangement of the nuclei of the LL is not well understood, as reports vary. Some investigators feel the tonotopicity of the VNLL and DNLL is very complex, while others believe it is naturally poorly defined (Oliver, 2004, p.c., Helfert et al., 1991). Both the VNLL and DNLL are sensitive to interaural time and intensity differences. As was the case in the SOC, excitatory and inhibitory responsive cells may contribute to localization cues (Brugge, Anderson, and Aitkin, 1970; see Helfert and Aschoff, 1997 for review).

The LL and its nuclei are major contributors to the ABR in humans (see Moller, 2000). Moller's work on generator sites of the ABR waveform in humans indicates that the predominate wave used in ABR applications, wave V, is generated (for the most part) from the LL.

Inferior Colliculus

● Anatomy

The IC is the next major structure in the ascending or afferent auditory pathway. The IC and the superior colliculus reside in the posterior aspect of the midbrain. The central nucleus, the dorsal cortex, and the external (or lateral) nucleus are the three main sections of the IC that will be discussed, with most focus being centered on the central nucleus. Practically all of the ascending fibers from lower auditory brainstem structures synapse at the IC (Morest and Oliver, 1984).

Ascending inputs to the IC include projections from the CN, SOC, and DNLL ipsilaterally and contralaterally. The VNLL also has ipsilateral projections to the IC (Ehret, 1997). The acoustic chiasm, mentioned earlier, has inputs from the LSO to the IC. The acoustic chiasm is depicted by the low-frequency fibers projecting ipsilaterally to the IC, and the high-frequency fibers crossing to the opposite IC (Glendenning and Masterson, 1983).

The two main types of cells in the IC (see Oliver and Schneiderman, 1991) are the disc-shaped cells, which are the most common, and the stellate cells.

The outputs of the IC are primarily fibers that course ipsilaterally to the MGB. There are also contralateral projections to the MGB, often through the commissure of the IC. The ipsilateral routes from the IC to the MGB are well defined by the brachium of the IC. This is a large neural tract that runs from the IC laterally and rostrally. The fibers from the central nucleus of the IC project to the ventral nucleus of the MGB. This connection is essentially the purest in terms of auditory neurons. The dorsal and lateral cortex of the IC project to the medial and dorsal segments of the MGB. This anatomical route has been considered the "nonclassical" pathway (see Winer, 1992; Moller, 2000).

● Physiology

The tonotopic organization of the IC runs dorsolaterally to ventromedially for low to high frequencies, respectively (Stiebler and Ehret, 1985). The TCs in the IC (central nucleus) are mostly sharp, but some are broad and some are even multi-peaked. These types of TCs indicate a relatively sophisticated frequency coding capability in the IC.

Intensity coding at the IC is associated with fibers that have both montonic and nonmontonic intensity functions. Some neurons increase their firing rates with intensity increases over a wide range of intensities (60–80 dB). On the other hand, some IC fibers "roll-over" in regard to their intensity functions, with intensity increases as little as 10 dB (Popelar and Syka, 1982).

Temporal processing studies of the IC have often been directed toward investigating phase-locking for amplitude-modulated signals and gap detection. The IC is the first level in the central auditory nervous system (CANS) that has sound duration sensitive neurons (Faure, Fremouw, Casseday, and Covey, 2003). These kinds of neurons are likely to play a key role in functions related to gap detection. In gap detection tasks the neural array that is involved must shut down and then turn back on with quickness and synchrony. Good correlations have been shown between behavioral gap detection values and those physiologically measured at the IC (Walton, Frisina, Ison, and O'Neill, 1997). Hence, from these measures the IC looks like a

CLINICAL CORRELATE

Damage to the IC and/or the brachium will yield contralateral deficits on central behavioral tests such as dichotic listening or low-redundancy speech tests. The ABR findings related to lesions of the IC remain somewhat controversial. Reports have been made of patients with damage to the IC who have normal ABRs (Jerger, Neely, and Jerger, 1980; Musiek et al., 1988). However, there have also been reports of some (but not total) compromise of wave V in patients with involvement of the IC (Musiek, Charette, Morse, and Baran, 2004). Lesion type, precise location, neural accommodation, and size of lesion could all be factors contributing to what appears to be disagreement in the literature regarding the effects of IC compromise on ABR results. ●

good temporal processor. However, the IC's phase-locking ability is not as good as that observed for lower-level neurons in the brainstem.

It has been known for some time that some IC neurons respond better to amplitude-modulated tones than to steady state tones (Erulkar, 1959). These modulation sensitive neurons are relatively common in the IC, with some of them capable of responding to 500 Hz (modulations per second) amplitude modulated (AM) signals.

The IC has neurons much like those in the SOC that are responsive to finite interaural time and intensity differences. Some sets of neurons respond to contralateral, monaural, and binaural inputs, and other neurons are responsive to monaural stimulation of either ear (Ehret, 1997). The vast majority of neurons in the IC are sensitive to binaural stimulation (Ehret, 1997). Given this neuronal network, it is clear that the IC plays a key role in sound localization and lateralization. This is supported by research on subjects with damage to the IC, which shows markedly decreased ability to localize sound sources in the sound field (Litovsky, Fligor, and Tramo, 2002).

The Medial Geniculate Body and Auditory Thalamus

● *Anatomy*

The next major structure in the ascending auditory pathway is the MGB. The MGB is located in the thalamus, on the dorsal and caudal aspect. It is now known that it is not only the MGB but also other structures in the thalamus, such as the pulvinar, the posterior nuclei group, and the reticular nuclei group that play a role in hearing at this level. The pulvinar is located in the dorsal (posterior) aspect, and the posterior and reticular nuclei are located in the lateral and ventral aspect of the thalamus. The MGB is divided into three main parts: the ventral, medial, and dorsal segments (Morest, 1964, 1965).

The main inputs to the MGB are ipsilaterally from the IC, with minor inputs from contralateral IC nuclei. The central nucleus of the IC inputs into the ventral division of the MGB, which is the main auditory pathway. Inputs from the dorsal and lateral IC connect to the MGB's medial and dorsal portions and form the nonclassical pathway.

The neural outputs from the MGB follow complex routes to the cortex. The ventral portion of the MGB takes a pathway through the internal capsule and then lateral to the primary auditory area. Fibers from the medial nucleus run along the inferior internal capsule and then proceed in an anterior direction alongside but medial to the optic tract before coursing laterally under the putamen to the external capsule from where they connect to the insula. The dorsal division fibers of the MGB run through the internal capsule route to secondary auditory (and possibly some primary) areas of the cortex, as well as the insula (Streitfeld, 1980).

Another MGB connection is from the medial division to the amygdala (LeDoux, 1986). This connection has not been studied a great deal by traditional auditory anatomists, but in general neuroscience it recently has received much attention. This connection seems to be a conduit to trigger the fear response in animals. This provides an auditory–emotional link in the brain.

The cell types in the MGB are highly varied. There are two main cell types in the ventral portion of the MGB: the large bushy cells and the small stellate cells. The dorsal and medial divisions of the MGB are highly diverse, with different types of stellate, bushy, tufted, and elongated nerve cells (Winer, 1992).

◉ Physiology

Rouiller, de Ribaupierre, and de Ribaupierre (1979) identified five types of responses from cells in the ventral portion of the MGB. The most common response type is the "on" response, which demonstrates activity only at the onset of an abrupt, short stimulus. There is also a "sustained" response, which responds for the entire duration of the stimulus, and an "off" response, which activates to the termination of the stimulus. Cells in the ventral MGB also provide a "late" response, which is delayed in regard to the onset of the stimulus, and a "suppressive response," which is inhibitory in nature.

The tonotopic organization comments here will pertain only to the ventral segment of the MGB. In the cat the low frequencies are located laterally and high frequencies, medially. Tuning curves from the ventral MGB have been classified as broad, narrow, multipeaked, and atypical (Morel, Rouiller, de Ribaupierre, and de Ribaupierre, 1987).

The MGB codes intensity similarly to the IC. There are both monotonic and nonmonotonic fibers in the MGB. There are far more nonmonotonic fibers than monotonic fibers (about a 3:1 ratio) (Rouiller, de Ribaupierre, Morel, and de Ribaupierre, 1983). Some fibers in the ventral MGB have a dynamic range in excess of 60 dB (Rouiller et al., 1983).

Temporal coding at the MGB, specifically the ventral segment, is slightly different than at the lower nuclei. Only about 10% of the neurons in the MGB (ventral) can phase-lock onto tones up to 1000 Hz. The majority of the neurons in the MGB can phase-lock only to tones under 250 Hz. It does appear that temporal coding is better preserved in the ventral portion than in the medial or dorsal portion of the MGB (Lennartz and Weinberger, 1992).

The MGB (ventral portion) is active in localization and lateralization tasks. As in the IC and lower brainstem auditory structures, the MGB has neurons that are sensitive to interaural time and intensity differences. Like in the IC, some sets of neurons respond to contralateral, monaural, and binaural inputs, and other neurons are responsive to monaural stimulation of either ear. The vast majority of neurons in the MGB are sensitive to binaural stimulation (Calford, 1983; Cetas, Price, Velenovsky, Crowe, Sinex, and McMullen, 2002). Interactions of excitatory and inhibitory neurons in reference to sounds coming from the ipsilateral or contralateral auditory field are noted at the level of the MGB (de Ribaupierre, 1997). Damage to the MGB in animals compromises localization and lateralization abilities (Jenkins and Masterton, 1982).

It seems likely that the MGB contributes to the middle latency response (MLR). Damage to the ventral and medial segments of the MGB in animals reduced the MLR considerably (McGee, Kraus, Littman, and Nicol, 1992).

Auditory Cortex and Subcortex

◉ Anatomy

The auditory cortex and subcortex receive input from the MGB (Figure 1.17b). The pathway between the MGB and the auditory cortex (and subcortex) is referred to as the thalamo-cortical pathway. This pathway courses through the internal capsule, but some fibers run beneath the lenticular process (putamen and globus pallidus). The internal capsule is a large white-matter tract connecting the subcortical areas to the cortex. The ventral portion of the MGB takes a pathway via the internal capsule and then courses laterally to the primary auditory area (Heschl's gyrus).

CLINICAL CORRELATE

Abnormal MLRs and 40-Hz potentials have been shown in patients with lesions of the MGB (Harada, Aoyagi, Suzuki, Kiren, and Koike, 1994). This is consistent with animal studies that identified generators of the MLR along the thalamo-cortical pathway (Kraus, Kileny, and McGee, 1994). Dichotic listening studies performed on patients with unilateral MGB involvement showed this procedure to be highly sensitive to lesions at this level of the CANS. Marked deficits were noted in the ear contralateral to the MGB involved (Berlin, Cullen, Berlin, Tobey, and Mouney, 1975; Hugdahl, Wester, and Asbjornsen, 1991). Therefore, from a clinical perspective, a central test battery that includes MLRs and dichotic listening tests would be good to use with patients with suspected dysfunction of the thalamic region of the brain. ◉

● **Figure 1.18**

Lateral view of the human brain showing the auditory areas at the brain's surface (area encircled).

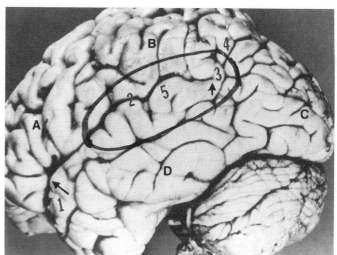

A = frontal lobe, B = parietal lobe, C = occipital lobe, D = temporal lobe, I = temporal pole of temporal lobe, 2 = Sylvian fissure with the beginning and end of this fissure marked by arrows, 3 = supramarginal gyrus, 4 = angular gyrus, 5 = superior temporal gyrus.

MGB fibers (probably from the suprageniculate or medial nucleus) run along the inferior internal capsule and proceed anteriorly alongside but medial to the optic tract before running laterally under the lenticular process to the external capsule, from where they connect to the insula. The dorsal division of the MGB takes the common internal capsule route to the secondary auditory areas of the cortex, as well as the insula (Rouiller, 1997).

The auditory cortex is composed of gray matter that is the nuclei of the nerve fibers. The subcortex is composed of both white matter (myelin) and gray matter.

● **Figure 1.19**

Looking down on the temporal plane of the right hemisphere (parietal and frontal lobes removed). I = Heschl's gyrus, 2 = planum temporale, 3 = insula, 4 = external capsule containing the claustruum.

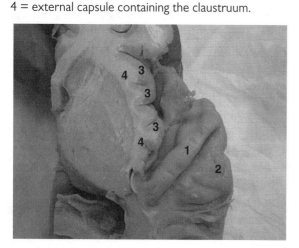

The sulci are the small grooves or folds in the cortex that enhance the total area of gray matter. The gyri are "bulges" of neural tissue, often located between sulci. The six layers of cortex in the human brain are defined by their cell types and are designated by the Roman numerals I to VI (Campbell, 1905; Winer, 1985).

The extent or boundaries of the auditory cortex awaits complete specification (Figures 1.17, 1.18). The boundaries vary across species, and animal cortices are different than human. As we learn more about these differences, our views of what constitutes the human auditory cortex will change. The auditory cortex from a lateral view exposes the **Sylvian or lateral fissure**. This fissure lies between the rostral part of the superior temporal gyrus and the inferior aspect of the frontal and parietal lobes. Located deep within the posterior half of the Sylvian fissure are two important auditory structures: Heschl's gyrus (often termed the primary auditory area) and the planum temporale (Figure 1.19). Also included in the auditory regions of the brain are the posterior inferior frontal lobe, the inferior parietal lobe, the angular gyrus, the supramarginal gyrus, and the superior temporal gyrus and insula (Rubens, 1977).

Heschl's gyrus courses medially and posteriorly on the superior temporal plane (STP). The identification of Heschl's gyrus and the planum temporale is difficult at times because there can be more than one Heschl's gyrus (Campain and Minckler, 1976; Musiek and Reeves, 1990). There have been reports of Heschl's gyrus being larger on the left than on the right side of the brain in humans (Campain and Minckler, 1976; Musiek and Reeves, 1990; Penhune, Zatorre, MacDonald, and Evans, 1996).

The planum temporale is located on the STP directly posterior to Heschl's gyrus. The planum temporale shares the acoustic (Heschl's) sulcus anteriorially and extends to the end point of the Sylvian fissure immediately anterior to the supramarginal gyrus. Perhaps one of the most famous neuroanatomical discoveries involving the planum temporale was when Geschwind and Levitsky (1968) reported that this structure was larger in the left hemisphere than in the right hemisphere. These investigators reasoned that if the left hemisphere was the dominant speech hemisphere and the planum temporale was in the region of **Wernicke's area**, then the planum temporale may be an anatomical correlate to receptive language functions in humans.

Recently, there has been a different view of the auditory cortex anatomy called the core and belt concept (Kaas, Hackett, and Tramo, 1999; Hackett, Preuss, and Kaas, 2001). The core refers to the center of active auditory substrate, whereas the belt(s) refers to the area surrounding the center or core of auditory fibers. The core and belt regions are essentially located on the superior temporal plane and gyrus (see Hackett et al., 2001) and encompass the planum temporale, Heschl's gyrus, and a region immediately anterior to Heschl's gyrus.

The primary auditory cortex or the core, belt, and parabelt areas need to communicate with other auditory (as well as nonauditory) areas of the brain. Two types of tracts connect auditory areas in the brain: intrahemispheric and interhemispheric. Intrahemispheric tracts include fiber pathways that are located within one hemisphere, and interhemispheric tracts are pathways that connect the two hemispheres. The classic intrahemispheric connection is from the primary auditory area posterior to Wernicke's area. Then via the arcuate fasciculus, which is part of the longitudinal fasciculus, the impulses are conveyed to the frontal lobe (in the region of Broca's area). Heschl's gyrus also has connections to the insula and other frontal lobe areas via the arcuate (and longitudinal) fasciculus (Streitfeld, 1980; de Ribaupierre, 1997). Interhemispheric connections will be discussed later with the corpus callosum.

The insula lies deep in the Sylvian fissure under the operculum and is covered by segments of the temporal, frontal, and parietal lobes. The insula can be observed directly by removing segments of these brain lobes. There are several gyri and sulci in the insula. There are anterior, medial, and posterior short gyri and anterior and posterior long gyri, all divided by distinct sulci (Ture, Yasargil, Al-Mefty, and Yasargil, 1999). Like Heschl's gyrus and the planum temporale, the insula is larger on the left than on the right side (Mesulam and Mufson, 1985). Recently the insula has garnered interest as an important structure in auditory function (Bamiou, Musiek and Luxon, 2003) (Figure 1.20).

● *Physiology*

The tonotopic organization of the primary auditory cortex (based on animal studies) indicates that the low frequencies are located rostro-laterally and the

CLINICAL CORRELATE

The insula, when damaged, appears to compromise central auditory function. A number of reports have shown deficits on both behavioral and electrophysiologic tests in patients with involvement of the insula (see Bamiou et al., 2003 for review). In one case, strokes to each insula resulted in temporary complete central deafness (Habib, Daquin, Milandre, Royere, Rey, Lanteri, Salamon, and Khalil, 1995). This case study did much to alert clinical and research professionals as to the potential role the insula plays in hearing. ●

● **Figure 1.20**

Magnetic resonance image (MRI) of the lateral view (left hemisphere) with the computer slice medially placed from the lateral surface about 1.5–2 cm so that only the most medial aspect of the temporal lobe is seen. The dotted arrows show the long gyri of the insula and the solid arrows show missing tissue of the superior temporal plane as a result of a stroke. This middle-aged patient showed marked contralateral ear deficits on dichotic listening tests and highly abnormal middle latency evoked responses for both ears. The patient had a normal audiogram but had extreme difficulty hearing in noisy background situations.

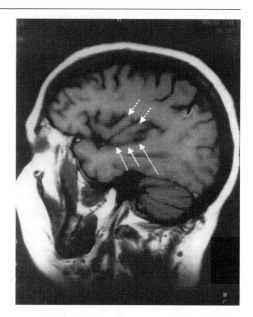

high frequencies are located caudo-medially (Merzenich and Brugge, 1973). Liegeois-Chauvel and colleagues showed that low and high frequencies were organized in humans in a manner similar to that found in functional imaging and primate studies (Liegeois-Chauvel, Giraud, Badier, Marquis, and Chauvel, 2001). However, the core-belt organization of the auditory cortex suggests a different tonotopic arrangement at the cortex, at least for primates (Hackett et al., 2001). The core is divided into three segments: anterior, middle, and posterior. The anterior and posterior segments run from low to high frequencies in a lateral to medial manner, and the middle segment courses from low to high frequencies in a posterior to anterior manner. The TCs in the auditory cortex are V-shaped for the most part, with sharpness increasing with increasing frequencies (Calford, Webster, and Semple, 1983). There are also multipeaked TCs at the auditory cortex (Onishi and Katsuki, 1965).

Auditory cortex fibers handle intensity representation in several ways. One is that as the intensity of the stimulus increases so does the firing rate of the fibers. Some fibers in the auditory cortex are monotonic and others are nonmonotonic in their responses to increasing stimulus intensity (Pickles, 1988; Phillips, 1989). As intensity increases, more auditory cortex fibers respond. This can be indirectly observed with both cortical EPs and functional imaging studies (Lasota, Ulmer, Firszt, Biswal, Daniels, and Prost, 2003). Intensity functions, however, may not be straightforward. Some increases in the intensity of the stimulus may result in more inhibitory responses rather than excitatory responses. This depends on the specific neurons involved and their unique functions (inhibition or excitation).

Interest in the responses of the auditory cortex to amplitude-modulated (AM) and frequency-modulated (FM) signals has increased recently because of introduction to the clinical arena of the auditory steady-state response (ASSR) procedure. The ASSR uses AM and/or FM stimuli to evoke a response from the CANS. Investigators have demonstrated that for FM signals the cortex yielded better (larger and more consistent) responses than for steady-state tones at the same frequency. This important finding was the basis for much basic and more recently clinical research on modulated signals (Whitfield and Evans, 1965). AM signals also result in stronger responses from the auditory cortex than a steady-state tone of the same acoustic characteristics. The cortex responds better to slow modulation rates (1–50 Hz), while brainstem neurons respond better to faster rates of modulation (>50 Hz) (Phillips, Reale, and Rugge, 1991).

Temporal processing in the auditory cortex is another topic of great interest. Two types of temporally based acoustic stimuli are relevant to this discussion of auditory cortex function. One is periodic stimuli, such as observed with pure tones or modulated tones, and the other is transient or single event stimuli, such as individual clicks. It is fairly well accepted that cortical neurons can only respond to periodicities up to approximately 100 Hz. Interestingly, cortical neurons can respond extremely well to rapid individual acoustic stimuli like clicks. Some, but not all, auditory cortex neurons can respond to click intervals of 1–2 msec—amazing temporal precision for these kinds of neurons (see Phillips and Hall 1990; Phillips et al., 1991). Gap detection requires much synchrony throughout the auditory system but clearly the cortex plays a major role. In animals with ablations of their auditory cortices, gap detection performance is markedly compromised (Kelly, Rooney, and Phillips, 1996). Neff (1961) demonstrated that cats with auditory cortex ablations could not recognize patterns of sounds created by frequency or intensity changes and attributed this deficit to temporal processing dysfunction.

There is general agreement that the auditory cortex is highly involved in the perception of speech stimuli. It has been known for some time that the auditory cortex area in animals responds to vocalizations from other animals (Wollberg and Newman, 1972). In primates and humans, speech or speech-like stimuli create neural activity along the posterior temporal plane (Steinschneider, Arezzo, and Vaughan, 1982; Giraud and Price 2001). Functional imaging studies have shown greater left than right superior temporal lobe activity for dichotic listening to speech. This is consistent with the right ear advantage often seen in human behavioral dichotic listening studies.

Localization and lateralization are dependent on proper auditory cortex function. Interaural intensity (IID) and time differences (IIT) serve as a basis for localization. These time and intensity factors relate to excitation and inhibition properties of cells in the auditory cortex as well as at other levels of the auditory system (Middlebrooks, Dykes, and Merzenich, 1980). Overall, there is a contralateral bias for increased cortical activity related to cues originating from the contralateral side (Aitkin, 1990). This is consistent with the clinical observation that damage to the auditory cortex on one side creates deficits in localization in the contralateral auditory field.

A number of auditory evoked potentials (AEPs) are associated with auditory cortex function. In general, AEPs are of slightly greater amplitude for contralateral recordings than for ipsilateral recordings; however, in our judgment this is a weak tendency. The earliest AEP associated with the auditory cortex is the middle latency response (MLR). It is likely generated by the primary auditory cortex, thalamo-cortical pathway, and reticular nuclei of the thalamus and is approximately 1 microvolt in amplitude (Kraus and McGee, 1994; for review see Musiek and Lee, 1999). The key waves of the MLR are Na and Pa, which occur around 12–20 and 21–32 msec after stimulus onset, respectively, when elicited at moderate intensity levels in adult humans.

CLINICAL CORRELATE

Studies have shown that auditory cortex lesions in humans can result in deficits in temporal discrimination. Both the discrimination of two acoustic clicks with variable silent interstimulus intervals and the discrimination of gaps in noise are compromised by auditory cortex lesions (Lackner and Teuber, 1973; Efron, Yund, Nichols, and Crandall, 1985). We also know that the appropriate sequencing of several acoustic events to perceive a pattern (e.g., frequency patterns) is compromised in humans when the auditory cortex is damaged (Musiek and Pinheiro, 1987). ●

CLINICAL CORRELATE

It is well known that lesions in either auditory cortex result in deficits for dichotic listening in humans. These deficits are usually noted in the ear contralateral to the involved hemisphere (see Hugdahl, 1988). ●

CLINICAL CORRELATE

Even simple tests of sound localization performed in an informal manner can implicate damage to the auditory areas of the cortex. The ability to locate a sound source or to track sound movement in an auditory field that is opposite the side of the lesion is very difficult for the patient with an auditory cortex lesion (Sanchez-Longo and Forster, 1958). ●

After the MLR, the late potentials, N1 and P2, sometimes referred to as the N1-P2 complex, are also likely to be generated by the primary auditory cortex (see Steinschneider, Kurtzberg, and Vaughan, 1992 for review). The N1 usually occurs in the 80–100 msec latency range and the P2 in the 160–220 latency range. These potentials are from about 1–5 microvolts in amplitude (see McPherson, 1996). The P300 is an event-related potential that follows the N1 and P2 in time. It is larger than the N1-P2 complex and occurs around 300 msec. It is considered an endogenous potential, meaning it is generated by internal processes in the brain (such as decision making and/or attention). The P300 is not as dependent on external stimuli as the other AEPs that have been discussed elsewhere in this chapter. The P300 or P3 probably has multiple contributors to its generation both intra- and interhemispherically. Although most investigations have not yielded information strongly implicating the auditory cortex in the generation of the P300, damage to the auditory cortex and/or the temporal parietal junction seems to compromise the P3 (Knight, Scabini, Woods, and Clayworth, 1989; Obert and Cranford, 1990).

The mismatched negativity (MMN) response, another late EP, is obtained by having subjects listen to standard and deviant sounds. The standard sounds are trains of the same stimuli and the deviants are stimuli that are different from the standards in some manner (i.e., frequency, intensity, duration, etc.). The deviant stimuli (if sufficiently different from the standard) result in a negative shift in the time region after the P2. Hence, this potential is an electrophysiological correlate to various types of auditory discrimination measures. The MMN is probably generated by or near the auditory cortex (Scherg, Vajar, and Picton, 1989).

CLINICAL CORRELATE

The AEPs that have just been discussed to various degrees have been used in clinical evaluation. The MLR has been shown to be sensitive to lesions of the auditory cortex and subcortex (Musiek, Charette, Kelly, Lee, and Musiek, 1999). The late potentials have also been employed clinically to determine central auditory dysfunction and are somewhat sensitive to lesions of the auditory cortex. In using these AEPs, it is important to consider using multiple electrode sites, or at least enough electrode sites to gain some insight into the function of each hemisphere. This is best done by comparing responses from electrodes placed over each hemisphere regardless of which ear is stimulated. Usually C3 and C4 or T3 and T4 are used as electrode sites for comparison. If one side's (electrode) waveform is significantly smaller or later than the other, it is termed an electrode effect. The responses from each ear, regardless of electrode site, can also be compared and if different, an "ear effect" results. Ear and electrode effects can occur separately or in combination. Ear and electrode effects can both occur with lesions to the auditory cortex.

The P300 and MMN are not as laterality specific as the late potentials or MLR. Hence the use of ear and electrode effects are not as relevant or useful. The P300 is sensitive to auditory cortex lesions, but little data has been generated to date about auditory cortex dysfunction and MMN. ●

One of the insightful experimental procedures from which we have learned a great deal about the auditory cortex is ablation studies. Ablating the auditory cortex and/or surrounding auditory structures has provided highly relevant information about dysfunction to the clinician and basic scientist. Although much controversy surrounds many ablation studies, there are trends that appear solid. Auditory cortex ablations compromise pattern perception and temporal discrimination. Less complex auditory tasks such as tonal detection may also be influenced by auditory cortex ablation. Unilateral auditory cortex ablation in Japanese macaques has demonstrated hearing loss in the ear contralateral to the ablation—at least for a period of time following the ablation (Heffner and Heffner, 1989). Frequency discrimination is decreased after cortical (auditory) ablation, although this finding has some disagreement surrounding it (Cranford, 1979). More agreement is seen regarding auditory cortex ablations and sound localization abilities, as most studies show a decrease in performance, although the degree of deficit noted varies (Kelly and Kavanagh, 1986; Beitel and Kaas, 1993).

Much of the information we have at our disposal about the auditory cortex is based on animal data, yet the most relevant data, especially to the clinician, is human data. Thanks to new functional imaging techniques such as functional magnetic resonance imaging (fMRI) and positron emission tomography (PET), we are now able to gain new insights as to the physiology and pathophysiology of the auditory cortex in humans. Functional imaging is not limited to the auditory cortex, but clearly considerable work has been focused on this structure. Both fMRI and PET reflect changes in metabolism in a designated area of the brain. This increased metabolism is related to blood flow into the designated area of the brain. Brain metabolism increases when brain tissue has to work hard. Therefore, by using sophisticated techniques of measuring increased metabolism, one can learn much about the functional anatomy of the human brain. In functional imaging studies, the amount of brain activity is color-scaled to indicate high (usually bright colors) to low (usually cool colors) activation of a particular region. Tonotopic organization of Heschl's gyrus, location of speech perception, tonal detection, and temporal processing are just a few of the key findings associated with functional imaging of the auditory cortex and surrounding regions of the brain (see Johnsrude, Giraud, and Frackowiak, 2002).

The Corpus Callosum

● *Anatomy*

It is interesting that only on occasion is the corpus callosum (CC) discussed as part of the auditory system. Clearly the CC plays an important part in transferring auditory information from one hemisphere to the other. Our knowledge about the CC, like most other auditory structures, comes from both animal and human data. However, a healthy portion of our understanding of the CC's structure and function comes from studies of humans who have had to have their corpus callosum sectioned surgically. These individuals are often termed "split-brain patients" because they have had their two hemispheres divided for medical reasons—usually intractable epilepsy.

The CC connects the two hemispheres of the brain. It is the largest fiber tract in the primate brain. The CC in adult humans is about 6.5 cm in length and varies from 0.5 to 1 cm in thickness (Musiek, 1986, for review). The CC is composed of large (among the largest in the brain) myelinated axons that course from one hemisphere to the other. Hence, the CC is not only a midline structure, but its axons cover the entire area from one cerebral cortex to the other. The fibers connecting the two hemispheres can be viewed as two main types: homolateral fibers (connecting to the same locus but in opposite hemispheres) and heterolateral fibers (connecting to different loci in each hemisphere) (Mountcastle, 1962). The callosal fibers course rostrally from the cortex, over the lateral ventricles, and toward the opposite cortex to form the base of the longitudinal fissure.

The CC is specifically organized to subserve different regions of the cortex. The posterior sixth of the CC is the splenium, which contains visual fibers that connect the two occipital lobes. Anterior to the splenium is a thinned portion of the CC termed the sulcus, which in essence is the auditory portion of the CC. The sulcus has fibers from the superior temporal gyrus and posterior insula. The trunk of the CC is anterior to the sulcus and has fibers from the parietal and frontal lobes. The genu is the most anterior part of the CC and contains fibers from the olfactory region and anterior insula. Finally, the anterior commissure is under the trunk following the inferior to posterior curve of the genu. It is thought that olfactory and possibly auditory fibers course through the anterior commissure (Figure 1.21).

● **Figure 1.21**

A midline section through a human brain showing the corpus callosum.

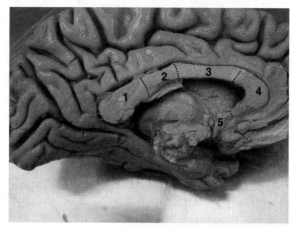

1 = splenium, 2 = sulcus, 3 = trunk, 4 = genu, 5 = anterior commissure.

● *Physiology*

One of the key aspects related to the function of the CC is the transfer time from one hemisphere to the other. There are excitatory fibers and inhibitory fibers. The excitatory fibers have a transfer time ranging from 3–6 msec, while what appear to be inhibitory fibers require in excess of 100 msec to transfer an impulse (Bremer, Brihaye, and Andre-Balisaux, 1956; Salamy 1978). This transfer time between hemispheres decreases with age in the human, reaching minimum values in the teenage years (Gazzaniga, Bogen, and Sperry, 1962). Interestingly, this change in transfer time correlates with the mediation of maturation of the CC. Myelin maturation increases in the CC until the teenage years. Hence, the correlation well known to physiologists is that as the myelin on the axon increases, so does the conduction velocity.

Much of our knowledge of the function of the CC has been the result of studying split-brain patients. Since the CC is primarily responsible for communication between the two hemispheres, tasks that require the two hemispheres to interact are important in testing the integrity of the CC. In the auditory domain one such task is dichotic listening. In dichotic listening the ipsilateral inputs to the auditory cortex are suppressed and audition becomes primarily a contralateral phenomenon (Kimura, 1961). Therefore, in the dichotic

CLINICAL CORRELATE

Individuals that are tested with dichotic listening tasks before and after commissurotomy (split-brain surgery) show left ear deficits of a marked degree on various dichotic tests. Competing sentences, dichotic digits, dichotic CVs, dichotic rhymes, and dichotic words all show good right ear performance and extremely poor left ear performance (Musiek et al., 1984b). If the speech test is not dichotic in nature, it is seldom affected by callosum abnormalities.

Left ear performance decrements (relative to right ear performance) on dichotic listening are noted in children under the age of 11 years, with the size of the decrements decreasing with increasing age. It is theorized with good support that the decreased performance in the left ear of young children may be related to the extent of myelin maturation of the CC (Musiek, Gollegly, and Baran, 1984a). Left ear dichotic listening deficits are also seen in the elderly, probably secondary to myelin breakdown in the CC (Bellis and Wilber, 2001). It appears that the degree of myelination of the CC at each end of the age spectrum influences performance on dichotic listening tasks.

Pattern perception tests requiring verbal responses also seem to be dependent on interhemispheric processing. These tests also show a maturational trend consistent with myelin maturation of the CC (see Musiek et al., 1984a). ●

mode, speech signals directed to the right ear are coursing directly to the left hemisphere. Since the left hemisphere is the speech hemisphere, the subject can engage the speech response mechanism and repeat the word. However, the speech stimulus presented to the left ear in a dichotic mode goes to the right hemisphere, and since the right hemisphere doesn't have speech capabilities, the information directed to the right hemisphere must travel across the CC to the left hemisphere, where a speech response can be initiated. When the CC is cut or in some way damaged, the speech signals from the left ear cannot cross from the right hemisphere to the left hemisphere. Therefore, the left hemisphere has no perception because no information is coming from the right hemisphere; the result is a marked left ear deficit (Musiek, Kibbe, and Baran, 1984b).

VASCULAR ANATOMY AND RELATED FUNCTIONS

Vascular Anatomy of the Peripheral System

Vascular anomalies are one of the main causes of hearing loss. Depending on the particular loci of the vascular disorder, various symptoms and dysfunctions may emerge. Therefore, understanding the vascular anatomy of the auditory system can be of considerable help with diagnosis and treatment.

The pinna and the EAM gain their blood supply from two main arteries: the superficial temporal artery (STA) and the posterior auricular artery (PAA). Both are branches of the external carotid artery. The STA courses immediately anterior to the pinna and sends branches superiorly, and the PAA is posterior to the pinna along the mastoid area. The deep auricular and maxillary arteries are key vessels that supply the middle ear and the tympanic membrane. They are branches of the subclavian and external carotid arteries. Other arteries are also involved in a complex manner in this blood supply. Not located in the middle ear, but rather immediately inferior to it, is the jugular bulb. This structure can result in a glomus jugulare tumor, which may compromise the middle ear structure and function (Anson and Donaldson, 1967).

The cochlea and AN receive their blood supply via the vertebro-basilar system (Portmann, Sterkers, Charachon, and Chouard, 1975; Moller, 2000). The vertebro-basilar system can be traced back to the vertebral arteries, which course up each side of the vertebral column. These vessels enter the cranium at the foramen magnum and course anteriorly to the ventral aspect of the medulla. The two vertebral arteries join to form the basilar artery. The basilar artery gives rise to the internal auditory artery (IAA) (often termed the labyrinthine artery) directly or via the anterior inferior cerebellar artery (AICA). The IAA branches in the inferior half of the pons and courses laterally across the CPA and into the IAM, where it supplies the facial, auditory, and vestibular nerves. The IAA then branches into the cochlear and vestibular arteries. The cochlear artery branches into two important vessels, the spiral modiolar and the cochlear-vestibular artery. The spiral modiolar vessel spirals around the modiolus and supplies the apical portion of the cochlea, while the cochlear-vestibular artery supplies the basal turns of the cochlea (see Axelsson and Ryan, 2001). As Smith (1973) describes, further branching of the cochlear vessels (radiating arterioles) in the cochlea eventually forms a network of arterioles.

CLINICAL CORRELATE

The glomus jugulare tumor arises from the jugular bulb and can invade the middle ear space. There it can create a conductive hearing loss and result in abnormal tympanograms. This is a serious condition requiring otologic care. ●

CLINICAL CORRELATE

Occlusion of the small arterioles can cause rapid and frequency-specific hearing loss depending on the vessels involved. The hearing loss would not be as devastating as if the cochlear artery or vestibular artery were occluded, which would probably result in severe hearing loss across most frequencies and dizziness. ●

Vascular Anatomy of the Central Auditory System

Two main vascular systems supply the CANS. One is the vertebral-basilar system, which is primarily responsible for the auditory structures in the brainstem (and the periphery). The other is the internal carotid system, which is key to the auditory structures in the cerebrum (Waddington, 1974). The basilar artery forms from the vertebrals. The basilar gives rise to AICA, which often supplies the CN. Along most of the length of the basilar artery, small arteries penetrate the pons (pontine arteries) to supply structures deep in the pons such as the SOC and the cochlear stria. At the most rostral aspect of the pons, the basilar artery provides the superior cerebellar artery, which supplies the cerebellum and circumferentially supplies the IC and LL. The basilar artery rostrally gives rise to the posterior cerebral artery, which supplies the splenium of the CC and also forms the posterior segment of the circle of Willis (Barr, 1972; Waddington, 1974).

The blood supply to the auditory cortex and subcortex is primarily derived from the middle cerebral artery (MCA), which is a branch of the internal carotid. The MCA may run a short or long distance along the Sylvian fissure, sending branches to the anterior middle and posterior temporal lobe and inferior middle parietal lobe. The angular artery continues as a posterior branch of the MCA, supplying the angular gyrus and surrounding region. The insula is supplied by the fronto-opercular artery, which is an early branch of the MCA (Waddington, 1974). This vascular anatomy supplies most of the auditory structures in the cerebrum, with the exception of the CC. The anterior four-fifths of the CC is supplied by the pericallosal artery (which is a branch of the MCA), and the posterior one-fifth is supplied by the posterior cerebral artery (Musiek, 1986).

THE EFFERENT SYSTEM

The Caudal and Rostal Systems

● *Anatomy*

The afferent or ascending auditory system has a counterpart known as the efferent or descending auditory system. Comparatively little is known about the efferent system, yet it attracts a major research effort. The efferent system can be viewed as two subsystems: the rostral and caudal. The rostral system is generally regarded as the efferent structures rostral to the superior olivary region, while the caudal system is considered to be the portions of the efferent system that include the structures in the superior olivary region and the more caudal efferent structures.

The efferent auditory pathway begins at the auditory cortex and association area and courses from these areas down through the internal capsule to the MGB and further courses along a similar route as the ascending pathway until it finally ends up at the cochlea. This system has fewer fibers associated with it and it is not as anatomically distinct as the ascending system. At certain points along the way the efferent system combines with the ascending system to form various **feedback loops**, making for a rather complex array of auditory fibers.

The rostral system has a series of feedback loops that involve the auditory cortex, MGB, and IC. There are also loop connections between the insula, superior colliculus, and medial geniculate (see Spangler and Warr, 1991; Warr, 1992; Sahley, Nodar, and Musiek, 1997). The caudal system is made up of the olivocochlear bundle (OCB) and its caudal connections—including the cochlea. The rostral segment is not as well studied as the OCB; hence, the amount of information available is much greater for the OCB segment. The OCB segment arises primarily around the SOC and has lateral and medial divisions. The lateral olivocochlear bundle (LOC) is primarily ipsilateral, and the medial olivocochlear (MOC) bundle is a crossed system. More specifically, the LOC bundle arises from the area around (periolovary nuclei) and including the LSO. This unmyelinated tract runs ipsilaterally connecting to the CN, exits the brainstem via the IAM, enters the cochlea, and connects to the afferent fibers immediately beneath the IHCs (Warr, 1980, 1992; Sahley et al., 1997).

The MOC bundle arises from around the MSO, crosses midline of the brainstem, and combines with the LOC fibers and takes a similar course to the LOC efferent fibers out of the brainstem and into the cochlea. The MOC fibers connect directly to the OHCs. The MOC fibers are mostly myelinated fibers (Warr, 1980, 1992; Sahley et al., 1997).

● Physiology

Little is known about the function of the rostral efferent system. Studies of stimulation of the auditory cortex have shown an inhibition and excitation at the MGB (Watanabe, Yanagisawa, Kanzaki, and Katsuki, 1966; Ryugo and Weinberger, 1976). Similarly, auditory cortex stimulation has resulted in both excitation and inhibition at the level of the IC (Mitani, Shimokouchi, and Nomura, 1983).

It is difficult to determine how the rostral efferent system affects hearing, but hypothetically it may play the role of a regulator of afferent input.

The functions of the OCB (caudal efferent system) have been studied more extensively than its rostral counterpart. This system can be activated by electrical stimulation of the bundle or by introducing sound to the contralateral ear. It has been shown in animals and humans that when stimulated, the OCB will result in decreased firing of the AN (Galambos, 1956). The general implication is that OCB stimulation may result in inhibitory actions in the auditory system. This phenomenon can be observed in humans measuring an EP or an OAE from one ear with and without noise presented to the contralateral ear (Folsum and Owsley, 1987; Collet, Kemp, Veuillet, Duclaux, Moulin, and Morgon, 1990).

The OCB activation appears to play an interesting role in hearing in noise. When the OCB is triggered (again by electrical stimulation or by introducing sound to the contralateral ear) and the test ear is stimulated by a signal imbedded in noise, there will be a release from masking or antimasking effect (Kawase and Liberman, 1993). This phenomenon is receiving much interest as at least a partial explanation of how humans hear in noise. A recent study by May, Budelis, and Niparko (2004) demonstrated with cats that localization accuracy in noise was decreased when the OCB was sectioned. This poorer localization was only manifested in a background noise situation. This study, like others before, demonstrated a key role for the OCB in hearing in noise.

CLINICAL CORRELATE

A clinical measure of OCB function is OAE suppression (Berlin, Hood, Cecola, Jackson, and Szabo, 1993; Hood, 2002). By measuring OAEs with and without noise presented to the contralateral ear, the amount of suppression can be measured. This is done by measuring the amount that the OAE amplitude decreases (in decibels) when the noise is present in the contralateral ear. The amount of attenuation when introducing noise is typically on the order of 1–3 dB. This suppression is considered to be an indicator of normal OCB function. The lack of suppression on the OAE is taken to mean the system may be impaired. Lack of suppression has been seen in patients with acoustic tumors and low brainstem involvement. This technique of measuring OCB function suffers from the subtleness of the effect and is therefore only marginally used as a clinical tool. ●

The inhibitory effects of the OCB seem to play a role also in protecting the auditory system from high-intensity sound (Reiter and Liberman, 1995). In guinea pigs, electrical stimulation of the OCB during exposure to high-intensity tonal stimuli resulted in a reduced amount of **temporary threshold shift (TTS)** compared to control conditions—hence a possible additional function of the OCB.

NEUROTRANSMISSION IN THE AUDITORY SYSTEM

Various chapters of this book briefly mention the neurotransmitters found in the auditory structures (the cochlea, AN, central auditory afferent and efferent systems). This section will provide some background into the neuropharmacology of the auditory system.

The manner in which neural systems work is based on communication between and among nerve cells. The site of this transmission is the synapse, which is the cleft between nerve cells where the communication between and/or among nerve cells takes place. This communication is accomplished by chemicals that cross the synaptic cleft from one nerve cell to the next. In the base of the nerve cell are vesicles that store and release the neurotransmitter. The neurotransmitter, once it crosses the cleft, binds to receptors in the adjacent cell membrane (postsynaptic site). This binding is a matching process between the neurotransmitter and the receptor that functions like a lock and key (Figure 1.22). If the neurotransmitter and receptor match, neurotransmission is accomplished. If they don't match, then the transmission is compromised.

Drugs can play an important role in neurotransmission. Some drugs can mimic the chemical characteristics of a given neurotransmitter and bind to and activate the postsynaptic receptor. This kind of drug is termed an agonist. It has the potential to

● **Figure 1.22**

The anatomy of a synaptic transmission showing the "lock and key" concept. The receptor site on the post-synaptic nerve cell must have a molecular accommodation for the chemical (neurotransmitter) that is released by the pre-synaptic neuron so that binding can take place. (From Sahley et al., 1997 and the Cleveland Clinic Foundation, with permission.)

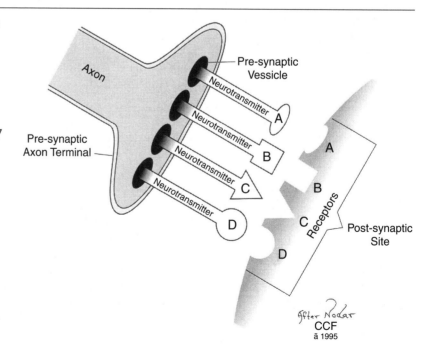

enhance the activity of the receptor. Other drugs can bind to the receptor but do not activate it. These drugs are called antagonists. They occupy the receptor site but do not do anything to facilitate a response in the adjacent receptor. They function, in essence, to block or prevent other natural transmitters from binding to the receptor, which prevents activation of the receptor. Thus, these antagonists can block neurotransmission. Agonists and antagonists are chemically very similar but have different (usually opposing) actions. The agonistic and antagonistic actions of chemicals can be viewed as excitatory and inhibitory phenomena, respectively (Musiek and Hoffman, 1990). In the auditory system there is a balance between inhibitory and excitatory activity that is accomplished by neurotransmitters either activating or not activating postsynaptic receptors along the auditory pathway.

SUMMARY

This chapter overviews the contents of this book. This can provide a quick reference for those in need of information. It also sets the stage for reading more detailed information in each of the chapters. One of the key goals of this book is to provide information on anatomy and physiology of the auditory system and relate this to the clinical situation in which it may be used. This type of orientation should be ideally suited for the student and practicing clinician.

Starting with the external ear, the structure and function of the peripheral and central auditory system is presented. The peripheral system, which includes the pinna, external auditory meatus, tympanic membrane, middle ear cavity, ossicular chain, cochlea, and auditory nerve is mostly housed in the temporal bone of the cranium. The periphery focuses sound, transforms it, transduces it to electrical impulses, and sends it to the brain with an intensity, frequency, and time code. The central auditory system (CAS) provides sequential and parallel processing of neural impulses that can be enhanced or inhibited from the cochlear nucleus in the caudal pons to the auditory cortex in the cerebrum. There is also an efferent pathway that courses from the auditory cortex caudally to the cochlea that may modulate afferent impulses. The processing in the CAS is complex and enables us to glean meaningful information from our acoustic environment.

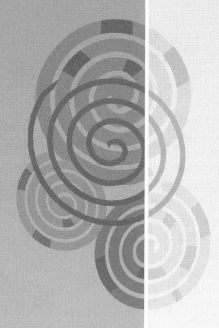

2

The External Ear: Its Structure and Function

Introduction

The external or outer ear constitutes the first portion of the auditory system. It consists of two main structures: the pinna (auricle) and the external auditory meatus (ear canal). This portion of the auditory system begins at the pinna and it ends at the tympanic membrane (eardrum). The outer ear collects the acoustic energy arriving at the head and funnels or directs this energy to the middle ear, where it is transformed into mechanical (vibratory) energy. The acoustic energy that arrives at the outer ear is modified somewhat by the resonant properties of the pinna and ear canal (Rose, 1978; Zemlin, 1998). As a result, the acoustic signal that is delivered to the middle ear by the outer ear is not identical to that which entered the ear.

In addition to having an auditory function, the structures of the outer ear also serve some protective functions. Ceruminous secretions (wax) by hair follicles and glands located in the ear canal have antibacterial and antifungal properties. Hence, these secretions help prevent the growth of some bacterial and fungal infections that might otherwise arise in the ear canal. In addition, since the earwax is a bitter sticky substance, it also protects against the intrusion of insects into the ear canal.

A number of medical conditions can affect the pinna and the ear canal. However, most of these conditions do not seriously compromise auditory function.

ANATOMY

Pinna (Auricle)

The **pinna** or **auricle** is the large flap-like structure of the hearing mechanism that is attached to the side of the head. In humans, the pinna protrudes away from the head at an angle of 15° to 30° (Zemlin, 1998; Yost, 2000). However, there is considerable variability in the actual degree of this angle in humans—as can readily be seen as one looks at the general population. Many individuals have ears that are tight to the head, while others have ears that protrude quite some distance from the head (i.e., at an angle significantly greater than 30°).

The pinna itself consists of several pieces of cartilage that are held together by ligaments. It also contains some extrinsic and intrinsic muscles,

● **F i g u r e 2 . 1**

A photo of the
human pinna
showing the major
structural landmarks.

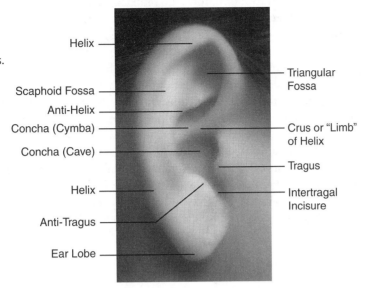

Helix ─────

Scaphoid Fossa ─────
Anti-Helix ─────
Concha (Cymba) ─────
Concha (Cave) ─────

Helix ─────

Anti-Tragus ─────

Ear Lobe ─────

───── Triangular
Fossa

───── Crus or "Limb"
of Helix

───── Tragus

───── Intertragal
Incisure

which appear to be largely vestigial muscles in humans. Although these muscles are largely nonfunctional in humans, they are functional in many animal species and play an important role in the keen, finely tuned localization abilities of these animal species. The cartilaginous foundation of the pinna is covered by an epidermis that is a continuation of the skin that covers the face and head.

The configuration of the cartilage within the pinna produces several ridges and depressions on the surface of the structure (Figure 2.1). Prominent landmarks of the pinna include the **tragus**, which is the protective flap originating from the front of the pinna and protruding back toward the rear of the pinna; this partially covers the entrance to the ear canal. The **concha** is a large cup-shaped depression to the rear of and below the tragus which forms the entrance to the ear canal. The concha has a diameter of 1 to 2 cm in the adult (Yost, 2000) and it forms the actual entrance to the **external auditory meatus** (EAM), commonly referred to as the ear canal. The ridged rim along the posterior and superior region of the pinna is the **helix**. The helix courses downward along the posterior perimeter of the pinna until it reaches the **lobe** (lobule); in the superior region of the pinna the helix courses in an anterior direction and then it turns in a caudal direction and ultimately a posterior direction to form the crux of the helix—a hook-shaped ridge on the pinna. Located immediately anterior to the helix is a groove that runs down the posterior portion of the pinna. This groove is referred to as the **scaphoid fossa**. Proceeding in an anterior direction from the scaphoid fossa is a prominent ridge, the **antihelix**. The antihelix essentially runs parallel to the helix; however, in its upper portion, this structure splits into two segments that are referred to as the **crura of the antihelix**. One crus of the antihelix continues to course in parallel with the helix, while the second segment courses in an anterior–superior direction. A prominent depression is observed in a triangular area that is formed by the branching of the antihelix into two crura. This region of the pinna is referred to as the **triangular fossa**. At the inferior-most region of the antihelix is a widening of the structure, known as the **antitragus.** The tragus and antitragus are separated by a notch referred to as the **intertragal incisure** (or intertragic incisure) (see Zemlin, 1998 and Yost, 2000 for reviews).

As mentioned above, the internal structure of the pinna consists of a cartilaginous foundation that has much the same shape as is seen in the external structure. Medially the cartilage is contiguous with the cartilage that serves as the foundation of the lateral portion of the ear canal. The cartilage of the pinna attaches via a cartilaginous spine to the zygomatic arch of the temporal bone and by a cartilaginous tail to the mastoid process of the temporal bone. In addition to the cartilaginous foundation, there are three muscles that attach to the pinna, and the anterior, superior, and posterior auricular muscles. In humans, these are vestigial muscles and they have no significant auditory function. In many animal species (e.g., cats, dogs, horses), however, these muscles are functional and afford the animal the ability to orient the pinna toward a sound source—an ability that is believed to significantly improve the animal's ability to quickly and effectively locate the source of a sound (Gelfand, 1997; Zemlin, 1998). Finally, there also are several small intrinsic muscles within the pinna itself. However, as is the case with the auricular muscles, these muscles appear to have little or no function in humans (see Zemlin, 1998 for review).

EXTERNAL AUDITORY MEATUS (EAR CANAL)

The ear canal, also referred to as the external auditory meatus (EAM), is a tube-like structure that measures approximately 2.5 to 3 cm in length and .75 cm in diameter in the normal adult (Rose, 1978). The diameter of the canal is larger at the auricular orifice and it gradually decreases in diameter along the length of the canal as it approaches an area in the canal referred to as the **isthmus**. Medial to this point in the EAM, the canal opens up and once again increases in diameter. The EAM is not a straight tube or cylindrical structure, but rather one that has two curves forming a somewhat elongated or lazy "S" (i.e., an "S" that would be lying on its side). The opening at the medial end of the EAM tends to be somewhat circular in configuration in humans, as does the opening at the outer end, at least in children. There is a tendency for the shape of the outer end of the canal to change with age; therefore, the configuration of the canal at this end of the EAM (i.e., the outermost end) is often observed to be more oval in shape in the adult. In addition, there is a tendency for the lumen of the canal to become smaller in size in adults and in avid swimmers (see Moeller, 2000, for review).

The axis of the EAM runs roughly perpendicular to the head (Figure 2.2). It does, however, take a slight downward direction at either end, at least in the adult human. This slight downward turn of the canal at its lateral, or outer, end prevents (or at least minimizes) the retention of water in the ear, as small amounts of water entering the ear are likely to drain out of the canal. The course of the ear canal in infants and young children tends to be more horizontal than in adults. As a result, there is an increased tendency for foreign objects to find their way into the ear canals of infants and young children.

● **F i g u r e   2 . 2**

A coronal section of the human ear showing the configuration and course of the external auditory meatus (adapted from Zemlin, 1998, with permission).

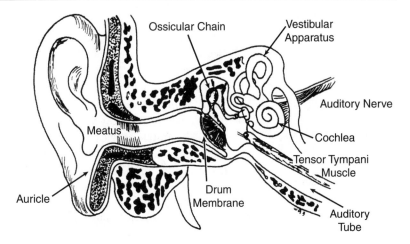

In the adult, the outer one-third to one-half of the EAM has a cartilaginous foundation, whereas the inner, or medial, portion has a bony (osseous) foundation that is part of the hard bone of the skull. Since the foundation of the medial portion of the EAM is bone, the diameter of the canal in this area is fixed in the adult. On the lateral end of the canal, however, there is often some dynamic variability in the diameter of the canal since the foundation in this region is cartilaginous. Thus, the diameter of the opening in this portion of the canal may change with movements of the mandible during a number of motor activities (chewing, yawning, talking, etc.). In addition, the shape and dimensions of the EAM in this region can be altered by pulling on the pinna—a strategy often employed by health-care professionals to achieve better visualization of the TM.

The bony portion of the canal is formed by three main structures: (1) the tympanic portion of the temporal bone, which forms the floor and anterior wall and the inferior–posterior wall of the canal; (2) the squamous portion of the temporal bone, which forms the roof and a portion of the posterior wall of the canal; and (3) the condoyle of the mandible, which contributes to the inferior–anterior wall of the canal at the temporomandibular joint (Gelfand, 1997, p. 43). At birth there is no osseous portion to the foundation of the EAM in the human species. This osseous portion develops from an incomplete cartilaginous ring (referred to as the tympanic annulus) in the human over a period of several years. The development of the osseous part of the EAM may not reach full maturation until around the end of the third year of life (see Zemlin, 1998).

The ear canal is covered by an epidermal lining that closely adheres to the supportive structures of the canal. This lining covers the length of the canal and eventually forms the lateral-most layer of the TM at the medial end of the EAM. The epidermal lining of the outer portion of canal contains hair follicles and glands that secrete a waxy substance, cerumen, which serves some protective functions for the peripheral hearing system; for example, this substance helps prevent the epidermal lining of the EAM from drying out. The wax-producing cells are concentrated in the cartilaginous portion of the external auditory canal (i.e., the outer portion of the canal), while the medial portion of the EAM is devoid of such hair cells.

Two types of cells within the EAM contribute to the secretion of cerumen: the sebaceous glands, located close to the hair follicles, and the ceruminous glands. The sebaceous cells produce an oily substance that lubricates the ear canal. These cells form their secretions by passive breakdown of cells since they are incapable of

CLINICAL CORRELATE

The ear canal is shorter in infants; hence, clinicians must be careful in placing such things as ear inserts and otoscopic speculums in the ear canal to avoid causing damage to the either the sensitive lining of the EAM or the TM. ●

producing active secretions. The oil secreted by the sebaceous glands mixes with the wax-like substance secreted by the ceruminous glands to form the ear wax (cerumen) that is found in the human ear. The consistency of cerumen varies from dry and flaky to wet and sticky, depending upon the relative contributions of the secretions from the two different types of cells. There are some differences in the consistency of cerumen that is produced by individuals from different racial backgrounds. Individuals of Asian descent are more likely to have the flaky type of cerumen, while Caucasians, Latinos, and individuals of African descent are more likely to have the wet, sticky variety (Moller, 2000).

The outer layer of skin that covers the ear canal migrates outward and transports the cerumen out of the ear. Therefore, in most individuals, cerumen will be found only in the outer region of the EAM as it is typically transported away from the medial portion of the canal. In some individuals, however, the cerumen may find its way down to the medial portion of the EAM and become hard and impacted. This is more likely to occur in individuals who have overactive ceruminous glands and in individuals who force or direct the cerumen into the medial portion of the canal while attempting to clean the ear canal with a Q-tip or other type of cleaning device.

As indicated above, the presence of cerumen provides some protective functions for the ear; for example, the secreted cerumen has a slight antibacterial and antifungal property and may repel or discourage insects from entering the ear canal. Therefore, the presence of cerumen in the ear canal is both normal and desirable. Although the presence of ear wax provides a protective function for the auditory system, if there is an excessive accumulation of this substance it can become a cause of hearing loss, especially if the ear wax migrates down the ear canal and covers the TM or blocks the transmission of sound through the EAM to the TM (a condition often referred to as impacted wax). Increased productions of cerumen are frequently noted in geriatric patients, particularly in older male patients, since there is often an increase in the growth of the hair cells in the concha and the EAM associated with normal aging processes. The build-up of excessive cerumen in the ear canal (from an overproduction of cerumen, the lack of normal epithelial migration in the ear canal, or from the misguided attempts to clean the ears with Q-tips or some other cleaning device) typically requires management with either an over-the-counter solution or direct intervention by a health-care professional.

The ear canal has a rich supply of nerves for tactile sensitivity and pain as it receives innervations from the Vth (trigeminal), VIIth (facial), IXth (glossopharyngeal), and Xth (vagus) cranial nerves. Stimulation (touching) of the inner part of the EAM can often result in a coughing response in some individuals since there is a rich supply of innervations offered to this region of the auditory system by the glossopharyngeal nerve. Also, mechanical stimulation of the ear canal can affect the heart and blood circulation in some sensitive individuals because of the innervations that the EAM receives from both the glossopharyngeal and vagus nerves. In a subset of these highly sensitive individuals, the effects of manipulation of the EAM can be strong enough to trigger a fainting episode (Moller, 2000).

CLINICAL CORRELATE

Impacted cerumen is a common cause of conductive hearing loss. It can also result in itching of the ear canal, tinnitus, vertigo, and external otitis. In severe cases of considerable impaction, the conductive hearing can reach 45 dB HL (Gelfand, 2001). ●

CLINICAL CORRELATE

The ear canal is innervated by a number of cranial nerves that provide for tactile sensitivity. As mentioned above, touching and mechanical manipulation of the EAM can result in coughing and, in some highly sensitive individuals, fainting responses because of this rich innervation. Although most audiological procedures do not require this type of manipulation of the ear canal, some cerumen management procedures (i.e., wax removal procedures) do require manipulation of the EAM to an extent that may trigger these responses in some individuals. ●

FUNCTIONS OF THE OUTER EAR

Pinna (Auricle)

The auricle functions most effectively as a sound collector for frequencies around 5000 Hz. This is because the wavelengths of frequencies in this range are smaller than the pinna and cannot easily pass around the pinna. On the other hand, the wavelengths of lower frequencies are larger than the dimensions of the pinna and they may pass around the pinna with relative ease. The configuration of the ridges and depressions on the surface of the pinna cause it to function as a complex resonator for high-frequency sounds (Figure 2.3). These high-frequency resonance patterns change as the location of the source of the sound changes, which provides cues for localization along the horizontal plane (Blauert, 1983). It appears that the pinna may also play a key role in providing cues for localization along the vertical plane in humans (Hofman and Van Opstal, 2003). The pinnae do this by providing spectral shape cues that contribute to elevation as well as back versus front sound source information. By applying binaural earmolds that compromise the pinnae's cavities, individuals lose much of their ability to localize changes in sound source elevation (Butler and Musicant, 1993).

External Auditory Meatus (Ear Canal)

The EAM carries the acoustic signal arriving at the entrance of the ear canal to the middle ear. Because of its anatomical configuration, the EAM functions as an acoustic resonator and thus it alters the sound that is being transmitted to the TM (Figures 2.3 and 2.4). The EAM is configured somewhat like a tube that is closed at one end and open at the other end. Such an arrangement provides for reinforcement of acoustic energy with wavelengths four times greater than the length of the tube. If the typical length of the EAM in the adult is 2.5 to 3 cm and the EAM were in fact a tube open at one end and closed at the other, the EAM should function as a quarter-wave resonator that would boost the level of those frequencies

● **Figure 2.3**

The average pressure gain that is contributed by different components of the head, body, and outer ear (concha, pinna plange, and ear canal/eardrum) as well as the combined effect of all of these components. Note: the sound source for these measurements was presented at in the horizontal plane at a 0° azimuth (from Shaw, 1974, with permission).

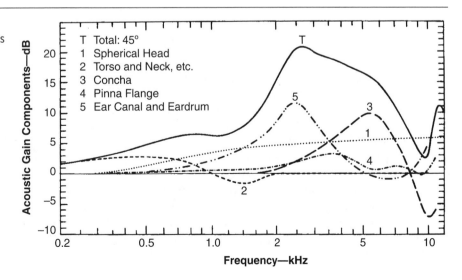

● **Figure 2.4**

Resonance effects of the EAM displayed as the ratio of the sound pressure at the eardrum to the sound pressure at the entrance of the ear canal. The measurements presented in this figure were obtained with a sound source presented at an azimuth of 0° (i.e., with the subject facing the sound source) (from data from Wiener and Ross, 1946, adapted by Zemlin, 1998, with permission).

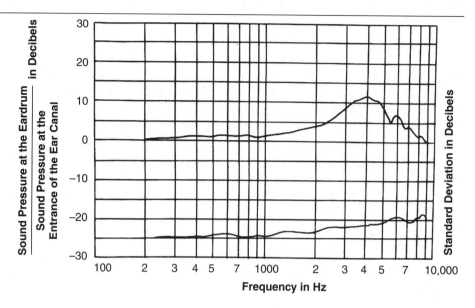

with wavelengths of 10–12 cm—these would typically fall in the frequency range of 3.5 to 4 kHz. Based upon direct measurements, Dallos (1973) demonstrated that the EAM has a broadly tuned resonance pattern providing for a 10 to 15-dB amplification of sounds in the frequency range of 3000 to 4000 Hz which closely matches the predictions based upon the model described above. Some deviation from the predictions is expected since the "closed end" of the EAM in this model is actually terminated by the TM, which is compliant and which transmits some acoustic energy to the middle ear, in addition to reflecting back some of the energy (i.e., the basis for the resonance). This results in a modification of the effective length (as opposed to the actual length of the EAM) and results in a damping effect. As a result, the EAM resonates over a relatively wide range of frequencies as opposed to the somewhat more restricted frequency range that would be predicted if the EAM were actually a tube or pipe with a closed end (i.e., hard wall closure) (Figure 2.4) (see Pickles, 1988 and Zemlin, 1998 for discussion).

CLINICAL CORRELATE

The resonance patterns for the auricle (pinna) and the ear canal provide a selective tuning of the peripheral auditory mechanism. In practical terms, this means that the spectrum of a sound being delivered to the ear would be shaped to provide an emphasis of 10 to 15 dB in the 3000 to 4000 Hz range and that there would be a complex pattern of emphasis and de-emphasis at the higher frequencies. This shaping of the spectrum of the sound is a natural experience for the listener, and its loss is a major consideration in the fitting of hearing aids and other amplification devices. When the outer portion of the ear canal is occluded by an earmold, the resonance patterns of the ear are altered and the natural resonance that typically occurs at 3000 to 4000 Hz is altered or eliminated. The experience for the listener who now has lost this natural augmentation of the sound in a restricted frequency region determined by his or her unique anatomy is that of a signal that is no longer natural sounding. Patients fitted with occluding earmolds (those that result in an extensive blocking off of the ear canal) often complain that amplified speech signal sounds "tinny or hollow"—a situation that needs to be addressed by the dispensing audiologist if the patient is to be pleased with the amplification device. ●

Directional Effects

Although not considered part of the auditory system per se, the head (and to some extent the torso) may play a role in how humans hear—at least in some situations (e.g., in the sound field or in normal conversational situations). Therefore, a brief discussion of this topic appears to be in order. As sound travels from a loudspeaker or other sound source in a free-field type of listening environment, the acoustic signal is affected by the path that it takes to reach the eardrum, or TM. As mentioned above, the acoustic signal is altered noticeably by the presence of an ear canal resonance and the properties of the pinna, but other factors external to the ear also affect the signal that reaches the ear. These factors include refractions and reflections of the sound caused by the presence of the head and body, as well as other environmental factors (e.g., room acoustics). The acoustical effects afforded by the head depend upon the direction of the sound (Figure 2.5). Different directions of a sound source are designated as angles around the head in a plane or axis that is relative to the position of the head. For example, in the horizontal plane, a signal that is presented at a 0° azimuth would be originating from a sound source directly in front of the listener. One that is presented at a 90° azimuth would be originating to the right side of the head, 180° to the back of the head, and 270° to the left of the head.

A sound presented in the sound field will not be the same sound when it reaches the two ears because of the influence of the head (Figure 2.5). Consider a sound source presented at an azimuth of 45° to the right. In this case the signal would arrive at the right ear at a slight angle to the entrance to the ear and would meet little interference; however, the head would offer a significant obstruction to the sound that is arriving at the left ear, and as a result, the level of the signal reaching the left ear is lower (i.e., softer). This is referred to as the head shadow effect. This effect, however, is not equal across frequencies. Frequencies with longer wavelengths (i.e., low-frequency sounds) can pass around the head more readily and have negligible head shadow effects, but frequencies with shorter wavelengths (i.e., high-frequency sounds) are more significantly affected by the head shadow effect.

CLINICAL CORRELATE

A collapsed ear canal, if not recognized and managed, can cause problems for the clinician. It can result in a conductive hearing loss (usually greater at high frequencies), which is associated with applying circumaural earphones to a patient. The pressure from the earphone on the outer ear can cause the canal to collapse in some individuals. The problem is most common in elderly patients who have lost elasticity in ear canal tissues. The best way around this problem is to use insert earphones (Gelfand, 2001). ●

● **Figure 2.5**

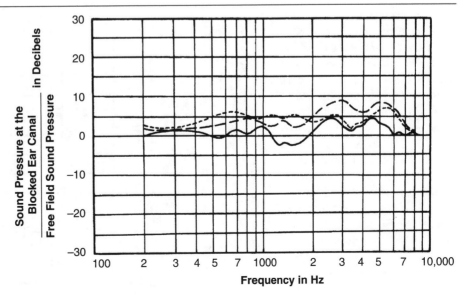

The effect of the head in the sound field when the angle of incidence is 0° azimuth (solid line), 45° azimuth (long dashes) and 90° azimuth (short dashes). At frequencies above 500 Hz, the effects exceed 5 dB when the azimuth is 90° (i.e., when the sound source is in the same plane as the ear), which helps to explain why we turn our ear toward the source of a faint sound rather than directly facing the source of the sound (from Zemlin, 1998, with permission).

This difference between the intensity levels of the signal reaching the two ears is referred to as the **interaural intensity difference**, a phenomenon that is important for normal localization abilities.

Another phenomenon that occurs when the signal is presented at an angle from the center of the head in the horizontal plane is a difference in the time of arrival of the signal at the two ears. In the example above, the sound would have a more direct and shorter route to the right ear than it would to the left ear. The difference in the time of arrival between the two ears is referred to as the **interaural time difference**. Although low frequency sounds do not typically result in significant interaural intensity differences, they do result in interaural time differences. These two interaural differences (time and intensity) provide important cues that are used by structures within the central hearing mechanism to identify the source of a sound (i.e., sound localization).

Combined Effects of the Head and Torso and Outer Ear on Pressure Gain

A number of factors interact to determine the level of the signal that reaches the eardrum. Some signals are reinforced, or enhanced, while others are attenuated, or depressed. These effects are determined by both the incidence of arrival (as the head shadow effects may alter the signal levels) as well as the resonance effects afforded by the outer ear structures (Figure 2.6). If one is listening in the sound field, it is important to take both of these factors into account.

Figure 2.3, which is based upon the work of Shaw (1974), presents a sequential model of the effects of the various factors that can affect or alter the gain of the signal that arrives at the eardrum. It is mentioned here again to highlight the fact that the signal that reaches the eardrum is not the same signal that is being delivered by the sound source. A number of individual elements shown in this figure alter the intensity of the signal as it continues along its path from its source to the eardrum. These individual effects combine to result in a significant overall change

● Figure 2.6

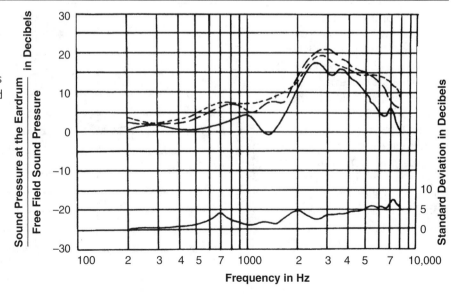

The combined effects of the ear canal resonance, the outer ear resonance (i.e., from the concha), and the head on the intensity level reaching the ear from sound sources at three different azimuths. The solid upper curve represents the data obtained with the signal presented at the 0° azimuth, while the curves with the long dashes and the short dashes represent the data obtained for signals presented at 45° and 90° azimuths, respectively (data from Wiener and Ross, 1946, adapted by Zemlin, 1998, with permission).

in the acoustic signal at the eardrum (represented by the T in the figure). A closer look at the figure shows a rather broad overall increase in acoustic pressure (i.e., gain) over a frequency range from approximately 2000 to 7000 Hz (see Pickles, 1988; Gelfand, 1997; Zemlin, 1998; and Moller, 2000 for reviews).

SUMMARY

The outer ear system functions as a collector of acoustic energy that is transferred to the middle ear for transduction to an alternate form of energy (vibrational). The acoustic signal reaching the middle ear is modified in the process. Because of some resonance characteristics associated with the functions of the pinna and the EAM, some frequencies are enhanced while others are depressed. The most prominent enhancement of the signal tends to occur in the higher frequency range and is the direct result of an ear canal resonance. Loss of this ear canal resonance results in a signal that no longer sounds normal. This may become a concern when one is fitting a hearing aid since if the ear canal is occluded, the ear canal resonance can be lost or significantly altered. The pinna appears to provide sound shape cues to the auditory system, which in turn helps in front versus back and elevation sound source localization.

The effect of the head can also influence the level of the sound that reaches the ear. The sound pressure arriving at the entrance to the ear canal depends on the frequency of the sound, the angle of incidence of the sound, and the unique characteristics of the individual's head and torso. Differences in intensity levels as well as time of arrival serve as the physical bases for directional hearing in the horizontal plane. The presence of the head can alter the level of a signal that originates from different locations in acoustic space. These changes, when coupled with the changes in the signal afforded by the resonance properties of the outer ear structures, result in an acoustic signal at the eardrum that is significantly different than the signal originating at the sound source (see Figure 2.3).

Although many medical conditions can affect the outer ear, most of them have little or no audiological consequence. There are, however, a few conditions that can result in significant hearing loss. One such disorder is atresia, which can be partial or complete. In cases of complete atresia, the ear canal is absent and a moderate to moderately severe hearing loss is common. Intervention may involve the surgical creation of a canal if the more medial portions of the auditory system are intact and there are no contraindications to surgery. Another option would include the fitting of a special amplification device called a bone conduction hearing aid. This type of hearing aid delivers a vibrational source of energy representing the sound stimulus directly to the skull of the individual, which then transmits the vibrational representations of the sound directly to the inner ear (cochlea), thus bypassing the need to be able to direct an acoustic signal down the EAM to the middle ear for conversion to mechanical energy (i.e., vibrational). Another condition that may result in hearing loss is impacted cerumen; fortunately, this condition can be resolved easily with appropriate management procedures.

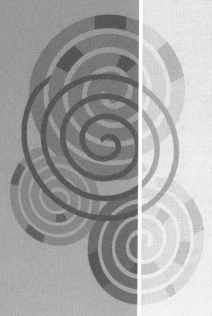

3

Anatomy and Physiology of the Middle Ear

Introduction

Sounds entering the auditory system pass through the outer ear to the middle ear, which is the second major portion of the auditory system. Here the acoustic energy that entered the outer ear strikes the eardrum (the first structure in the middle ear system) and is converted to mechanical energy (vibrational energy). This energy is then passed on through the ossicular chain to the inner ear. The ossicular chain is a series of three small bones (the malleus, the incus, and the stapes) that are suspended in the middle ear space by a number of ligaments and muscle tendons. The vibrational patterns of the eardrum are readily passed to the ossicular chain, as there is a direct attachment of a portion of the first bone in the ossicular chain (i.e., the malleus) to the eardrum itself. Since the three bones are connected by an encapsulated joint (malleus to incus) and a flexible joint (incus to stapes), the vibrational patterns are then transmitted through the chain to an opening into the inner ear (oval window).

The middle ear is a hard-walled cavity located in the temporal bone. It is normally filled with air that is refreshed by the functioning of a small tube located in the inferior region of the cavity. This tube, the Eustachian tube (ET), connects the middle ear space and the nasopharynx. It is normally closed, but opens during motor activities such as yawning and swallowing. When the tube opens, air can travel either into or out of the middle ear space so that the pressure in the middle ear can be maintained at a level that is equal to that of the air in the environment or atmosphere. The air pressure in the ear canal (located on the lateral side of the eardrum) is equal to the pressure of the air in the environment. If the pressure on the medial side is equal to that in the ear canal, no pressure differential across the eardrum exists and the eardrum is in its normal position (i.e., the position or condition in which the eardrum would move most readily). If, on the other hand, the pressure on the medial side of the eardrum (i.e., in the middle ear space) is not equal to the pressure on the lateral side, the eardrum will be displaced toward the region of lesser pressure and the individual may experience some discomfort in the ear—an experience that anyone who has flown will quickly recognize.

The following is a brief explanation for this pressure differential. As the airplane makes its ascent, the air pressure in the cabin drops, which means there is less pressure in the cabin (and in the ear canal) than there is in the middle ear (at take-off the pressure would have been equal to the atmospheric pressure on the ground). Until such time as the ET opens (during swallowing or yawning), the pressure in the middle ear space is greater than that in the ear canal; hence, the greater pressure in the middle ear pushes on the eardrum, displacing it toward the outer ear. Motor activities such as swallowing or yawning cause the ET to open, and some of the air from the middle ear passes out of the ET until the pressure is once again equal on either side of the eardrum. The reverse set of circumstances occurs on descent.

The middle ear plays an important role in hearing in that it functions as an impedance matching device. Without this unique function, our hearing sensitivity would not be nearly as keen or sensitive as it actually is. This is because of the large impedance differential (i.e., difference in the opposition to the flow of energy) that exists between the air, which is a low impedance medium, and the fluid contained in the inner ear, which is a high impedance medium. Without a special mechanism to "match" the impedances of these two mediums, most of the acoustic energy entering the ear would be reflected back by the high-impedance fluids of the inner ear.

Two muscle tendons enter the middle ear space and connect to two of the bones in the ossicular chain (specifically the first and last bones in the series). When these muscle tendons contract, they pull the ossicular chain in roughly opposite directions, thus stiffening the ossicular chain. The end result is that greater opposition is offered to the flow of energy through the middle ear system. These muscles, but especially the stapedius muscle, contract in response to intense sounds in normally hearing individuals. It is believed that this response to intense sounds may play some role in protecting the inner ear from the damaging effects of high intensity noise. However, some debate exists about the role of this response in hearing protection.

ANATOMY

Middle Ear Space (Cavity)

The middle ear is an air-filled space that is situated between the outer ear and the inner ear (Figure 3.1). It is also referred to as the tympanum or the tympanic cavity (Gelfand, 1997; Zemlin, 1998; Yost, 2000). It is a relatively narrow, elongated space that is encased within the temporal bone of the skull. In the adult, it has a width that varies from 2 to 4 mm along the horizontal plane, a vertical dimension of about 13 mm, and a volume of approximately 2 cm^3. The middle ear cavity includes two main areas: (1) a large area in the lower portion of the cavity referred to as the **tympanic cavity proper** and (2) a smaller upper area (in the posterio–superior portion of the cavity) that is referred to as the **attic**, the **epitympanum**, or **epitympanic recess** (Figures 3.1 and 3.2). This latter area of the cavity houses significant parts of the two larger ossicles (i.e., the head of the malleus and a significant portion of the incus) (Gelfand, 1997; Zemlin, 1998; Yost, 2000).

The lateral boundary of the middle ear space is formed in large part by the tympanic membrane (TM);

● **Figure 3.1**

Schematic of the middle ear (right side of the head) as seen from the front (from Zemlin, 1998, with permission).

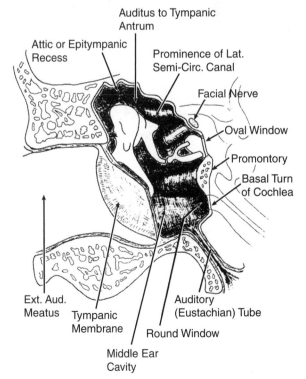

● **Figure 3.2**

Lateral view of the medial wall and parts
of the anterior and posterior walls of the
tympanic membrane (human).

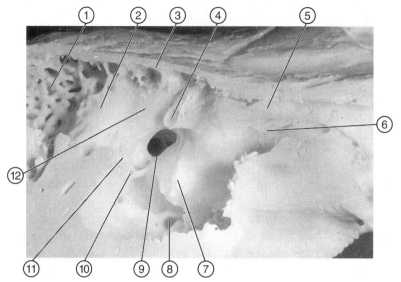

KEY: 1 = tympanic antrum, 2 = aditus to tympanic antrum, 3 = tegmen tympani, 4 = cochleariform process, 5 = septum canalis musculotubarii, 6 = bony part of the ET, 7 = promontory, 8 = niche of the round window, 9 = oval window, 10 = pyramidal eminence, 11 = epitympanic recess, 12 = prominence of the lateral semicircular canal (from Zemlin, 1998, with permission).

however, a portion of the lateral wall above the TM (in the epitympanic recess) is formed by a section of the squamous portion of the temporal bone (Figure 3.1). The superior boundary of the middle ear cavity is formed by a thin plate of bone (**tegmen tympani**), which separates the middle ear space from the cranium (Figure 3.2). This bone continues in a posterior direction to form the roof of the **tympanic atrium**, where there is an indirect communication between the middle ear space and the mastoid air cells. The inferior boundary is formed by the **tympanic plate** of the temporal bone. This plate separates the middle ear cavity from the **jugular fossa** (a groove in the temporal bone through which the jugular vein passes). The anterior wall, often referred to as the **carotid wall**, is a thin plate of bone that is perforated in its superior region by an opening for the **Eustachian tube** (ET) (Figure 3.2) and an orifice for the tendon of the **tensor tympani muscle**. The posterior wall (or mastoid wall) is also formed by portions of the temporal bone. This wall has a number of landmarks, including an entrance to the tympanic atrium (referred to as the **tympanic aditus**) (Figure 3.2), the **fossa incudis** (a small bowl in the epitympanic recess that accommodates the short process of the incus), and the **pyramidal eminence** (a bulge in the bony foundation of the posterior wall that houses the stapedius muscle) (Figure 3.2). There is additionally one small aperture that opens into the posterior wall near the juncture of this wall with the lateral wall through which a branch of the facial nerve enters the middle ear (Figure 3.1) and courses through the middle ear to exit the cavity near the **tympanic sulcus**. Finally, the medial wall of the cavity is formed by a dense portion of the temporal bone, which houses the inner ear (Figures 3.1, 3.3, and 3.4). Significant landmarks on this wall include the **promontory** (a rounded prominence formed by the lateral projection of the basal turn of the cochlea), the **round window** (an opening into the basal turn of the scala tympani), the **oval window** (an opening into the vestibule of the inner ear that accommodates one of the middle ear bones, the stapes), and the **prominence of the facial nerve** through which the facial nerve courses (Figures 3.1 and 3.2).

Zemlin (1998) provides a comprehensive review of the boundaries of the middle ear space for the reader who is interested in more detailed information on the boundaries of this part of the auditory system. Other sources of information can be found in Pickles, 1988; Gelfand, 1997; and Yost, 2000.

Tympanic Membrane (Eardrum)

The tympanic membrane (TM) is oval in shape, and although it is often compared to the skin of a drum, it is not a flat membrane. Rather, the TM has a concave configuration that makes it appear somewhat cone-shaped, with the point of the cone being located more medially than its rim (Figure 3.1). In the adult, the TM has a diameter of approximately 8 to 9 mm along the horizontal axis and 9 to 10 mm along the vertical axis. On average, it is about 0.1 mm thick and it contains three layers. However, there is variability in these dimensions, as well as in the number of layers that are present in the TM (see Rose, 1978; Gelfand, 1997; Zemlin, 1998; Yost, 2000 for reviews).

The outer layer of the TM is formed by an extension of the epidermal lining of the external auditory meatus (EAM), while the inner layer is a continuation of the membranous lining (mucosal lining) of the middle ear space. The middle layer is composed of a fibrous material that is believed to provide support for the TM. Within the fibrous center layer (or layers) are two sets of fibers that are closely interconnected. One set radiates from the center of the TM to the periphery in much the same manner as the spokes of a wheel (radial fibers), while the second set is composed of concentric rings of fibers (circular fibers). It turns out that the

● **Figure 3.3**

The middle ear of a cat. The inner surface of the drum membrane (T), the manubrium of the malleus (M), the promontory (P), and round window (R) are all clearly seen (from Zemlin, 1998, with permission).

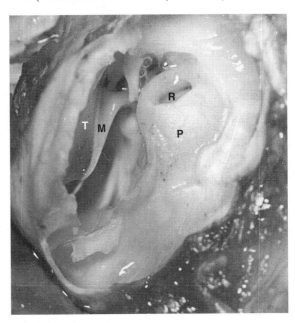

● **Figure 3.4**

The ossicles and cochlea of a 4-month-old human fetus. The apex (A) can be seen at the top of the cochlea, and the round window (R) can be seen at the basal turn (B). Also seen are the head of the malleus (HM), the manubrium of the malleus (MM), the long arm of the incus (I), the head of the stapes (S), and the footplate of the stapes (F), along with the ligament of the stapedius muscle (L) (dissection by Patricia Gauper, from Zemlin, 1998, with permission).

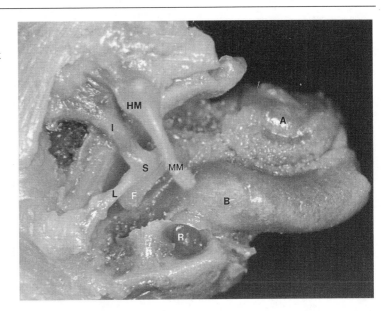

Schematic of the tympanic membrane and some associated structures (from Zemlin, 1998, with permission).

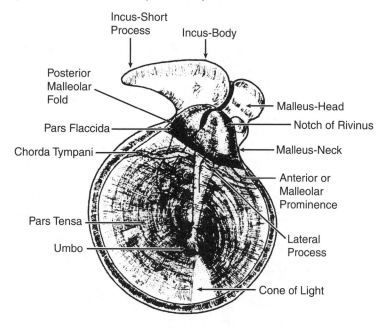

Incus-Short Process
Incus-Body
Posterior Malleolar Fold
Malleus-Head
Notch of Rivinus
Pars Flaccida
Chorda Tympani
Malleus-Neck
Anterior or Malleolar Prominence
Pars Tensa
Umbo
Lateral Process
Cone of Light

fibers within this middle or center layer are not equally distributed throughout the TM (Zemlin, 1998; Moller, 2000). Increased densities of the fibers are noted toward the periphery of the membrane and in the region where the manubrium of the malleus attaches to the TM (Figure 3.5). There is another region of the TM where the fibers are quite sparse. This region is found in the upper superior portion of the TM (above the manubrium of the malleus) in an area that is in close proximity to the epitympanum. Here the fibers are not only fewer in number, but they are also not arranged in as orderly a fashion as they are in other parts of the TM. This particular area of the TM is referred to as the **pars flaccida**, also referred to as **Schrapnell's membrane** (Zemlin, 1998). There is a greater density of supportive fibers outside of this area of the TM, where the TM tends to be stiffer and tenser (as opposed to flaccid). Hence, this larger region of the TM is referred to as the **pars tensa**. The fibers (radial and circular) are composed of collagen and provide for a lightweight, stiff membrane that is ideally suited for converting sound energy into mechanical or vibratory energy (Moller, 2000).

The periphery of the TM is thickened to form a fibrocattilaginous ring, or annulus, which is located in a groove within the auditory meatus and is referred to as the **tympanic sulcus**. The **tympanic annulus** has an opening or deficiency at its superior aspect (**notch of Rivinus**) that is caused by a tiny interruption in the tympanic sulcus (Figure 3.5) (Zemlin, 1998). The manubrium of the malleus attaches in a vertical direction to the TM. This attachment is referred to as the **malleal prominence** (Figure 3.5). Ligamentous bands called the **anterior and posterior malleolar folds** run from both sides of the malleolar prominence to the notch of Rivinus, forming a triangular area, which is the location of the pars flaccida region of the TM (Gelfand, 1997; Zemlin, 1998).

As mentioned above, the TM forms a deep cone, which is the result of the attachment of the ossicular chain to the TM in its upper portion. The TM is displaced inward in the vicinity of its center by about 2 mm. The tip of the cone of the region of maximal concavity is referred to as the **umbo** (Figures 3.1 and 3.5).

The TM develops early, reaching its full size during fetal development. It is positioned obliquely in the external canal, forming an acute angle at the lower wall (40°) and an obtuse angle at the upper wall (140°). At birth the TM is in such a position that it is almost lying on the canal floor. As the EAM lengthens, the TM gradually becomes more erect until it approaches its adult position. The TM in the infant is very thin and highly compliant (Zemlin, 1998).

The outer layer of the TM migrates from the center out; this results in the elimination of small imperfections, injuries, or scars. Therefore, small perforations in the TM are likely to heal spontaneously and may not require reconstructive surgery (Moller, 2000).

When looking at the TM, several important landmarks can often be noted (Figure 3.5). The manubrium of the malleus and the long process of the incus often can be seen through the TM, especially if the observer has experience in viewing the

TM. The rim of the TM (the annular ligament) can also be observed, and in addition, it may be possible to differentiate the pars tensa and pars flaccida areas of the TM. In addition to these landmarks, when the normal TM is viewed with an otoscope, the light from the otoscope is reflected back in a characteristic way. The reflection of light is referred to as the cone of light and is seen as a bright area on the anterior-inferior surface of the eardrum, radiating from the tip of the manubrium to the periphery of the TM. In the right ear, this light radiates from the tip of the manubrium to the 5 o'clock position, while in the left ear it radiates from the tip of the manubrium to the 7 o'clock position (Figure 3.6) (Gelfand, 1997).

● **F i g u r e 3 . 6**

Major otoscopic landmarks of the tympanic membrane (from Gelfand, 1997, with permission).

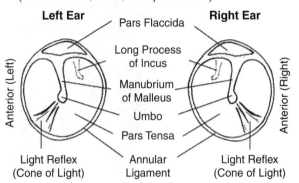

Ossicular Chain

Suspended in the middle ear cavity is a series of three small bones that form a bridge between the TM and the inner ear (i.e., the oval window). These three bones, the malleus, the incus, and the stapes, are the smallest bones in the human body and collectively are referred to as the **ossicular chain** (Figure 3.1). These three bones reach their adult size late during the fetal period, and their overall size and shape do not change substantially following birth (Gelfand, 1997; Zemlin, 1998).

● *Malleus*

The **malleus** is the first of the three bones in the ossicular chain. It is about 9 mm in overall length and it weighs anywhere from 23 to 37 mg (Yost, 2000) (Figures 3.1, 3.3, 3.4, 3.7, 3.8 and 3.9). This bone consists of a head, a neck, and three processes (Figure 3.7). The **manubrium**, which is one of the three processes, attaches firmly to the TM, with the most intimate attachment occurring toward the middle of the eardrum as described above. The **head** of the malleus is a large bulb-shaped portion of the ossicle that projects in an upward direction from the manubrium into the epitympanic recess (Figure 3.1). The posterior surface of the bone contains an **articular facet** (Figure 3.7) that serves as the point of connection with the second bone in the series, the incus. The **neck** of the malleus is a constriction in the bone located between the manubrium and the head. At the point where the manubrium joins the neck there is a small projection that forms the point of attachment for the tensor typmpani muscle. Besides the manubrium, the malleus contains two other processes. The **anterior process** is a spine-like process that can be seen in the region of the juncture of the manubrium and the head. Also in this area is the **lateral process**, which is directed laterally and attaches to the upper portion of the TM.

● *Incus*

The **incus** is the middle of the three bones in the ossicular chain (Figures 3.1, 3.4, 3.7, 3.8, and 3.9). It is composed of essentially three parts: a body and two crura, or processes. On the anterior surface of the body is an articular facet that serves as the contact point for the incus' connection to the malleus (Figure 3.7). The two processes of the incus both arise from the body of this bone at approximately right angles to each other. One of these, the **short process**, is directed backward in a roughly horizontal plane and it shares some of the epitympanic recess with the head of the malleus. The long process courses in a vertical direction that is somewhat

● **F i g u r e   3 . 7**

Various views of the disarticulated human ossicles (from Zemlin, 1998, with permission).

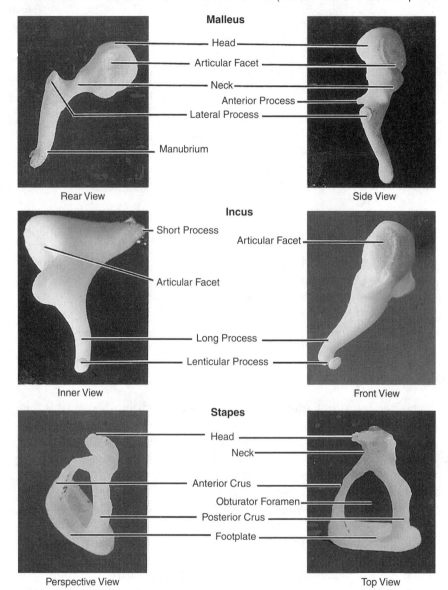

parallel to the manubrium. At its inferior-most end the long process turns abruptly in a medial direction and it terminates as a rounded projection referred to as the **lenticular process**. The medial end of this process is covered with cartilage and articulates with the head of the third and final bone in the ossicular chain, the stapes. In the human, the short process tends to average about 5 mm in length and the long process tends to measure about 7 mm in length; and the weight of the incus averages between 23 and 32 mg (Yost, 2000).

● *Stapes*

The third bone the ossicular chain and the smallest bone in the human body is the **stapes** (Figures 3.1, 3.4, 3.7, 3.8, and 3.9). It consists of a head, a neck, two crura and a footplate (Figure 3.7). The head of the stapes contains a concave articular facet that forms the point of connection for the lenticular process of the incus.

● **Figure 3.8**

Various views of the articulated human ossicles (from Zemlin, 1998, with permission).

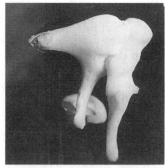
As Seen from the Side

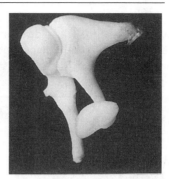
As Seen from Within

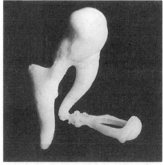
As Seen from the Front

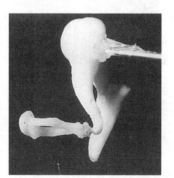
As Seen from Behind

The head (or neck, as it's sometimes called) has a small spine where the tendon of the stapedius muscle attaches. Proceeding medially from the neck are the two crura, which connect the **footplate** of the stapes to the neck. These two crura (the anterior and posterior) tend to connect to the footplate more toward the inferior margin of the footplate than to the posterior margin, and there is a slight difference in the dimensions and shape of the crura, with the anterior crus being shorter, somewhat more slender, and less curved than the posterior crus (Zemlin, 1998). The height of the stapes varies from 2.5 to 3.8 mm and its weight from 2.1 to 4.3 mg (Yost, 2000). The dimensions of the footplate are approximately 1.4 × 3.2 mm and its area is estimated to be 3.2 mm^2 (Rose, 1978).

The medial surface and the periphery of the footplate are covered by a thin layer of hyaline cartilage that is fastened to the bony wall of the oval window (cochlea) by the **annular ligament** (Figure 3.10). The dimensions of this ligament are not constant across the footplate; that is, there is a tendency for this elastic ligament to be larger in the anterior region than in the posterior region. As a result, the footplate tends to be held more rigidly in place in its posterior connection, which affects the displacement of the stapes into the oval window (i.e., rather than functioning as a piston, it tends to pivot or rock a bit, with greater displacement occurring more along the anterior ridge than along the posterior ridge (Zemlin, 1998).

Support for the Ossicular Chain

The ossicular chain is suspended in the middle ear cavity by the tendons from two muscles (**tensor tympani** and **stapedius**) and a number of ligaments (Figure 3.10). The tendons of the two muscles will be discussed in greater detail below. The reader interested in additional discussion of the ligaments is referred to Zemlin, 1998.

● **Figure 3.9**

(a) The middle ear cavity with the ossicular chain removed. The oval window (OW) and promontory (P) are visible. The arrow shows the niche of the round window. (b) The middle ear space with the stapes in place (see upper left-hand portion of photograph. (c) The middle ear cavity with the stapes, incus, and malleus in place. (d) The middle ear structures as seen from within a reconstruction of the tympanic cavity. The structures shown include the head of the malleus (HM), the chorda tympani (CT) (branch of the facial nerve), the tensor tympani muscle (MTT) , the short process of the incus (ISP), the long arm or process of the incus (LP), and the drum membrane (DM) (from Zemlin, 1998, with permission).

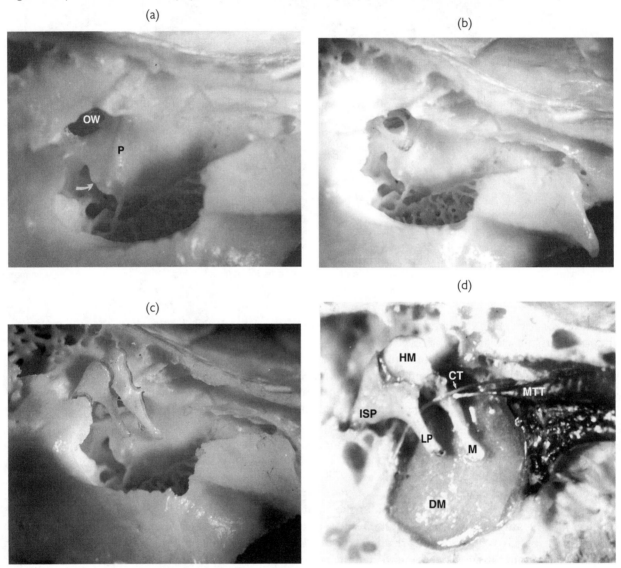

(a)

(b)

(c)

(d)

Eustachian Tube

The **Eustachian tube** runs from the anterior wall (about 3 mm above the floor) of the middle ear cavity and courses to the posterior wall of the nasopharynx in an inferior, medial, and anterior direction at a angle of approximately 45° in the adult (Figures 3.1, 3.2). The first third of the tube (approximately 12 mm) has a bony foundation, while the remaining two-thirds have a cartilaginous foundation (approximately 18 to 24 mm) (Zemlin, 1998). The point where the bony and cartilaginous foundations meet is referred to as the isthmus, which is the narrowest point in the tube (1 to 2 mm) compared to 3 to 6 mm in the remainder of the tube (Gelfand, 1997). The lumen through the bony portion is normally open, or patent,

● Figure 3.10

Schematic of the middle ear ligaments and the tendon of the stapedius muscle (from Zemlin, 1998, with permission).

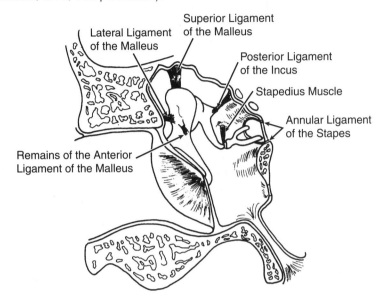

and varies from about 3 to 6 mm in diameter. At rest, the cartilaginous portion of the tube is closed, but it opens upon action of the levator veli palatini and tensor veli palatini muscles (Rose, 1978). The cartilaginous portion begins as a rounded shelf located above the lumen and gradually opens to form an incomplete ring that folds back upon itself laterally—forming somewhat of a hook shape when viewed in the transverse section (Zemlin, 1998). The tube is completed by soft connective tissue.

Middle Ear Muscles

The tendons of two muscles can be found within the middle ear cavity. These two muscles include the tensor typmpani and the stapedius muscles. The tendon of tensor tympani muscle enters the middle ear space through the anterior wall of the middle ear cavity and it inserts into the malleus at the point where the manubrium meets the neck. The tensor tympani muscle is innervated by the fifth cranial nerve (trigeminal nerve), which when innervated pulls the malleus in an anterior and posterior direction. The muscle courses through a semicanal that runs in parallel, but superior to the osseous foundation of the ET. The ET and the semicanal of the muscle are separated by a thin plate of bone (**septum canalis musculotubarii**). This plate and the **cochleariform process** (the curved lateral terminal of the muscle) can be viewed in Figure 3.2.

CLINICAL CORRELATE

The ET in young children is about half as long as it is in adults and it is both wider and somewhat more horizontally positioned; it tends to lie in a plane that is almost parallel with the pharyngeal ostium. All of these factors make the child more susceptible to the spread of infection from the nasopharyngeal regions to the middle ear. As the child matures, the ET assumes a somewhat more vertical position and it becomes narrower. As a result of these changes in the position and dimensions of the ET, the potential for the spread of infection from the nasopharyngeal areas to the middle ear is decreased. This factor can account for the commonly known fact that middle ear infections are much more common in young children than in older children and adults. It is also one of the reasons that even children with frequent recurrences of otitis media in infancy and early childhood tend to "outgrow" these problems as they age (Giebink, 1988). ●

The second muscle is the stapedius muscle. This muscle originates in a bony canal behind the middle ear space, and its tendon enters the cavity through a small opening on the posterior wall of the cavity referred to as the **pyramidal eminence** (Figure 3.1, 3.2). The stapedius muscle attaches to the head of the stapes and is innervated by a branch of the seventh cranial nerve (facial nerve). When this muscle contracts, it pulls the stapes in a posterior direction (Zemlin, 1998).

The tensor tympani and stapedius muscles are antagonistic muscles; that is, when they contract, they each exert a force that is opposite in direction to that of the other muscle. This force is also perpendicular to the primary rotational axis of the ossicular chain (Zemlin, 1998).

Physiology

A concept that will be important to several of the discussions that follow is that of acoustic impedance. **Impedance** is the opposition to the flow of energy or the reluctance to accept energy. It is determined by a number of factors including a **resistance factor** and two reactance factors (**mass reactance** and **stiffness reactance**). These factors interact in complex ways to determine the total impedance of a system (see formula below).

$$Z = \sqrt{R^2 + (2\pi Mf - k/2\pi f)^2}$$

where Z represents the total impedance value, R is the resistance offered by an object (i.e., the loss of energy caused by friction), M is the mass of the object, k is the measure of stiffness of the object, and π is a constant (i.e., 3.14).

Resistance is the loss of energy caused by friction and is independent of frequency. The other two factors are influenced by the frequency of the signal; hence, the term *reactance* is used to define these two factors. Mass reactance is the factor within the formula that is related to the mass of the object or system. It interacts with frequency in a direct proportional manner; that is, if either the mass of the object or the frequency of the signal that is being applied to the system is increased, the contribution of this factor to the overall impedance is increased. The stiffness reactance (sometimes referred to as the elastic reactance factor) is related to the stiffness of the system or object and this factor is also affected by the frequency of the signal being delivered to the system or object. Here, however, there is an inverse relationship with this factor and frequency. That is, as the frequency of the signal is increased, the contribution of this factor to the overall impedance is decreased (see Berlin and Cullen, 1975 for additional review of these principles).

Related to these variables are some important concepts. These can be briefly summarized as follows: massive objects tend to be preferential to low-frequency sounds and offer greater resistance to high-frequency sounds, while the reverse holds true for stiff objects (i.e., stiff objects are preferential to high-frequency sounds and offer greater resistance to low-frequency sounds). As will be discussed, all systems offer some impedance to energy. The amount of opposition to the flow of energy offered by a system, however, depends upon the specific characteristics of the system. Changes to either the mass or stiffness of the system affect the impedance of the system, but the effects are not equal across all frequencies. For example, if the stiffness of the system is increased (as often occurs in some otologic conditions), the increase in impedance would affect the low frequencies. Hence, a low-frequency hearing loss would be predicted, at least in the early stages of the pathology. In many pathologies as the disease process progresses, more frequencies become involved and the hearing loss may begin to affect progressively higher frequencies until a relatively flat configuration of the hearing loss may be observed.

The opposite pattern would be expected if the mass of an object or system is affected. That is, as mass increases, hearing loss should affect the high frequencies first and then the low frequencies. However, most pathologies that increase the mass of the system also tend to affect the stiffness of the system as well; therefore, both high- and low-frequency effects are often noted on the audiogram.

CLINICAL CORRELATE

Tympanometry is a clinical test that assesses changes in the stiffness at the TM (which would also reflect changes in the stiffness of the middle ear system). As will be discussed in greater detail later, the TM/middle ear system has an inherent stiffness associated with it; however, the stiffness of the system can be changed by the presence of certain otologic conditions, as well as by varying the air pressure in an ear canal that has been sealed off with a hermetic seal (a procedure that allows one to maintain different levels of air pressure within the closed or sealed off cavity).

During this test procedure, a stimulus of a given intensity and frequency (most often a 226-Hz tone at around 80 dB SPL) is introduced into the hermetically sealed cavity through a special probe assembly, and the level of the sound that remains within the ear canal as pressure is varied is monitored by a small microphone (also contained within the probe assembly). The remaining or reflected SPL levels are compared to a standard and are then interpreted by a computer-based program as representing either an increase or a decrease in compliance (i.e., the reverse of stiffness). As the air pressure is varied, typically from a positive value relative to what is present in the environment through a negative value relative to the pressure in the atmosphere, changes in compliance are plotted on a graph displaying a pressure/compliance function (see Harford, 1975 for review).

In an individual with normal middle ear function, the initial increase in air pressure within the ear canal results in a pressure differential across the TM (i.e., greater pressure in the ear canal than in the middle ear space). As a result, the TM becomes stiffer and vibrates less readily. Since the frequency of the probe tone is relatively low (e.g., 226 Hz), this increase in stiffness offers increased opposition to the flow of energy for this stimulus and more of the sound will be reflected back from the TM and remain in the ear canal. This reflected sound is picked up by the microphone, and the instrumentation displays this as a decrease in compliance. As the pressure within the canal is reduced to the level that is present in the atmosphere, the TM becomes increasingly more compliant. As the TM vibrates more readily, more of the sound that is being introduced into the ear canal passes through the TM to the middle ear

Figure 3.11

Examples of five major types of tympanograms. Type A is a normal tympanogram; Type A_s is the tympanogram often noted with fixation of the ossicular chain, Type A_d, with ossicular disarticulation, Type C, with negative middle ear pressure, and Type B, with fluid build-up in the middle ear cavity.

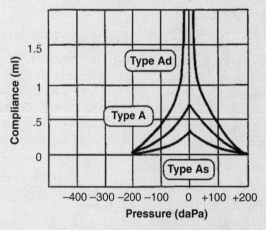

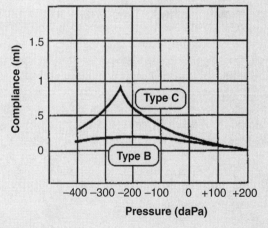

(less remains in the canal) and the result is displayed as increased compliance. At the point where the pressure in the ear canal is equal to that of the middle ear, then a point of maximum compliance is seen. This would typically occur at atmospheric pressure (which is designated as 0 daPa) on the x-axis of the function that is automatically plotted by the instrumentation. A normal tympanogram is shown in Figure 3.11. ●

CLINICAL CORRELATE

Any pathology that affects the volume of air within the middle ear cavity is likely to affect the acoustic impedance of the combined middle-ear/outer-ear system. For example, the accumulation of fluid within the middle ear space effectively reduces the volume of the middle ear and results in a net increase in stiffness. As the stiffness increases, so does the reluctance of the system to accept low-frequency energy. If a hearing test were completed, then one would likely see a low-frequency hearing loss that becomes increasingly severe as the fluid continues to accumulate. ●

CLINICAL CORRELATE

Cholesteatoma is a tumor-like growth, or cyst, in the epithelium in the middle ear, epitympanum, mastoid, or petrous apex (Glasscock, Haynes, Storper, and Bohrer, 1997). The most common type of cholesteatoma is primary acquired or attic. This type of cholesteatoma is often related to long-standing negative middle ear pressure that results in a retraction pocket in the posterior-superior quadrant of the TM. The TM is drawn into the attic area and forms an epithelial-lined cyst that accumulates keratin and increases in size rapidly. These growths can erode bone (Glasscock et al., 1997). Cholesteatomas are at times difficult to see on otoscopic exam. Tympanograms are often abnormal with negative pressure and/or reduced compliance, and a conductive loss can often be noted on the audiogram. ●

Middle Ear Space

The middle ear cavity is a hard-wall cavity that contains a small amount of air. This small amount of air is much less compressible than is the large volume of air found in the environment. When contained, as is the case in the middle ear, this small quantity of air has an acoustic impedance that is governed by its stiffness; that is, it tends to be quite stiff. Stiff objects tend to be responsive to high-frequency sounds and offer increased resistance to low-frequency sounds.

The enclosed air in the middle ear space provides for a general tuning of the ear, and the volume of air in the middle ear space acts as a filter that limits low-frequency sounds from passing through the system. In practical terms, this means the TM would also be governed by the stiffness characteristics of the middle ear system. The end result is that the middle ear system, because of its anatomical construction, alters an incoming signal so as to attenuate low-frequency sounds (Rose, 1978).

Combined Effects of the Outer Ear and Middle Ear on Sound Transmission

The filter effect of the middle ear when coupled with the characteristic resonances of the outer ear (pinna and ear canal) significantly affects the transmission of sound across the frequency range. As discussed above, the filter effects of the volume of air within the enclosed middle ear cavity dampen the transmission of low-frequency sounds, while the resonances of the pinna (a small effect) and the ear canal (a larger effect) result in a complex pattern of emphasis and de-emphasis of high-frequency sounds over a rather broad frequency range (from around 2000 to 7000 Hz). What this means in practical terms is that the signal that reaches the cochlea is altered in a number of ways and that it is not the same as or identical to the signal that enters the ear. For example, if a white noise (i.e., a noise source having equal energy at all frequencies) is delivered to the ear, the output at the cochlea would no longer be white noise. The amplitudes of the frequencies in the low-frequency region of the noise spectrum would have been reduced, while the energy in the mid to high frequencies would have been enhanced by as much as 15 dB in some areas. Above the resonance frequency of the EAM, there would also have been some frequencies that would have been de-emphasized because of the complex patterns of emphasis and de-emphasis associated with the ear canal resonance and other anatomical properties of the outer ear system. This example (as provided by Rose, 1978) discusses the response of the ear at suprathreshold levels, but the same principles would apply to threshold measures. In other words, because of the unique configuration of the human auditory system (outer ear and middle ear), hearing sensitivity across the range of frequencies that humans can

● Figure 3.12

Plot of the hearing threshold in decibels (dB) SPL for the audiometric test frequencies. (Note: these SPL values are the values used for calibration of pure-tone signals to be delivered through TDH 49/50 earphones. Slight variations in these SPL levels are seen for other earphone types).

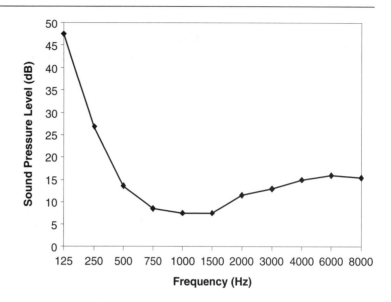

hear is not equal. Human hearing is most sensitive in the mid- to high-frequency range and it is somewhat poorer in the very high-frequency range and poorest in the low-frequency range. Figure 3.12 plots absolute hearing threshold in dB SPL for the average ear as a function of frequency. In this figure the data are plotted at the audiometric frequencies from 125 through 8000 Hz. As can be readily seen in this figure, which is based on information provided in the ANSI S3.6-1989 standard, the lowest thresholds in dB SPL are in the 1 to 4 kHz range, while the highest threshold in dB SPL is found at 125 Hz.

Tympanic Membrane (Eardrum)

As sound reaches the middle ear, it impinges upon the TM and sets this structure into vibration. The vibrational patterns of the TM have been the interest of much study and speculation. In the late 1800s, Helmholtz proposed a theory to account for the efficient transfer of energy from the outer ear to the inner ear (see Zemlin, 1998 for review). One of the factors he discussed was the vibrational pattern of the TM in response to acoustic energy. Helmholtz's theory suggested that the pressure applied to the curved sides of the cone-shaped eardrum would be transformed into a greater pressure value at the eardrum's apex because of a principle referred to as the catenary principle (as shown in Figure 3.13).

Other researchers have built upon Helmholtz's early work and have shown that

CLINICAL CORRELATE

The ear is not equally sensitive to all frequencies. In order to plot hearing relative to normal expectations, audiometers are typically calibrated to reflect these differences in audiometric thresholds. The referent typically used during pure-tone testing is dB HL, where HL stands for hearing level, which is referred back to audiometric zero (0 dB HL). At each audiometric frequency, the SPL of the signal presented is boosted or adjusted to the average hearing threshold for normal hearing. In this way the audiogram, the graphic display of hearing sensitivity as a function of frequency, represents "normal hearing" as a straight line. Any decreases in hearing sensitivity are then interpreted as a number of dB of hearing loss (dB HL) from the normal or average hearing level. Thus, it is easier to interpret the amount of hearing loss across the audiometric frequency range. ●

the displacement of the TM is not uniform and can often be quite complex (von Bekesy, 1941 [as cited in Zemlin, 1998]; Tonndorf and Khanna, 1968). Von

● **Figure 3.13**

(a) Illustration of the curved drum membrane as required for the catenary principle of Helmholtz. (b) Schematic of the catenary principle. Helmhotz theorized that this principle was responsible for an increase in force (F) at point H (from Zemlin, 1998, with permission).

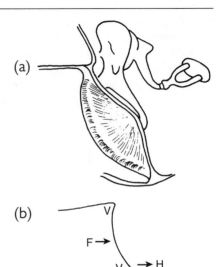

● **Figure 3.14**

Mode of transmission of the tympanic membrane for a 2000-Hz tone. Lines delineate isoamplitude regions, while the numbers represent relative amplitude (after von Bekesy, from Zemlin, 1998, with permission).

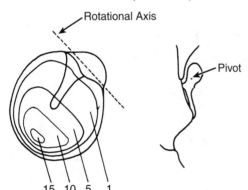

Bekesy (1941) plotted the response of the TM to different frequencies. Figure 3.14 shows the plot for a 2000-Hz stimulus. As can be seen in this figure, at 2000 Hz, the membrane vibrates like a disc around an axis in its superior aspect (see rotational axis indicated in the figure) and the maximum displacement tends to occur toward the inferior edge of the membrane. Surrounding this point of maximal displacement is a series of closed circles that represent areas of the TM where the amplitude of the displacement is roughly equal in magnitude. Similar patterns of displacement are seen for frequencies up to approximately 2500 Hz, above which the relatively organized pattern breaks up and the membrane vibrates segmentally (see Zemlin, 1998 for review).

Later Tonndorf and Khanna (1968) examined the pattern of TM vibration using a procedure known as time-averaged holography (an example of which can be found in Figure 3.15). As Zemlin explained in his review of this data, the isoamplitude contours for 525 Hz presented at 120 dB SPL show maximum displacement in the upper rear quadrant. As was the case in Figure 3.14, the curves represent the isoamplitude areas and the numbers, the relative movement of the TM in these regions. If the numbers in this contour are multiplied by 10^{-5}, then the extent of the displacements (in centimeters) in each section can be closely determined (or at least closely approximated).

Ossicular Chain

The ossicular chain is firmly attached to the TM on its lateral end and it is situated at its medial end within the oval window of the cochlea and is supported there by the annular ligament. As a result, the ossicular chain has its own characteristic impedance that is largely dominated by stiffness reactance. The ossicular chain transmits the vibrational

Figure 3.15

Holographic representation of the tympanic membrane vibration for a frequency of 525 Hz at 120 dB SPL. Maximum vibration occurs in the upper rear quadrant. If the numbers assigned to each isoamplitude region are multiplied by 10^{-5}, the displacement can be determined (after Tonndorf and Khanna, 1968, from Zemlin, 1998, with permission).

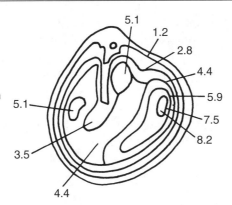

response of the TM to the fluids of the inner ear; however, the response of the ossicular chain is not uniform across intensities. von Bekesy (1936) showed that at low to moderate intensities, the stapes rotates around an axis that runs through the posterior region of its footplate (Figure 3.16a), whereas at high intensities the stapes began to rotate around an axis that ran horizontally across the wider dimension of the footplate (Figure 3.16b). The result was that the latter rotation resulted in less fluid movement. There have been some conflicting studies showing that the stapes' response to intensities as high as 130 to 140 dB SPL continued to be more piston-like than the titling or swinging-door type of response that would have been indicated if the rotational axis had changed (Guinan and Peake, 1967; Dankbar, 1970). A subsequent study using time-averaged holography showed a tilting response for a 600-Hz tone at high intensity levels (Hogmoen and Gundersen, 1977), which was in at least

Figure 3.16

Changes in mode of vibration of the stapes because of an increase in sound intensity (according to von Bekesy, from Zemlin, 1998, with permission).

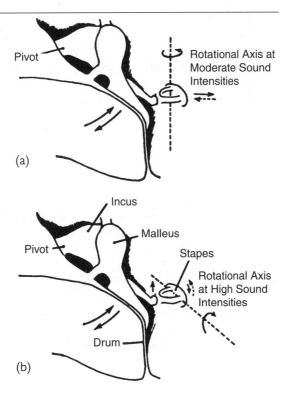

partial agreement with von Bekesy's early findings. In spite of the differences in these studies, it appears likely that there may be some alternation in the response of the stapes to high intensity sounds (probably away from a piston-like response to more of a tilting or rocking response). These changes in response patterns may occur coincidently with the activation of a stapedial reflex that is triggered by high-intensity signals, which may provide some protection against damage to the delicate cochlear structures. This reflex is mediated by structures within the brainstem (up through the level of the superior olivary complex) and will be discussed in greater detail in subsequent chapters following a review of the afferent and efferent pathways that play a role in the mediation of this reflex.

CLINICAL CORRELATE

A number of pathologies and disorders can affect the normal function of the ossicular chain. One of these is otosclerosis. This is an otologic condition that is a varying and active pathology that typically begins with vascular otospongiosis, which then becomes reabsorbed and replaced with sclerotic plaques. Over time, the stapes becomes "fixed," or less mobile, and the normal vibratory response of the ossicular chain is altered and an increase in stiffness is noted. Coincident with the increase in stiffness is a loss of hearing in the low-frequency range that will likely begin to involve more frequencies as the condition progresses. In the early stages of the disease, visualization of the TM may reveal a reddish-blue tint to the membrane that is the result of the increased vascularization to the region of the middle ear near the promontory of the cochlea. Also during bone conduction testing (see discussion that follows), a characteristic notch in the audiometric configuration of the bone conduction thresholds is often noted at 2000 Hz. This has been referred to as Carhart's notch and is attributed to the mechanical effect of the stapes anklyosis (Carhart, 1950; see Derlacki, 1996 for discussion). A characteristic tympanogram is noted with otosclerosis (see Figure 3.11). This tympanogram reflects the increased stiffness of the TM/middle ear system that is caused by the restricted movement of the stapes' footplate.

Although otosclerosis is the most common pathology that results in increased stiffness of the ossicular chain, it is not the only pathology. Fixation or restriction of movement anywhere along the ossicular chain can have similar results. The audiological findings are usually similar to those seen with otosclerosis, making it difficult to differentiate the site of lesion solely on the basis of the audiometric profile of the patient. Otologic factors (e.g., the reddish-blue blush to the TM) and the age of the patient are more helpful in identifying the etiology of the pathology. Otosclerosis is rare in children. Its onset is most common in the third or fourth decade of life (Derlacki, 1996). On the other hand, mallear fixation is often noted early in life and is often a congenital condition. ●

CLINICAL CORRELATE

A middle ear condition that results in increased mobility of the TM since the inherent stiffness of the system is significantly reduced by the presence of the middle ear condition is ossicular disarticulation. This is a condition in which the integrity of the ossicular chain is compromised and as a result, the ossicular chain is not held taut. This allows the TM to vibrate freely. Such compromise of the ossicular chain is often the result of a traumatic incident such as a fall or a blow to the head, but it can also be the result of a congenital malformation of the ossicular chain (Huang and Lambert, 1997). In cases with a disarticulation of the ossicular chain, a Type A_d tympanogram will often result (Figure 3.11). ●

Eustachian Tube

The ET is normally closed in the regions of the cartilaginous portion but opens by the function of two muscles (tensor veli palatini and levator veli palatini). Contraction of these muscle tendons causes the cartilage that is hooked around the ET to uncurl and the lumen of the tube to open. When this happens, (1) fresh air is supplied to the middle ear cavity, (2) any pressure differential that exists across the TM is equalized, and (3) small amounts of fluids that may have collected in the middle ear space drain down the tube into the nasopharynx (if large amounts of fluid are present, usually the ET will not be an avenue for drainage and either the fluids will need to be reabsorbed by the middle ear tissues or medically managed). This unrolling of the cartilaginous hook occurs routinely, during a number of activities throughout the day that cause contraction of the veli palatini muscles (yawning, swallowing, and other motor actions) that help to maintain normal middle ear function (Zemlin, 1998).

CLINICAL CORRELATE

The action of the levator veli palatini and tensor veli palatini muscles is to open the lumen of the ET. When this happens, the air supply in the middle ear is refreshed, the pressure in the middle ear is either increased or decreased to equalize pressure across the TM, and any fluid in the middle ear space is permitted to drain out of the middle ear space to the nasopharynx. If the ET fails to open, then a negative middle ear condition develops (i.e., the pressure of the air in the middle ear space is less than that which is present in the environment) and a sense of blockage is experienced by the individual. An example of a typical tympanogram (Type C) associated with this condition is shown in Figure 3.11. The maximum compliance in this example occurs at −250 daPa, which suggests that the pressure in the middle ear is 250 daPa less that than in the atmosphere where the testing was conducted.

If this condition persists, middle ear fluid may begin to invade the middle ear space. This is a sterile fluid from the surrounding membranes, which can be a fertile breeding ground for bacterial infections. As fluid builds up, there will be increases in both the mass reactance and stiffness reactance components of the TM/middle ear system, and a characteristic tympanogram is observed (see Type B tympanogram shown in Figure 3.11). Here little or no change in compliance of the TM is noted since the fluid build-up behind the TM severely restricts its mobility. If audiometric testing were conducted in the individual developing this fluid buildup, early audiograms would likely reveal hearing loss in the low frequency range caused by an increase in the stiffness factor afforded by the fluid buildup and a decrease in the higher frequencies caused by changes in the mass of the middle ear system, which is now increased by the presence of the fluid. As the condition progresses, the hearing loss is likely to flatten out somewhat as more frequencies become involved. ●

The Middle Ear Transformer

The acoustic signal that reaches the eardrum travels through the air, which is a relatively low-impedance medium, and is directed toward the inner ear, a fluid-filled structure that has an impedance that is significantly greater than that of the air. If the energy in the airborne acoustic signal were to be delivered directly to the ear, much of the energy would be reflected back out of the ear and little of the energy would be transmitted to the inner ear. It has been established that if this were in fact the case, that about 99% of the energy would be reflected back away from the cochlea and only 1% would reach the cochlea. This is obviously a highly undesirable and inefficient situation that would seriously compromise hearing sensitivity; that is, it would require considerable amounts of energy to overcome the impedance mismatch between the low impedance of the air and the high impedance of the cochlear fluids. The middle ear has an important role in hearing—it functions as an impedance matching device. A number of mechanisms within the middle ear work in tandem to overcome the impedance mismatch and to transform the acoustic energy arriving at the TM into a mechanical energy for efficient transfer to the inner ear.

This transformer action of the middle ear is achieved by the combination of three mechanisms: (1) the area differential that exists between the surface of the TM and the size of the stapes' footplate/oval window, (2) the lever action of the ossicular chain, and (3) the buckling effect of the curved membranous structure of the TM (Gelfand, 1997). The largest contribution to the transformer action comes from the area differential that exists between the TM and the stapes' footplate (Figure 3.17). Force that is applied over the TM is directed toward a smaller structure, the stapes' footplate, thus increasing the force per unit area (p = F/A). The effective surface area of the TM (largely the pars tensa) is approximately 55 mm^2, while the area of the stapes footplate is approximately 3.2 mm^2. This converts to a size ratio of 55:3.2, or 17:1 (Rose, 1978; Zemlin, 1998). The total area of the TM is much closer to 83 mm^2 (Gelfand, 1997), but only a portion (about two-thirds) of the membrane vibrates effectively (von Bekesy, 1960).

The lever action within the middle ear is afforded by the manner in which the malleus and the incus function together to form a lever (Figure 3.18). This lever is formed by the manubrium of the malleus and the long process of the incus, which are held tightly together at their articulation by an encapsulated joint; as a result the two ossicles move as a unit, with the manubrium being slightly longer than the long process of the incus (Figure 3.18). The lever provides a gain in force that is proportional to the ratio of the long handle (manubrium) to the short handle (long process of the incus). In humans this has been estimated to be about 1.3:1 (Rose, 1978).

Figure 3.17

A schematic showing the area advantage, which involves the concentration of the force applied over the larger tympanic membrane to the smaller area of the stapes footplate (from Gelfand, 1997, with permission).

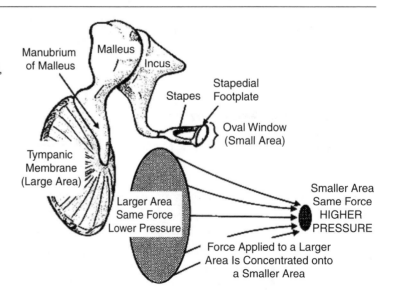

Schematic of the ossicular chain lever system as described by Helmholtz. The fulcrum is at point C, with the lever arms being the distances CA and CB (from Zemlin, 1998, with permission).

The third and final mechanism is related to the buckling of the curved TM (Gelfand, 1997). The TM curves from its attachment to the rim of the EAM at both ends to the point where the manubrium attaches to the TM. As a result of this curvature in the membrane, vibrations directed to the TM result in greater movement of the curved membranes, with less displacement for the manubrium (this is what has been referred to as the buckling effect). A boost in force accompanies the smaller displacement of the manubrium since the product of force must be equivalent on either side of a lever (that is, $F1 \times D1 = F2 \times D2$). The combination of the previous two mechanisms (area differential and lever effect) results in a total advantage on the order of 23:1 (if the effective area of the TM is considered to be approximately 56.7 mm^2 and the area of the stapes footplate is 3.2 mm^2). If the buckling factor is added into the equation, then the total advantage ratio becomes 46:1. Converting this to decibels of pressure, the total advantage would be 33 dB (i.e., $20 \times \log[46/1]$) (Gelfand, 1997). Similar, but slightly different measurements (i.e., a total advantage of 31 dB, due in part to slightly different dimensions for the TM used in the calculation), have been reported by Rose (1978). As Gelfand and others have pointed out, this increase in sound pressure is only an approximation. Its actual amount depends upon a number of factors, for example, individual differences in the vibrating area of the TM, the exact relationship of the TM area to the area of the stapes footplate, potential individual differences in the lever effect, and differences in the stimulus characteristic (e.g., frequency).

Bone-Conduction Mechanisms

The discussion thus far has focused on air-conducted signals. These signals start as airborne signals that are conducted down the ear canal to the TM where the acoustic energy is transformed into vibrational energy. This vibrational or mechanical energy is then passed on to the cochlea, where it causes displacement of the fluids in the inner ear, which then triggers a number of biological responses in the cochlea (these will be discussed in Chapters 6 and 7). Although this is one way that an acoustic signal can reach the cochlea and cause the necessary responses needed to generate the neural responses that will be used by the central nervous system for processing and ultimately for recognition of the signal, there is an alternate way in which these cochlear responses can occur. This is by a process called bone conduction and it occurs when the intensity of the acoustic signal reaching the head is intense enough to cause the head to vibrate in response to the acoustic signal. There is a significant difference in the impedance of bone compared to air. As a result, this mechanism does not play a major role in hearing, at least at low to moderate intensities (for additional information see clinical correlate below). If, however, a bone vibrator is applied to the head and a signal is delivered to the bone vibrator, the head can be set into a vibratory pattern that will follow the pressure changes (condensation and rarefaction) of the stimulus. Since the skull of the head is formed by rigid bones, it tends to vibrate as a whole, whereas structures that are loosely connected to the skull may tend to lag behind the skull when a force is applied. For example, if one were to apply a 500-Hz tone at a high enough intensity to right side of the head, the skull would move to the left during the compression phase(s) of the signal and to the right during the rarefaction phase(s). As the head moves to the left, the ossicular chain, which is loosely connected to the temporal bone of the skull, would initially lag behind because of the effects of inertia and then eventually catch up. The end result is that this causes a displacement of the stapes in and out of the oval window that sets up the necessary fluid movements in the inner ear to cause the biological changes needed to trigger a hearing response. What has just been described is referred to as inertial vibrational forces. This is the vibratory response that predominates for low-frequency sounds. At higher frequencies, more complex vibrational patterns may occur. This vibratory response is called compressional hearing. Here the skull begins to vibrate in segments (e.g., the forehead is driven backward and the back of the head moves

CLINICAL CORRELATE

When a signal reaches an intensity of 40 to 50 dB above an individual's threshold (as determined by the cochlear sensitivity), the intensity of the sound may be sufficient to trigger a response by an alternate method of stimulation (i.e., bone conduction). This has some implications for assessment of hearing in individuals who do not have symmetrical hearing losses, as well as for the administration of some audiological procedures that are presented at suprathrehsold levels, for example, in the extreme case of the patient with a unilateral profound hearing loss. If one were to place a bone vibrator (which has been calibrated) on the ear with the profound loss, the patient would likely provide normal responses to the test stimuli because the vibration of the skull has triggered responses in the normal cochlea on the opposite side of the head. Likewise, if one were to place an earphone on the impaired ear during air-conduction testing and deliver an acoustic signal to the earphone, once the intensity of the signal reached a level that was sufficient to set the individual's skull into vibration, then a hearing response would be triggered in the normal ear (this is referred to as cross hearing).

In other patients with significant asymmetries in their hearing thresholds, it is possible to obtain hearing threshold results when the poorer ear is stimulated that underestimate the hearing status of the test ear. This is because the thresholds being measured are not originating from the hearing mechanism on the side of the stimulus, but are coming from the responses of the normal, or better, ear. If the difference between the two ears is great enough to cause this to happen, one may observe what is referred to as a shadow curve, that is, if the threshold responses of the two ears are plotted on an audiogram. Here the configuration of the hearing loss in the poorer ear is parallel the configuration of the hearing levels obtained for the better ear; generally the difference between the two functions is at least 40 to 50 dB (see Yost, 2000 for review).

If one is attempting to establish a threshold measure for the poorer ear (test ear) in an individual with asymmetrical hearing loss, then the participation of the better ear (nontest) can often be eliminated by introducing a masking signal into this ear while reestablishing the threshold in the test ear. The use of masking is usually not indicated during air-conduction testing until the difference between the two ears exceeds 40 to 50 dB. ●

forward, and vice versa). This produces compressional or flexural forces within the skull that are related to the differences in the mobility of the oval and round windows. When these compressional forces are delivered to the inner ear, they act upon the noncompressible fluids of the inner ear, which then cause these fluids to move either toward or away from the more flexible round window, depending upon the phase of the signal (Rose, 1978). This fluid movement causes basilar membrane displacement, which in turn sets up the necessary biological changes in the cochlea to cause a response to the vibrational energy. Although inertial forces tend to predominate for low-frequency sounds (up to around 800 Hz) and compressional forces for high-frequency sounds (above 8000 Hz), all frequencies tend to have components of both forces. This is a brief overview of bone-conduction hearing mechanisms; for additional information, the reader is referred to Rose (1978), Gelfand (1997), Zemlin (1998), and Yost (2000).

SUMMARY

The middle ear is an air-filled cavity that begins at the TM on its lateral-most side and ends with the bony wall of the cochlea on its medial side. It houses the ossicular chain, which is a series of three bones. These three bones, the smallest in the human body, bridge the gap between the TM and the cochlea and transmit the energy that was delivered to the TM to the cochlear fluids. The acoustic energy that strikes the TM sets this membrane into motion and thus transduces the acoustic energy to mechanical energy. The TM vibrates in response to the sound and faithfully reproduces the acoustic characteristics of the acoustic signal (e.g., compressions and rarefactions) at least at low frequencies. In higher frequencies, a more complicated pattern of vibration occurs at the TM. Since there is a sizeable impedance difference between the relatively low impedance of the air where the acoustic signal is carried and the relatively high impedance of the cochlear fluids, the middle ear functions as an acoustic transformer or impedance-matching device to improve the transmission flow of energy from a region of low impedance to one of high impedance. It does this through a number of mechanisms, including an area difference between the TM and the stapes' footplate, a lever effect that is provided by the ossicular chain, and the buckling effect of the ossicular chain. These three features combine to result in an increase in energy at the oval window of 46:1, or an approximately 33 dB increase. This increase is frequency dependent and will also vary somewhat with the unique dimensions and functions of each individual's middle ear system.

The tendons of two muscles (tensor tympani and stapedius) enter the middle ear space and attach to the ossicular chain at its two ends. One attaches to the head of the malleus and the other to the neck of the stapes. When these muscles contract, they result in a stiffening of the ossicular chain. Contraction of the muscles occurs at high intensity levels in many species. However, in humans, it appears that the contraction of the stapedius muscle is the major response to high-intensity sounds. When either the stapedius muscle or both muscles contact, an increase in the stiffness of the ossicular chain results, which in turn causes an increase in the reluctance of the chain to accept or conduct mechanical energy. The end result is that the stapes' excursion into the oval window is reduced compared to what it would normally be when stimulated at high intensities. This response to high intensity signals is presumed to be a protective mechanism that helps prevent damage to the delicate structures within the cochlea.

An important structure that opens into the middle ear space is the ET. This tube maintains a fresh air supply to the middle ear tissues to maintain equal pressure across the TM and to allow drainage of fluids that may collect in the middle ear space (i.e., if the tube is able to open). The ET connects the middle ear space to the nasopharynx and is opened by two muscles during normal motor activities such as yawning and swallowing. If the ET does not function normally, significant middle ear pathology may result—a common occurrence in young children who frequently experience a buildup of fluid in the middle ear space.

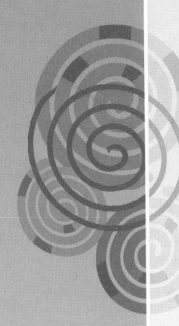

4

Functional Anatomy of the Cochlea

Introduction

The anatomy of the cochlea is represented by osseous or bony structures, membranous structures, fluids, and specialized sensory and supporting cells. The bony morphology of the cochlea provides the frame upon which the membranous and cellular structures rest either directly or indirectly. The cochlea is housed within the **temporal bone**, and an understanding of the anatomy of this bone is important to the understanding of the structure and function of the cochlea. The position of the cochlea in the temporal bone and the fact that the temporal bone is composed of a hard and rigid bony foundation provides protection for this extremely delicate and complex organ of hearing.

OVERVIEW OF THE TEMPORAL BONE

The temporal bone is an osseous structure that is part of the cranium and houses a portion of the external ear, as well as the middle ear, the inner ear including the cochlea and the vestibular apparatus, and the seventh and eighth cranial nerves. The temporal bone is a hard, rigid bone located within the skull and has a myriad of cavities, channels, and canals that subserve the end organs of hearing and balance; hence, the term **labyrinth** is used to describe this bony structure. The main purpose of the **bony labyrinth** is to provide support and protection for the delicate anatomical structures of hearing and balance. Within the bony labyrinth are membranous structures that line the channels and canals of the temporal bone and form the inner ear. These membranous structures, referred to as the **membranous labyrinth**, contain the fluids that bathe the sensory cells for hearing and balance. Within the membranous labyrinth are a number of structures, including the cochlea, or the end organ for hearing, and five sensory structures that are part of the vestibular end organ (three semicircular canals, the utricle, and the saccule).

The temporal bone is the focus of much training for otologists. Not only is it necessary for otologists to understand the anatomy of the temporal bone, but they also need to develop refined skills in drilling out areas of this bone so they can gain access to the anatomy of the ear that is required for surgical intervention. High proficiency in temporal bone drilling skills correlates with surgical expertise in the field of otology.

The temporal bone helps form the base of the human skull. It also forms the middle and posterior fossa of the cranial vault. The posterior fossa houses the cerebellum and the brainstem and is the area that is approached by the surgeon to remove acoustic tumors and other brainstem tumors, such as meningiomas of the cerebellopontine angle. The middle fossa accommodates the anterior-inferior aspect of the temporal lobe.

The four main parts of the temporal bone are the **squamous, mastoid, petrous, and tympanic** portions. Using the external auditory meatus as a reference point, the squamous portion is superior, the mastoid portion is posterior, the petrous segment is medial, and the tympanic segment is anterior and inferior (Anson and Donaldson, 1967).

The squamous portion of the temporal bone is positioned superior to the ear canal and is semicircular, or fan-shaped, in its orientation relative to the ear canal. Its lateral surface is smooth and its superior surface serves as the attachment for the temporal muscle. The superior part has a small sulcus, which accommodates the middle temporal artery. The inferior, lateral aspect of the squamous portion is characterized by the zygomatic process, which is a bony arch running posteriorly and anteriorly. The masseter muscle attaches to the zygomatic arch. The medial surface of the squama helps form the lateral aspect of the middle cranial fossa. Also, on the medial surface of this structure is a sulcus for the middle meningeal artery (Anson and Donaldson, 1967).

The mastoid part of the temporal bone is posterior to the ear canal and the squamous bone (Figure 4.1). The lateral aspect of the mastoid portion serves as the attachment for the occipital and postauricular muscles.

The mastoid has a sulcus that accommodates a branch of the occipital artery. Located on the mastoid part of the temporal bone is an eminence that projects outward. This part of the bone, which lies directly posterior to the pinna, is where the bone conduction oscillator is frequently placed on the skin covering this eminence for bone conduction testing. The medial aspect of the mastoid has a notable sulcus. This sulcus houses the sigmoid venous sinus and is called the sigmoid sulcus.

The petrous portion of the temporal bone is probably the most anatomically complex of all of the portions of this bone. This segment of the temporal bone houses most of the peripheral hearing mechanisms (Figures 4.2 and 4.3).

The petrous part of the temporal bone is triangular, allowing an anterior and posterior surface. The anterior surface forms part of the middle cranial fossa. Laterally the petrous bone fuses with the squama. The anterior surface has a

● **Figure 4.1**

Lateral view of the cranium showing the squamous portion of the temporal bone. S = squamous portion, ZA = zygomatic arch, e = external auditory meatus (opening), T = tympanic portion, M = mastoid portion, sp = styloid process, mb = ramus of the mandible.

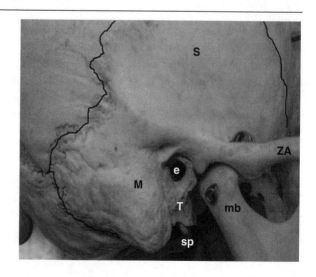

● **Figure 4.2**

Looking down onto the base of the cranial vault. PF = posterior fossa, P = petrous portion of the temporal bone, FM = foramen magnum, MF = middle fossa.

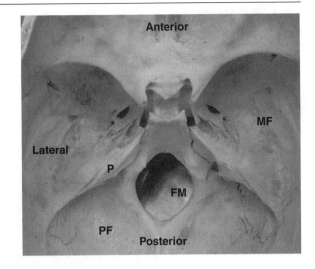

● **Figure 4.3**

Posterior view of the petrous bone. PF = posterior fossa, VA = opening to the vestibular aqueduct, ss = sigmoid sinus recess, iam = internal auditory meatus, ae = arcuate eminence (superior semicircular canal), MF = middle fossa.

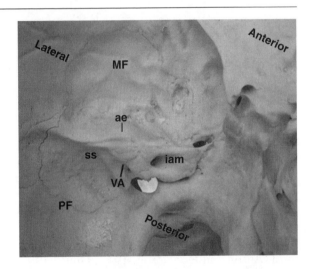

CLINICAL CORRELATE

Temporal bone fractures are a major clinical entity for both otologists and audiologists. The two types of temporal bone fractures are longitudinal and transverse. The longitudinal fracture courses along the long axis of the temporal bone and is far more common than the transverse fracture. Over 70% of temporal bone fractures are longitudinal in nature (Huang and Lambert, 1997) (Figure 4.4).

Longitudinal fractures may extend from the medial aspect of the temporal bone to the superior posterior aspect of the ear canal. These fractures often are a result of a severe blow to the temporal or parietal area of the head. This kind of fracture can result in sensorineural and conductive hearing loss, as well as balance problems. Facial nerve damage resulting in facial paralysis can also occur. Hemotympanum and blood in the ear canal can also be characteristic of longitudinal fracture. This results from laceration of the ear canal, the eardrum, or the middle ear (Fisch, 1974; Huang and Lambert, 1997). The symptoms associated with a longitudinal fracture are variable and depend on the precise locus of the fracture. Fractures anterior or posterior to the petrous pyramid may not yield as much auditory, facial, or balance dysfunction as do breaks that occur in close proximity to the otic capsule.

(continued)

Transverse fractures occur only 20 to 30% of the time. However, they generally extend across the petrous pyramid through the otic capsule and/or the internal auditory meatus (IAM) (Huang and Lambert, 1997). This can result in profound sensorineural hearing loss and severe vertigo. Facial paralysis also results in about 50% of the cases with transverse fractures (Fisch, 1974; Huang and Lambert, 1997) (Figure 4.4). ●

● **Figure 4.4**

Examples of longitudinal (left) and transverse (right) fractures of the temporal bone (based on Huang and Lambert, 1997).

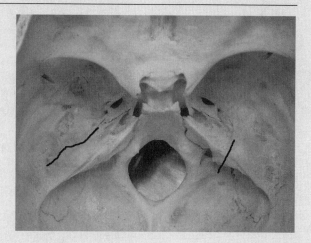

semicanal structure for the tensor tympani muscle, which is innervated by the fifth cranial nerve. It also contains a semicanal for the Eustachian tube. This surface of the temporal bone is characterized by two small openings toward the apex of the petrous segment. The first opening is for the facial nerve and the second is for the petrosal nerve and superior tympanic artery (Anson and Donaldson, 1967).

The posterior surface of the petrous bone makes up part of the posterior fossa (Anson and Donaldson, 1967; Gulya, 1997). Midway between the base and apex of the petrous bone is the opening of the IAM (Figures 4.2 and 4.3). This structure is important for hearing, balance, and facial function. Running through the IAM are the facial, auditory, and vestibular nerves. The IAM can be divided into four quadrants that accommodate these important nerve routes. If one were facing the opening of the IAM, the upper left area would contain the facial nerve, while directly inferior to the facial nerve would be the auditory nerve. Across from the facial and auditory nerves are the vestibular nerves. The superior quadrant houses the nerve fibers from the superior semicircular canal. The inferior quadrant of the IAM provides the route of the nerve fibers from the saccule, the utricle, and the semicircular canal. The singular foramen is a small opening in the inferior lateral aspect of the IAM that provides the route for the fibers of the posterior semicircular canal.

Also located on the posterior surface of the petrous part of the temporal bone is the bony accommodation for the vestibular aqueduct (VA). This sulcus is located about halfway between the opening of the IAM and the sigmoid sinus area (part of the mastoid). The VA is a channel that contains endolymph and communicates with the endolymphatic sac and duct. Both of these structures are part of the vestibular end organ (see Figure 4.3).

The inferior surface of the petrous bone in combination with the occipital bone forms the jugular foramen. Also located on the inferior surface of the petrous bone is the jugular fossa and jugular bulb. (The clinical significance of the jugular tumor will be discussed in Chapter 14).

OSSEOUS (BONY) COCHLEA

The cochlea is perhaps the hardest bony structure in the body. It is located in the petrous portion of the temporal bone, immediately medial to the tympanum, or middle ear cavity. The cochlea's position in the head is sometimes difficult to realize. The apex, or cupola, of the cochlea (representing the apical turn) is oriented anterior and slightly lateral within the head pointing toward the cheekbone (Figure 4.5). The portion of the cochlea that is opposite the apex points medial and posterior toward the back of the head. The bony cochlea resembles a spiral cone with auditory nerve fibers emanating from inside the cone in a spiral.

● **Figure 4.5**

Sketch of the bony inner ear (from Perkins and Kent, 1986, with permission).

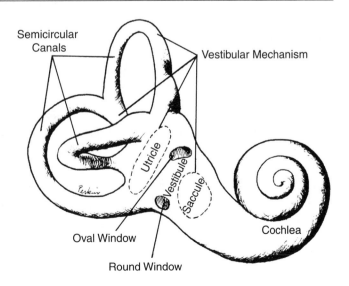

The bony cochlea resembles a snail shell, and in humans, it has between 2.2 and 2.9 turns (Buser and Imbert, 1992). These turns are smaller at the apex than at the base of the cochlea. The entire bony cochlea measures about 1 cm wide and about 5 mm from base to apex (Pickles, 1988). The **modiolus** is a central, perforated bony core that accommodates nerve fibers from the hair cells, as well as blood vessels (Figures 4.6, 4.7, and 4.8). At its medial end the modiolus is continuous with the IAM. The modiolus is also the central structure around which the cochlea is wrapped. Specifically, the **osseous spiral lamina** is a shelf-like structure that winds around the modiolus from base to apex (Figures 4.6, 4.7, 4.8, and 4.9). This

● **Figure 4.6**

The bony cochlea (apex at the top and base at the bottom) of the chinchilla, with part of the bony capsule removed revealing the osseous spiral lamina. Note the stapes and oval window in lower left of the picture (courtesy of Richard Mount, Hospital for Sick Children, Toronto).

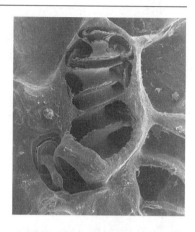

● **Figure 4.7**

The coils (osseous spiral lamina) of the human cochlea from base to apex. Note the difference between the chinchilla (see Figure 4.6) and the human (courtesy of Marilyn Pinheiro).

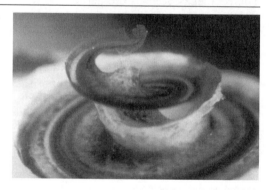

● **Figure 4.8**

Drawing of the bony cochlea (longitudinal section through the modiolus) (from Zemlin, 1998, with permission).

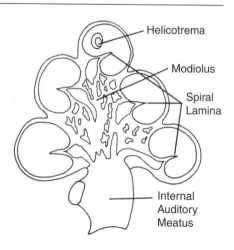

Helicotrema

Modiolus

Spiral Lamina

Internal Auditory Meatus

spiral lamina is composed of two thin plates between which auditory nerve fibers pass from the hair cells in the cochlea to eventually connect to nuclei within the brainstem. The spiral lamina is narrower at the apex than at the base of the cochlea (Zemlin, 1998). It is interesting to note that the human bony cochlea is wider at the base and flatter than the bony cochleae from many small animals. This is depicted well in Figure 4.7, which shows a human specimen.

The spiral lamina's lower shelf also serves as the support point and connector for the inner aspect of the **basilar membrane** (BM) and with the scala media or cochlear duct; it divides the cochlea into the scalae vestibuli (superior) and the scalae tympani (inferior). The upper shelf of the spiral lamina is continuous with a structure known as the **spiral limbus** and serves as an attachment and support point for the **tectorial membrane**. The medial aspect of the tectorial membrane along with the end of the spiral limbus, which is concave in shape, forms the internal **spiral sulcus**.

The bony cochlea has two windows located at the basal turn on its lateral aspect. The more superior of the two windows is the **oval window,** which interacts with the stapes of the middle ear and opens into the scala vestibuli. The oval window in humans ranges from about 1.2×3 mm to 2.0×3.7 mm (for review of measurements, see Yost, 2000).

● **Figure 4.9**

Membranous and bony cochlea (from Zemlin, 1998, with permission).

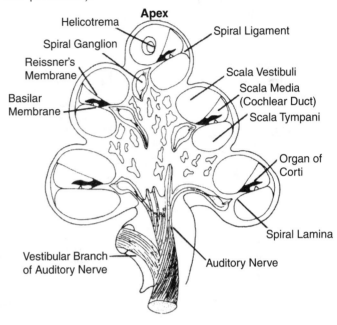

CLINICAL CORRELATE

Otosclerosis is a disease process in which a lamella forms around the footplate of the stapes. This lamella, or spongy growth, limits the proper movement of the stapes, which increases the overall impedance of the ossicular chain (see previous chapter for additional information on this topic). Otosclerosis that involves only the stapes bone within the middle ear is the most common variant of this disease, but cochlear otosclerosis can also occur. Cochlear otosclerosis occurs when the spongy growth (lamella) growing from the stapes infiltrates the cochlea, resulting in a sensorineural hearing loss in addition to the conductive loss created by the stapes fixation (Figure 4.10). It is difficult to make a definitive diagnosis of cochlear otosclerosis, and its existence is often presumed in many cases. Usually cochlear otosclerosis is present when there is also evidence of middle ear otosclerosis—whether or not cochlear otosclerosis can exist in isolation is a topic of considerable debate (see Schuknecht and Kirchner, 1974). Cochlear otosclerosis usually starts unilaterally and then progresses to the other ear. This disease has a strong genetic correlate. Audiologically, otosclerosis has an insidious onset and although it often begins in the second decade of life, it often isn't noticed or diagnosed until the third or fourth decade of life. The hearing loss is depicted by an audiogram that has a stiffness tilt (i.e., greater hearing loss at the low frequencies), an air–bone gap, possibly a Carhart's notch (i.e., a bone conduction threshold at 2 kHz that is more depressed than those noted at the other audiometric frequencies), and good to excellent speech recognition scores. ●

(continued)

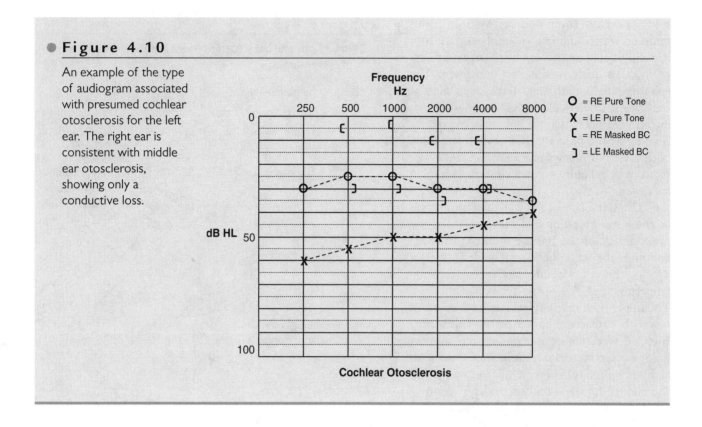

● **Figure 4.10**

An example of the type of audiogram associated with presumed cochlear otosclerosis for the left ear. The right ear is consistent with middle ear otosclerosis, showing only a conductive loss.

Cochlear Otosclerosis

O = RE Pure Tone
X = LE Pure Tone
[= RE Masked BC
] = LE Masked BC

The **round window** is inferior to the oval window and opens into the scala tympani. In humans the round window's dimensions are 2.25 × 1.0 mm. Between the oval and round windows is a bony eminence known as the **promontory**. The promontory is positioned to protect the oval and round windows in that it directly faces the middle ear cavity. Foreign bodies entering the middle ear would first strike the promontory. The promontory is the anatomical site for needle placement in transtympanic electrocochleography. For this procedure, a transtympanic needle electrode is placed in and through the lower portion of the eardrum, which allows alignment with the promontory. The round window is covered by a membrane that retains cochlear fluids within the cochlea.

MEMBRANOUS COCHLEA AND RELATED STRUCTURES

Scalae and Cochlear Fluids

Following the spiral shape of the bony cochlea from its base to its apex is the membranous cochlea. The membranous cochlea is highly elastic, allowing it to move easily within the bony cochlea. There are three ducts within the cochlea: the **scala vestibule,** which is superior; the **scala media** (often called the cochlear duct), which is located in the middle; and the **scala tympani,** which is the most inferior of the three ducts (Figures 4.11, 4.12, and 4.13). The oval window is at the opening of the vestibule, which is the site of the stapes footplate. The round window membrane is at the basal-most aspect of the scala tympani.

● **Figure 4.11**

The membranous labyrinth. SSC = superior semicircular canal, LSC = lateral semicircular canal, PSC = posterior semicircular canal.

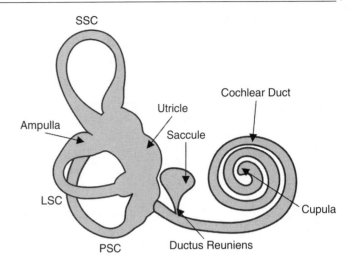

● **Figure 4.12**

A schematic of the cochlear scalae (canals) (from Perkins and Kent, 1986, with permission).

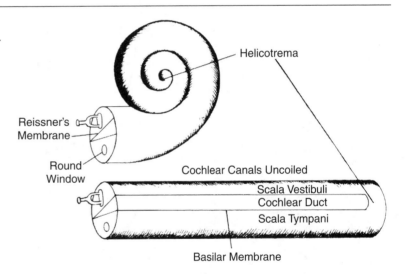

The three scalae are divided by two membranes: the **basilar membrane** and **Reissner's membrane**. The basilar membrane (BM) is connected to the spiral ligament on the outer wall of the bony cochlea and to the osseous spiral lamina to form the floor of the scala media or cochlear duct (Figures 4.12 and 4.13). Reissner's membrane forms the roof of the cochlear duct and the floor of the scala vestibuli. The three scalae spiral the length of the cochlea and are separated from one another, with a single exception. At the apex of the cochlea the scala vestibuli and scala tympani communicate, and this point of communication is termed the **helicotrema** (Figure 4.12). The cochlear duct (scala media) communicates at its basal region with the vestibular region (specifically the saccule) of the inner ear by way of the **ductus reuniens of Hensen** (Figures 4.11 and 4.14). This is a narrow passageway, which may be obliterated in the adult, although this point remains controversial.

● Figure 4.13

Cross section of the cochlea.

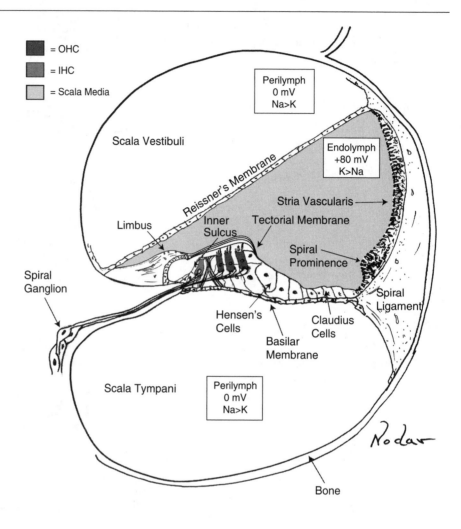

● Figure 4.14

Schematic of the membranous inner ear, emphasizing the cochlear and vestibular aqueducts. A = endolymphatic sac, B = vestibular aqueduct, C = endolymphatic duct, D = saccule, E = utricle, F = semicircular canals, G = ductus reuniens, H = cochlear aqueduct, I = round window, J = stapes (oval window), K = scala vestibuli, L = scala media, M = scala tympani.

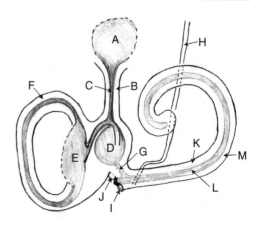

CLINICAL CORRELATE

The ductus reuniens may play an important role in the communication of endolymphatic disorders between the auditory and vestibular systems. For example, if the ductus reuniens were blocked, it might prevent a hydropic condition of the cochlea from spreading to the vestibular system. However, if the ductus reuniens were not blocked, then the hydropic condition could affect the vestibular portion as well as the cochlear portion of the inner ear.

The three scalae are filled with fluids (Figure 4.13). The scala tympani and vestibuli are filled with perilymph (16 to 23 μL in human) and the scala media with endolymph and cortilymph (2.7 μL in human) (Yost, 2000). Perilymph has essentially the same chemical composition as cerebral spinal fluid (CSF). Perilymph is low in potassium (K) and high in sodium (Na). Interestingly, however, it appears that the sodium and potassium concentrations in the perilymph are not uniform throughout the cochlea (Wangemann and Schacht, 1996). The scala vestibuli and scala tympani have slightly different Na+ and K+ concentrations. Cortilymph is similar to perilymph in its chemical composition, as it is high in sodium and low in potassium (Engstrom, 1960). The cortilymph bathes the hair cells and fills the spaces of Nuel, the external tunnel, and the main tunnel of Corti. Cortilymph is segregated from the endolymph by the reticular lamina. ●

● *Vestibular and Cochlear Aqueducts*

Contributing to the fluid systems of the cochlea are two fluid pathways: the **vestibular aqueduct** (VA) (endolymphatic) and **cochlear aqueduct** (CA). The VA (containing endolymph) is the bony channel that encompasses the endolymphatic duct (ED). The ED courses from the posterolateral wall of the vestibule to the endolymphatic sac, which is located on the posterior surface of the petrous pyramid of the temporal bone (Figure 4.3). The endolymphatic sac's opening in the temporal bone is 10 mm posterolateral to the opening of the IAM (Gulya, 1997). The ED is thought to help regulate endolymphatic pressure to avoid the effects of overproduction or under-absorption of endolymph. Because of the role it may play in the hydrodynamic function of the inner ear, dysfunction of the ED has been implicated in hydrops (Figures 4.11 and 4.14).

CLINICAL CORRELATE

Endolymphatic hydrops has been described as an overproduction or under-absorption of endolymph. In attempts to alleviate symptoms of meniere's disease, endolymphatic shunt surgery was developed. This procedure is often recommended for meniere's patients, but its use remains highly controversial. Theoretically, this surgery is used to open up a potentially blocked ED or to decompress the endolymphatic sac (Schwaber, 1997; Thai-Van, Bounaix, and Fraysse, 2001). This surgery, in turn, should reduce the endolymphatic pressure in the cochlea and the vestibular apparatus and stop the hydropic symptoms of dizziness, hearing loss, and tinnitus. Reported results from endolymphatic sac surgery are highly variable (see Schwaber, 1997 for review). One of the indications for suggesting endolymphatic sac surgery is an increased summating potential (SP): action potential (AP) ratio noted when electrocochleography is conducted (see discussion in next chapter). ●

The CA (containing perilymph) courses from the basal turn of the scala tympani only a few millimeters from the round window to the subarachnoid space near the jugular fossa. It runs parallel to the inferior margin of the IAM (Gulya, 1997). The CA allows transfer of cerebrospinal fluid (CSF). The CA is patent early in life, but in many individuals the channel becomes closed in later life. At 50 years of age, it is estimated that only 50% of individuals will have a patent CA (Wlodyka, 1978) (Figure 4.14).

CLINICAL CORRELATE

The CA has received considerable clinical attention recently. Some clinicians believe that an enlarged CA could be the basis for abnormal hydrodynamics in the cochlea, resulting in hearing loss, while others feel this is not the case (see discussion by Jackler and Wang, 1993). Another consideration regarding the CA is CSF hypertension, which may also affect cochlear function. This concern has given rise to the development of a noninvasive system for measuring inner ear fluid pressure. This system, called the tympanic membrane displacement (TMD) system, is based on the concept that if the perilymphatic pressure is high, it could reflect increased intracranial pressure (Krast, 1985). When the perilymphatic pressure is high, the stapes is pushed outward; when the pressure is normal, this is not the case.

The TMD assessment procedure is similar to measuring the acoustic reflex. The ear canal is sealed with a probe, and tonal stimuli are presented 20 dB above the acoustic reflex threshold. When the stapes is displaced outward and the stapedius muscle contracts, the stapes moves inward because it cannot move outward because of the maximal displacement in that direction (from increased perilymph pressure). This inward movement is recorded. When the stapes is normally positioned, the stapedius contraction results in an outward movement, which is recorded (Marchbanks, 2003). The application of TMD measurements requires more study, although early reports indicate reasonable correlations for changes in cochlear fluid pressure and its association with a variety of CSF and perilymphatic disorders. ●

The endolymph has high potassium concentration and is low in sodium. It is believed that this chemical relationship is maintained by an active process in the stria vascularis (Buser and Imbert, 1992). Endolymph is most likely produced in a complex manner, but the stria is certainly the main player (see Pickles, 1988). The high concentration of K+ in the endolymph is especially important to cochlear function because a considerable portion of the transduction current in the hair cells is carried by the K+ ions (Wangemann and Schacht, 1996). This is related to the high K+ and low Na+ concentrations in the endolymph and the K+ selectivity of ion channels in the membranes of the hair cells. The low K+ concentration in the perilymph also contributes to this ion action. Changing the K+ ion concentration in the inner ear fluids influences the cochlear potentials (Marcus, Marcus, and Thalmann, 1981).

CLINICAL CORRELATE

Endolymphatic hydrops, or meniere's disease, potentially involves a number of cochlear structures and fluid. It has been suggested that the excess endolymph may have several pathologic consequences in regard to cochlear structures. The increased endolymph may restrict the mechanics of the cochlea. If the increased pressure in the scala media is great enough, it could result in the tearing of Reissner's membrane and the mixing of cochlear fluids. Cochleae from individuals with meniere's disease have commonly shown ruptured or severely distended Reissner's membranes (see Schuknecht, 1993). The increased pressure in the scala media, over a period of time, could result in the distention of the BM in the apical end where it is less stiff. These suggested

pathological mechanisms could be the basis of the symptom complex known as meniere's disease. Low-frequency hearing loss and low-pitched roaring tinnitus may be related to the pressure effects in the apical end of the cochlea. The increased endolymph and associated pressure carries over to the vestibular system to result in vertigo. The aural pressure frequently reported by meniere's patients could be secondary to the increased pressure in the cochlea and vestibular apparatus. Why these symptoms of hearing loss, vertigo, tinnitus, and aural fullness, which characterize meniere's disease, come and go is still unknown. This disease is one that, at least in its early stages, does not permanently damage hair cells.

(continued)

The audiology related to meniere's disease is typically a unilateral low-frequency sensorineural hearing loss (see Figure 4.15). In some cases (estimated 20%) the disease becomes bilateral. Speech recognition can be compromised, but usually not to any significant degree. Recruitment can be demonstrated. Electrocochleography can be employed to help with the diagnosis of meniere's disease. The ratio of the SP compared to the AP of the auditory nerve is considered indicative of meniere's disease if the ratio of the amplitude for the SP approaches 50% of the AP amplitude (see review by Durrant and Ferraro, 1999) (see next chapter). The variability surrounding this measurement, however, has compromised its clinical use. Further discussion of the use of electrocochleography in meniere's disease is offered in Chapter 7.

Another clinical entity that affects the hydrodynamics of the cochlea is that of perilymph fistula (see Maitland, 2001 for review). This disorder exists when the membranes of the oval or round window are torn. Such compromises of the membranes of either window can result in the leaking of perilymphatic fluid into the middle ear space. This leaking may decrease the fluid pressure within the scala tympani and scala vestibuli, resulting in relatively more pressure in the scala media—similar to the mechanisms proposed for meniere's disease. If not treated, or if the fistula does not spontaneously heal, progressive hearing loss and vestibular symptoms often result (Weider, 1992). ●

● **Figure 4.15**

Audiogram from a patient with meniere's disease, showing bilateral involvement.

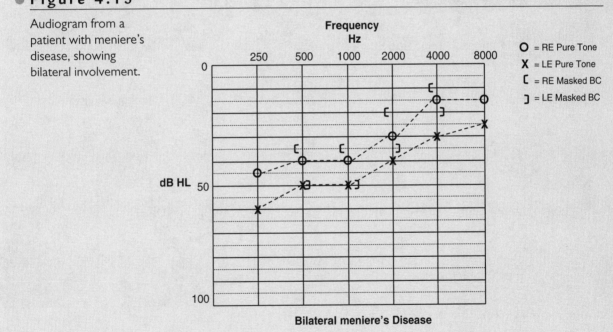

Bilateral meniere's Disease

Basilar and Reissner's Membranes

The BM is from 25 to 35 mm in length in the adult human. Its breadth is greater at the apex than at the base, with the base measuring about 0.04 mm and the apex 0.36 mm in the adult (Buser and Imbert, 1992). The base of the BM is thicker than the apex (Keiler and Richter, 2001). The BM is composed of approximately 24,000 fibers and is orientated transversely relative to the long dimension (Figures 4.13, 4.16a, and 4.17a,b,c). It has shorter fibers at the base than at the apex and is stiffer at the base than at the apex. This allows better tuning for high frequencies at the base and low frequencies at the apex. The BM has

● Figure 4.16

(a) Anatomy of the organ of Corti (based on Polyak, 1946). (b) The Human Ear The Sonotone Corporation Elmsford, New York pp 93–99 (b) A section of the organ of Corti. 1 = inner hair cell, 2 = cilia of inner hair cells, 3 = reticular lamina, 4 = outer pillar cell, 5 = tunnel of Corti, 6 = space of Nuel, 7 = outer hair cells, 8 = cilia of outer hair cells, 9 = phalangeal process of outer hair cell, 10 = nerve fibers. (c) Region of the tunnel of Corti (courtesy of Richard Mount, Hospital for Sick Children, Toronto).

(a)

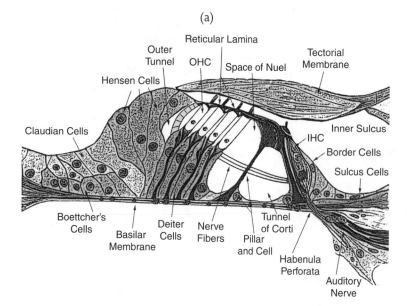

(b)

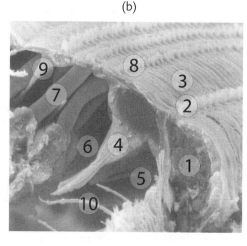

(c)

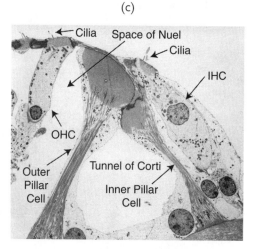

two sections. The inner section, which courses from the spiral lamina to the outer pillar cells, is thinly structured and is termed the **arcuate zone** (Figure 4.13). The second section extends to the spiral ligament and is structurally much thicker and is termed the **pectinate zone** (Raphael and Altschuler, 2003). The arcuate zone, because it is partly enclosed in the osseous spiral lamina, vibrates little, while the pectinate area moves more freely. The stiffness of the BM decreases and the mass increases as it progresses from the base to apex of the cochlea.

The structure of **Reissner's membrane** includes two layers of cells, termed epithelial and mesoepithelial cells (Figures 4.13 and 4.18). This membrane is avascular. It is permeable, by most accounts, but is responsible for maintaining a separation of endolymph and perilymph. The BM (and Reissner's membrane) has some interesting relationships with the cochlea in general. Progressing from the base to the apical region of the cochlea, the scala media becomes smaller, the spiral lamina narrower, and the BM (and hence Reissner's membrane) wider (Duvall and Rhodes, 1967; Flock and Flock, 2003).

● **Figure 4.17**

(a) A drawing looking down on the basilar membrane. (b) Showing the relative dimensions of the basilar membrane in regard to the bony cochlear shell. (c) A side view depicting changes in the thickness of the basilar membrane along the length of the cochlea.

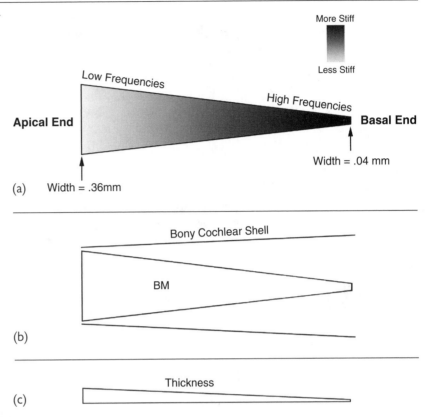

CLINICAL CORRELATE

In disorders such as endolymphatic hydrops, Reissner's membrane can become distended and even ruptured. Flock and Flock (2003) experimentally induced hydrops in the cochleae of guinea pigs and examined Reissner's membrane in these animals. Under increased pressure, Reissner's membrane became slack and its surface area increased. When the pressure was released, the membrane was found to be somewhat floppy and folded, but 15 to 30 minutes following the induced increase in pressure the membrane regained its normal shape and size. For short periods of pressure increases, ruptures in the membrane were not seen; however, in long-standing cases, ruptures were likely. When Reissner's membrane reached its limit of compliance, further pressure increase caused displacement of Corti's organ toward the scala tympani. This in turn affected cochlea function, such as reduced cochlear microphonics. This study supports many of the earlier observations made by Schuknecht (1975) of the temporal bones of humans diagnosed with hydrops. Schuknecht had shown that in cases of hydrops, Reissner's membrane is distended to the point where it is pushed to near the top of the scala vestibuli. ●

ORGAN OF CORTI

Tectorial Membrane

The organ of Corti, which is known as the organ of hearing, lies on the top of the BM. The organ of Corti runs the entire length of the cochlear duct and consists of supporting structures, sensory cells, and nerve fibers. The **tectorial membrane** is

● **Figure 4.18**

Photomicrograph of Reissner's membrane showing its filamentous composition (courtesy of Marilyn Pinheiro).

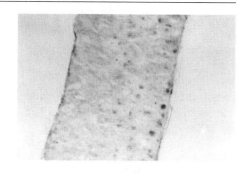

● **Figure 4.19**

View of the top of the tectorial membrane from above the structure. The limbus would be to the left (courtesy of Marilyn Pinheiro).

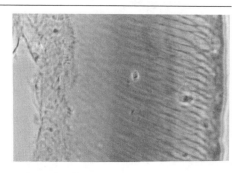

● **Figure 4.20**

Photomicrograph of the tectorial membrane (TM) and its connection to the vestibular lip of the limbus (L) (from Zemlin, 1998, with permission).

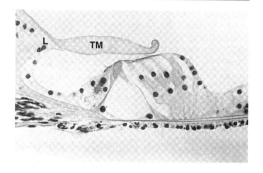

situated immediately above the organ of Corti and covers its entire length (Figures 4.16a, 4.19, and 4.20) (Lim, 1972; Steel, 1983). This structure plays an important role in articulating with the stereocilia of the outer hair cells (OHCs) (see the next chapter). The underside of the tectorial membrane has notches that accommodate the tallest of the OHCs (Slepecky, 1996). These notches allow the tectorial membrane to articulate without becoming decoupled. The stereocilia tips are firmly imbedded in the underside of the tectorial membrane (often termed Kimura's membrane). There do not seem to be any notches on the medial tectorial membrane that accommodate the inner hair cell (IHC) stereocilia; in fact, the IHCs may not contact the tectorial membrane (Slepecky, 1996). This area on the underside of the tectorial membrane above the IHCs is termed Hensen's strip. Hensen's strip is a bulge on the underside of the tectorial membrane directly above the IHCs that restricts the area between the IHC cilia and the tectorial membrane (see next chapter for related physiology). The relative mass and dimensions of the tectorial membrane increases from base to apex. The tectorial membrane is not really a membrane, but rather a gelatinous flap composed of collagen and proteins (Steel, 1983). The tectorial membrane is attached to the spiral limbus on one side and is thought to be attached to Hensen supporting cells on the other (see Geisler, 1998).

Reticular Lamina

The **reticular lamina** forms the ceiling of the sensory and supporting cells of the organ of Corti. This ceiling separates the endolymph from the internal structures of the organ of Corti, as the fluid around the cells and in the tunnel of Corti is cortilymph, which is similar to perilymph (Figure 4.16b and 4.21). The reticular lamina is formed by the phalanges of the Deiters' and inner phalangeal cells, as well as by the inner and outer pillar cells, which all form tight junctions. These phalanges mushroom out at their tops and contact the top margin of the sensory cells (termed the cuticular plate) as well as the inner and outer pillar cells, which all form tight junction complexes to compose the reticular lamina (Leonova and Raphael, 1997). The reticular lamina provides support for the upper portion of the hair cells. It is important to understand that the cilia of the hair cells penetrate the reticular lamina. This means that only the cilia are bathed in endolymph; otherwise the reticular lamina forms a barrier to the endolymph compartment (scala media) and separates the hair cells proper from the endolymph. Therefore, the cilia are bathed in a high-potassium concentration that has a +80-mV charge. On the other hand, the hair cells are bathed in perilymph, which is low in potassium and has a 0-mV charge.

Figure 4.21

View of the organ of Corti looking down on the reticular lamina. Note the tightly packed cells and connective membranes (courtesy of Marilyn Pinheiro).

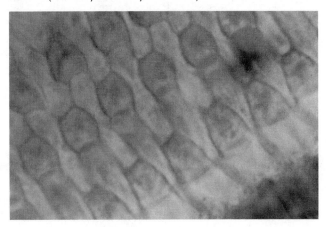

Lateral Wall of Cochlear Duct

Positioned on the outer edge of the cochlear duct are the **spiral ligament** and the **stria vascularis** (see Figures 4.13, 4.16a, 4.22, and 4.23). The spiral ligament is situated between the otic capsule wall and the stria vascularis. It covers the entire

Figure 4.22

Close-up of the stria vascularis showing many vessels packed with red blood cells (courtesy of Marilyn Pinheiro).

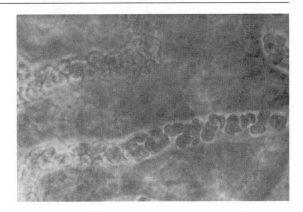

● **Figure 4.23**

Scanning electron microscopy showing a turn of the cochlea with a composite view of numerous structures previously shown. I = bony wall, 2 = spiral ligament, 3 = stria vascularis, 4 = Claudian cells, 5 = Hensen cells, 6 = cilia of the outer hair cells, 7 = region of the tunnel of Corti, 8 = cilia of the inner hair cells, 9 = tectorial membrane, 10 = limbus, 11 = Reissner's' membrane (courtesy of Richard Mount, Hospital for Sick Children, Toronto).

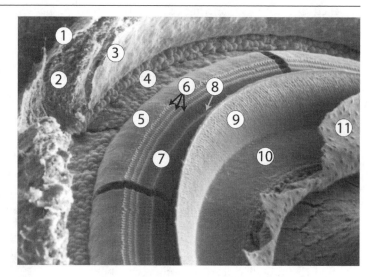

lateral wall of the scala media and extends inferiorly into the upper part of the scala tympani. The spiral ligament is composed of connective tissue cells and provides overall support to the BM and Reissner's membrane and anchors the lateral aspect of the BM. The spiral ligament has a prominent capillary bed for the supply and drainage of blood (see Chapter 14). The spiral ligament may also help maintain ionic balance in the cochlea (Slepecky, 1996; Raphael and Altschuler, 2003). There is some thought that the spiral ligament may play a role in regulating the tension of the BM (Henson, Henson, and Jenkins, 1984). The stria has the potential for secretory and absorptive functions. It is composed of three cell types: marginal cells, intermediate cells, and basal cells, which all play roles in this structure's metabolism (Slepecky, 1996). The marginal cells are epithelial cells that form a single layer and line the lateral wall of the scala media. These cells are associated with ion channels and pumps (Raphael and Altschuler, 2003). The intermediate cell layer is lateral to the marginal cells and contains melanin. When melanocytes are absent, the stria becomes dysfunctional and an endocochlear potential cannot be generated (Steel and Barkway, 1989). Interestingly, Albinos can and do have normal hearing. The basal cell layer is just medial to the spiral ligament and forms a tight junction with intermediate cells (Raphael and Altschuler, 2003). The stria supplies blood and nutrients to the cochlea and probably manufactures endolymph (Zemlin, 1998). The stria is characterized by a rich network of capillaries (Figure 4.22). It is commonly considered to be the source of the +80-mV endolymphatic resting potential (Crouch and Schulte, 1995; Geisler, 1998).

Hair Cells

The gross anatomy of the organ of Corti reflects sensory cells of two main types: **inner hair cells** (IHCs) and **outer hair cells** (OHCs) (Figures 4.16a,b,c and 4.20). Multiple rows of OHCs and a single row of IHCs are arranged on opposite sides of the Pillar cells (which define the tunnel of Corti). In the human, a single row of IHCs course the length of the cochlea and number about 3,500 cells. Three to five rows of OHCs course the length of the cochlea and number about 12,000 cells (Moller, 2000). There may be, in some cases, more OHCs at the apical end of the cochlea. At the top end of the hair cells are **stereocilia (or cilia)**, while at the base of the hair cells are afferent and efferent auditory nerve fibers. The IHCs and OHCs are very different in their structures, which is a prime indication that their functions are quite different (Figures 4.24 and 4.25a,b).

The OHCs are cylinder-shaped and are about 10 μm in diameter. The length of the OHCs may range from 10 to 90 μm. In regions along the BM that are tuned to low frequencies, the OHCs are relatively long, whereas in regions tuned to high frequencies, the OHCs are shorter (Geisler, 1998). Within the OHCs are contractile proteins such as actin, myosin, prestin, and tubulin, as well as cylindrical components near their lateral outer shells called cisterns (Forge, Zajic, Li, Nevill, and Schacht, 1993). These chemical and cellular elements are necessary for the rapid expansion and contraction of the OHCs (see the following two chapters for additional information on this topic). The OHCs have a −60-mV electrical charge (Geisler, 1998) and have K+ (potassium) channels for ion flow out of the cells after partial depolarization (see further discussion below).

The OHCs have stereocilia (on top of the cuticular plate that anchors them) that are attached to the underside of the tectorial membrane. There are three rows of stereocilia on each cell. The rows are graded in length and form a W-shape on each OHC. There are more stereocilia for the OHCs located at the base than for those situated at the apex of the cochlea. Wright (1981) reported about 150 stereocilia for hair cells at the base and about 50 for hair cells at the apex. It appears that the stereocilia are relatively stiff and remain stiff when they are displaced. However, He and Dallos (2000) have shown in isolated OHCs that their axial stiffness changes when the membrane potential changes. They also have shown that overall cell stiffness decreases with depolarization and increases with hyperpolarization.

The IHCs are structurally stronger than the OHCs. They are ovoid or flask-shaped and are about 35 μm in length. The IHCs have more mitochondria than the OHCs. There is a −40-mV electrical charge in the IHCs and these hair cells have both potassium and calcium channels (Geisler, 1998).

● **Figure 4.24**

Sketch of an outer hair cell. 1 = stereocilia, 2 = cisternae, 3 = mitochondria, 4 = cross–links, 5 = tip-links, 6 = pores, 7 = nucleus, 8 = efferent nerve terminal, 9 = afferent nerve terminal.

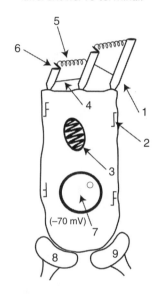

● **Figure 4.25**

(a) Sketch of an inner hair cell. 1 = stereocilia, 2 = nucleus, 3 = mitochondria, 4 = tip–links, 5 = cross-links, 6 = afferent nerve terminal, 7 = efferent nerve terminal. (b) Sketch of an outer hair cell (OHC) and its Deiters' cell.

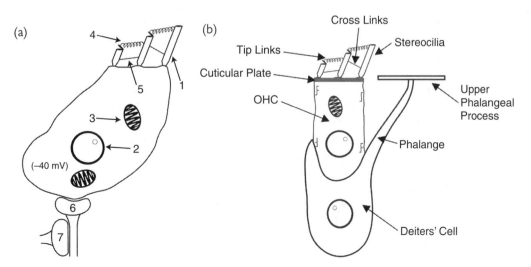

The IHCs have about 50 to 70 stereocilia per cell, and these are not W-shaped like the OHCs, but rather flat U-shaped. The IHC's stereocilia are probably not imbedded in the tectorial membrane. This has significant implications as to how these cilia are deflected (see next two chapters for additional information on cilia deflection). The IHC's stereocilia are arranged in three rows and are graded in length. The cilia also increase in length from the basal to apical region of the cochlea (4 to 5 μm at the base; 7 to 8 μm at the apex) (Wright, 1984). It is generally agreed that IHC's cilia are courser, thicker, and stronger than the cilia of the OHCs.

The stereocilia in both the IHCs and OHCs have a core of actin filaments and an electron dense base that is inserted in the cuticular plate. The stereocilia are longest at the apex and progressively become shorter toward the base of the cochlea (Raphael and Altschuler, 2003). The **kinocilium** (in vertebrates) is the tallest of the stereocilia for each hair cell and is located at the array of cilia. It has its own base, unlike the other cilia that are anchored to the cuticular plate (Geisler, 1998). The stereocilia have **pores** that open upon excitation (allowing K ions in the cell). Recall that the cilia are bathed in endolymph, a fluid that has a high potassium concentration and a +80-mV charge, while inside the cell a −40 to 60-mV charge exists. These differences in charges permit the K+ ion flow into the cell and depolarization to occur. Related to these pores' openings are **tip-link** structures. These pores are openings to mechanotransducer channels and are located toward the tips of the stereocilia or just below the stereocilia tips. Tip-links are small filaments that have several orientations in their connections to other cilia and hair cells. These tip-links connect to mechanotransduction channels and open these channels when the cilia move. Also, tip-links, when connected to the top of the stereocilia, may open the pores to allow the K+ ions into the cells (Gillespie, 1995). Each cilium has only a few ion channels (Howard and Hudspeth, 1988). The tip-links open the "gates" of the channels quickly, perhaps on the order of 50 μsec (Hudspeth, 1989).

Cross-links are similar to tip-links; however, they are located at the sides of the cilia. The cross-links help the cilia move in concert when stimulated. Specifically, when the tallest cilia move in one direction, because of the cross-links, all the cilia move in that direction.

The hair cells are tuned along the length of the BM. Those hair cells that are located at the basal part of the cochlea respond to high-pitched acoustic stimuli, and those at the apical end, to low-pitched sounds. The **characteristic frequency** (CF) of the hair cell (the frequency to which the hair cell best responds, which is generally determined by the hair cell's lowest threshold or greatest magnitude of response to a tone) systematically becomes lower in frequency as one moves from the basal to apical part of the cochlea (Gelfand, 1998; Hudspeth, 2000b). If successive hair cells along the BM were analyzed by their CFs, there would be on average about a 0.2% frequency change from cell to cell. By comparison, adjacent piano strings differ in frequency by 6% (Hudspeth, 2000a). A cochlear hair cell is sensitive to a restricted range of frequencies that are higher or lower than its CF (Hudspeth, 2000a). This means that frequencies other than the CF have to be more intense to result in a response from the hair cell. Generally, the more distal the frequency of a tone from the hair cell's CF, the more intense the stimulus needs to be to trigger the hair cell to fire. This relationship is the basis of (physiological) **tuning curves**, that is, the plotting of the intensity needed to make a hair cell (or neuron) fire across a range of frequencies (see Figure 4.26).

Figure 4.26

Sketch of a tuning curve that might be obtained from an inner hair cell.

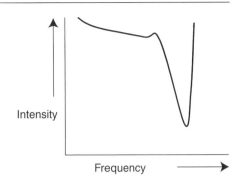

CLINICAL CORRELATE

One of the best clinical models for studying hair cell dysfunction is damage to the hair cell from intense noise. In cases of noise exposure (and other OHC disorders), it is often the OHCs and their stereocilia that are first and most seriously damaged. The OHCs seem to incur more damage than the IHCs from high-intensity noise. In noise and ototoxic damage, there is a systematic progression of damage to the OHCs, with the first row showing more damage than the second row and the second more than the third (Harrison and Mount, 2001). The IHCs are much more resistant to noise damage, as has been shown in cases in which the OHCs are essentially absent while the IHCs remain intact following noise exposure (Figures 4.27, 4.28, and 4.29).

It has been known for many years that the basal part of the cochlea is more susceptible to damage from high-level noise exposure. Even with exposure to low-frequency noise, there is damage at the basal end and throughout the cochlea (Bohne and Harding, 2000). Exposure to high-level noise results in sensorineural hearing loss with maximum hearing loss occurring around 4 kHz, reduced speech recognition, and flattened psychophysical tuning curves for the involved frequencies (Figure 4.30). In addition, tinnitus, poor

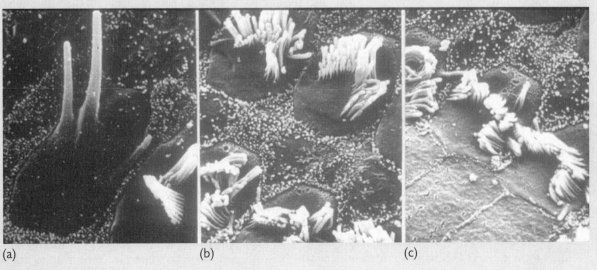

(a)   (b)   (c)

Figure 4.27

Scanning electron microscopy showing damage to the stereocilia of outer hair cells 30 days after intense noise exposure. (a) Fused stereocilia; (b) and (c) collapsed stereocilia (courtesy of Donald Henderson, University of Buffalo).

(continued)

● **Figure 4.28**

Small lesion area (see arrow) of the stereocilia of the outer hair cells 30 minutes after impulse noise exposure (courtesy of Donald Henderson, University of Buffalo).

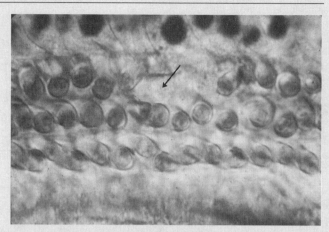

OHCs—30 Minutes after Traumatic Noise Exposure

● **Figure 4.29**

Damage to the pillar cells within the organ of Corti following intense noise exposure. Note that these cells are detached at their base (courtesy of Donald Henderson, University of Buffalo).

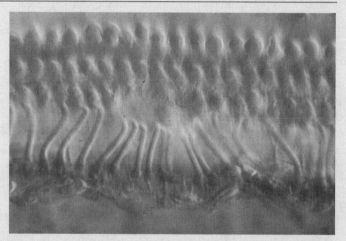

Pillar Cells after Impulse Noise Exposure

hearing in noise, intolerance to loud sounds, and aural fullness are common consequences of high-intensity sound exposure.

The damage that high-intensity noise creates is related to alterations in the organ of Corti. One of these is disruption of the stereocilia. Noise exposure can result in the decoupling of the OHC's stereocilia from the tectorial membrane. The stereocilia can then become fused or collapse (Harrison, 2001). When this happens, whether from noise, ototoxicity, or some other disorder, the tip-links become nonfunctional and the pores cannot open and close appropriately. Another alteration of cochlea anatomy and function that can result

from noise exposure is the loss of hair cell bodies, which has been shown for many years. A third alteration can arise from damage to the supporting cells (Bohne and Harding, 2000). All of these conditions can result in noise-induced sensorineural hearing loss.

The pathogenesis of noise-induced hearing loss seems elusive. Bohne and Harding (2000) overview four leading hypotheses: (1) reduced blood flow during exposure resulting in hypoxia, (2) metabolic exhaustion of the hair cells, (3) excessive neurotransmitter release during exposure, possibly leading to nerve fiber damage, and (4) intermixing of cochlear fluids secondary to reticular lamina damage. All of these pathological actions could

(continued)

play a role in causing cochlear damage and associated hearing loss from noise. However, a relatively new and popular view includes the role of free radicals in the pathophysiology of noise-induced hearing loss. It is well known in the pharmacological literature that free radicals are dangerous to proper cell function. ●

● **Figure 4.30**

Audiogram of a patient with long-term noise exposure. Speech recognition scores were 92% for the right ear and 80% for the left ear.

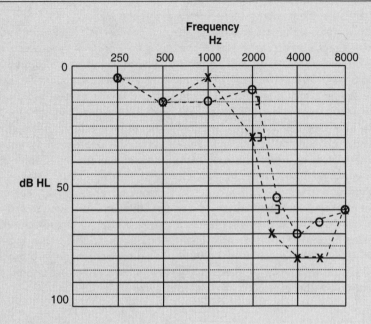

CLINICAL CORRELATE

It appears that both noise damage and ototoxicity could share a damaging agent—free oxygen radicals (FORs) (Henderson, McFadden, Liu, Hight, and Zheng, 1999). FOR damage is a distinct possibility for a pathogenesis for noise-induced hearing loss. High noise levels tax mitochondrial respiratory processes, leading to FOR generation (Hyde and Rubel, 1995). Also, intense exposure to noise may lead to ischemia, which can eventually result in FORs being released from the stria vascularis. FOR damage is likely to result in hair cell death. Of great interest here are the studies that show that antioxidant enzymes appear to partially protect against noise-induced hearing loss (see Henderson et al., 1999 for review). These studies suggest that there may be ways in which the damaging effects of intense noise exposure on the cochlea can be moderated.

The primary classes of ototoxic drugs include aminoglycosides, chemotherapeutics, loop-diuretics, and salicylate analgesics (aspirin). The aminoglycosides are a class of drugs that include many of the '-mycins,' and of all of this class is clearly one of the most toxic. Cisplatin is a chemotherapeutic agent that is presently the most ototoxic medication currently used in clinical practice. It demonstrates potent and irreversible effects on both the cochlear and vestibular systems (Fausti, Henry, Schaffer, Olson, Frey, and Bagby, 1993). Although the damaging and permanent effects of ototoxic agents are known, the incidence of ototoxicity remains unclear.

Aspirin results in sensorineural loss, which is reversible upon stopping the drug. Because of its reversibility, aspirin is often used to study hair cell function (see Monsell, Teixido, Wilson, and Hughes, 1997).

Ototoxic damage is primarily focused on the basal and medial portions of the cochlea, with damage spreading toward the apex as the ototoxic effects progress. As a result, audiological findings generally demonstrate high-frequency sensorineural hearing loss.

(continued)

This hearing loss often begins above the 8-kHz range with a downward progression to the lower frequencies with continued treatment. Within the organ of Corti, the OHCs experience the first sign of pathology, with damage occurring to the IHCs following destruction of the OHCs (Hawkins, 1976). Morphological changes are also evident in Reissner's membrane, the supporting cells within the cochlea, and the stria vascularis (Ruedi, Furrer, Luthy, Nager, and Tschirren, 1952; Estrem, Babin, Ryu, and Moore, 1981; Komune and Snow, 1981; Schweitzer, 1993). In addition, evidence suggests that the spiral ganglion cells demonstrate destruction (Hawkins, Beger, and Aran, 1967), which may progress for some time following discontinued treatment (Webster and Webster, 1981; Zappia and Altchuler, 1989). There are also some instances in which ototoxic agents may attack the vestibular organs.

Little is known regarding the mechanism that contributes to the trauma that is initially seen in the basal region of the cochlea. Several hypotheses have been proposed; however, work by Sha and colleagues (2001) provides the most logical hypothesis for the primary mechanism associated with the damage gradient that occurs within the organ of Corti. They attribute the base-to-apex sensitivity to the formation of free radicals. In the animal model, it appears to be that different levels of susceptibility to free radicals exist along the gradient and that cellular death may be more susceptible to aminoglycoside toxicity in the basal portion of the cochlea.

There is a significant body of research investigating the effects of otoprotectorants, such as glutathione, glutathione ester, and d-methionine, in preventing and minimizing ototoxic effects. Evidence suggests that these agents protect against some of the destructive effects of ototoxic damage. Research indicates that glutathione ester, and not glutathione alone, provides significant protection against damage associated with cisplatin treatment (Campbell, Larsen, Meech, Rybak, and Hughes, 2003). However, the most promising agent currently appears to be d-methionine. In rats, d-methionine was found to provide complete protection against cisplatin ototoxicity (Campbell, Meech, Rybak, and Hughes, 2003). This research provides promise of a possible mechanism to protect against the devastating effect of ototoxicity on the auditory and vestibular systems. ●

Supporting Cells

Along the organ of Corti are not only hair cells but supporting cells (Figure 4.31). These include **phalangeal cells, Deiters' cells, pillar cells, Hensen cells, Claudian cells, Bottcher's cells,** and **inner and outer border cells** (Slepecky, 1996; Raphael and Altschuler, 2003). Progressing medial to lateral along the BM, the inner border cells are encountered first. These cells separate the IHCs from the cells of the spiral sulcus. The phalangeal cells support the IHCs and have a stalk that separates the lateral sides of the IHCs. Lateral to the IHCs are the Deiters' cells, which have three main parts: the cell body, the stalk, and the apical plate, also termed the phalangeal process. The inner and outer pillar cells form the **tunnel of Corti** and also contribute to the reticular lamina apically. The base for the pillar cells is on the BM and is broad and supportive. These cells are located between the OHCs and IHCs and are oriented at approximately a 45° angle that allows the composition of the tunnel of Corti. The pillar cells contribute to the rigidity of the BM. These cells also help maintain a strong structural attachment between the reticular lamina and the BM (Gelfand, 1998; Raphael and Altschuler, 2003). Immediately lateral to the outer pillar cell is the **space of Nuel.** This structure varies in size, sometimes being as large as or larger than the tunnel of Corti (see Figure 4.16).

The Deiters' cells are next in the medial to lateral progression along the BM and they support the OHCs that rest on the "seats" of these cells. The apical or cuticular plate helps form the reticular lamina. Each Deiters' cell may contact as many as five OHCs (the one it supports as well as adjacent OHCs both in the same row

Schematic of the organ of Corti, without hair cells to better show the supporting cells (from Zemlin, 1998, with permission).

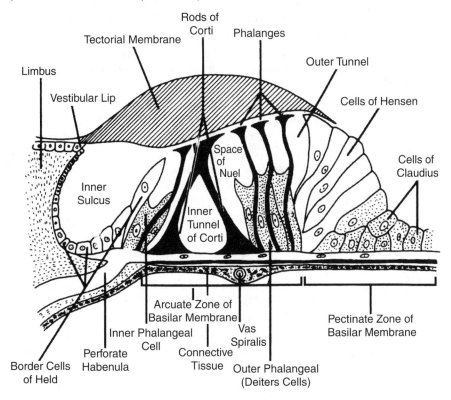

as well as in adjacent rows). The outer tunnel is a space between the stalk of the most lateral Deiters' cells and the OHCs (see Figure 4.16).

The Hensen cells are lateral to the Deiters' cells and on their medial sides; they help form the outer tunnel of Corti. The cells of Hensen probably provide lateral support to the OHCs and support to the tectorial membrane. Interestingly, Deiters' and Hensen cells appear to have synaptic connections to type II nerve fibers and possibly some efferents, as shown in the guinea pig (Fechner, Nadol, Burgess, and Brown, 2001). Moving more laterally, the cells of Claudius extend from the Hensen cells to the outer border or sulcus cells at the base of the stria vascularis covering the BM. The Claudian cells probably add strength to the BM. There are also Bottcher's cells, which are interspersed between the BM and the Claudian cells. It is currently thought that these supporting cells do more than just support the hair cells and the BM. They may function actively to help maintain the ionic balance in the cochlea (Kikuchi, Adams, Miyabe, So, and Kobayashi, 2000; Raphael and Altchuler, 2003).

SUMMARY

The cochlea is located in the temporal bone, which is divided into squamous, mastoid, petrous, and tympanic portions. The temporal bone houses and protects the peripheral hearing mechanism. The cochlea is located in the petrous portion of the temporal bone, and its outer framework (otic capsule), which resembles a snail-shaped spiral cone, is composed of hard bone and serves as a shell that surrounds the membranous cochlea. The center of the cone is the modiolus, which is a perforated bony core that accommodates nerve fibers and blood vessels that course through small openings. The osseous spiral lamina is a shelf-like structure that winds around the bony modiolus and supports the organ of Corti. The oval and round windows are openings with membranes into the bony cochlea.

The membranous cochlea has three scalae that run its length. The scalae vestibuli, media, and tympani define much of the structure of the membranous cochlea. The BM separates the scala tympani from the scala media, and Reissner's membrane separates the scala media from the scala vestibuli. The scalae vestibuli and tympani join together at the apex. The scalae vestibuli and tympani are filled with perilymph (Na > K), which probably originates from the CSF spaces in the brain via the CA. The scala media (or cochlear duct) is filled with endolymph (K > Na). Excess endolymph may result in meniere's disease, and it is believed that the vestibular aqueduct that encompasses the endolymphatic duct and sac may play a role in regulation of endolymph. The lateral wall of the cochlear duct houses the stria vascularis, which likely produces endolymph and plays a role in maintaining the endocochlear potential, as well as the spiral ligament that supports the BM.

The BM is narrower and stiffer at the basal end compared to the apical end and therefore is tuned for high frequencies at the basal end and low frequencies at the apical end. The organ of Corti rests on this membrane. It is composed of supporting and sensory cells. The IHCs and OHCs are located on the medial and lateral sides of the A-shaped tunnel of Corti that is composed of pillar cells. There is one row of IHCs (3,500 cells in total) and three rows of OHCs (12,000 cells in total) in the human cochlea. The IHCs are flask-shaped and OHCs are cylinder-shaped, the latter appropriate for expansion and contraction. The cilia (stereocilia) are located on top of the hair cells and are anchored to the cuticular plate, which along with phalangeal processes from the Deiters' and phalange cells, form most of the tightly sealed reticular lamina. The stereocilia of the OHCs appear W-shaped, while those of the IHCs are flat and U-shaped. Tip-links (microstrand-like filaments between and connecting cilia) open pores on the cilia when they are deflected. Cross-links, which are structured like tip-links, are connected to cilia and help the cilia move in unison upon deflection. These cilia are covered by the tectorial membrane that contacts the cilia of the OHCs but not those of the IHCs. The OHCs' cilia are often the first structures damaged by high-intensity sound exposure. The key remaining structures in the organ of Corti are supporting cells. The phalange and Deiters' cells support the IHCs and OHCs, respectively, and the Hensen and Claudian cells support the more lateral aspect of the BM.

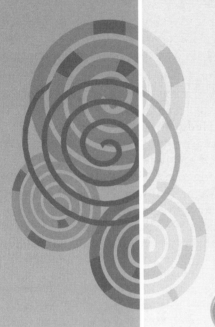

5

Cochlear Physiology I: Mostly Mechanics

Introduction

The mechanics of the cochlea begin with the vibratory input of energy from the stapes, which in turn causes the oval window membrane to vibrate in response to sound energy that is being transferred from the middle ear to the inner ear (Figure 5.1). This mechanical input from the stapes to the oval window membrane is accommodated by expansion of the round window membrane when the stapes moves inward. The opposite happens when the stapes moves outward. In small animals, compression waves in the cochlea also affect the flow resistance of the cochlear aqueduct, which contributes to the equalization of pressure along with the round window (Wit, Feijen, and Albers, 2003). Thus, this may indicate that not all of the displacement at the oval window is transferred to the round window.

CLINICAL CORRELATE

Both the footplate of the stapes at the oval window and the round window membrane must be able to move freely for proper functioning of the cochlear mechanics to occur. It is well known that conditions such as otosclerosis can result in a situation in which the stapes at the oval window does not move appropriately. If this condition exists, then a conductive hearing loss is likely to result. What is not as widely recognized is that a number of other otologic disorders can affect the movement of the round window membrane as well as that of the oval window. For example, fluid in the middle ear can restrict round window membrane movement. This, in turn, can impede the input to the cochlea originating at the oval window and result in a conductive hearing loss. ●

Subsequent to the input from the middle ear, there are a variety of complex interactions in the cochlea that involve the cochlear fluids, various membranes within the cochlea, and the hair cells that combine to define cochlear mechanics. The cochlear mechanics discussed in this chapter operate in the same manner whether the incoming signal is produced via an air-conducted or bone-conducted mechanism. The entire cochlear operation is highly dependent on the mechanical properties of the basilar membrane (BM), and these mechanical properties vary continuously along the entire length of this membrane. The width of the BM is far greater at its apex

● **Figure 5.1**

Schematic diagram showing the input from the stapes causing an inward movement of the oval window and an outward movement of the round window (arrows). This input also results in the deflection of the basilar membrane (based on von Bekesy, 1960).

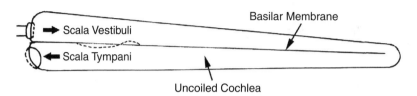

than it is at its basal portion. This progression in width is the opposite of those noted in the cochlear chambers, which are larger at the base than at the apex of the cochlea. At the apex the BM is rather loose and floppy, whereas at the base it is rather tight and stiff (Hudspeth, 2000a). As Hudspeth suggests, the BM could be viewed as a number of strings varying in characteristics from those that are very thick and coarse (such as the strings seen on a bass instrument) to those that are thin and stiff (such as the highest-pitched string on a violin) (Hudspeth, 1989, 2000a,b). Longer, thicker strings tend to move more slowly than shorter, thinner strings and as such result in the generation of lower-frequency sounds. Further, the longer strings have greater movement excursions (which require more time) than the shorter strings. These basic principles of physics are well played out in cochlear mechanics.

THE TRAVELING WAVE (TW)

Perhaps the key process in the mechanics of the cochlea is the generation of the **traveling wave** (TW). The TW in essence is the movement of the cochlear partition in which the key player is the BM. The cochlear partition and the BM movements are fundamental to the transduction process. Because BM movements are rapid, complex, and extremely small, they have been and continue to be difficult to study. Perhaps the major technical advance in the study of BM movement was the introduction of the **Mossbauer** technique by Johnstone and Boyle (1967). This technique allowed indirect measurements of BM movements in vitro, which in turn markedly advanced the knowledge of cochlear physiology. The Mossbauer technique involves the placement of a radioactive source (substance) on the BM. When the BM moves or vibrates, some of the gamma rays that were absorbed by the structure are modulated in a manner that is directly related to the vibration excursions of the BM. This allows the accurate calculation of BM displacement (see Geisler, 1998 for additional information). This technique has been used in numerous studies of cochlear mechanics since its inception and it has helped expand and extend the 1961 Nobel Prize–winning efforts of the late **George von Bekesy** (von Bekesy, 1960), who first defined the mechanics of the TW. More recently, laser inferometry has been used in studying fine movements of the BM. This technique involves a superior submicron measurement methodology that produces even more definitive results than those afforded by the Mossbauer technique (Geisler, 1998).

The development of the TW along the BM is dependent on the vibratory input to the cochlea that is provided by the stapes. Since the cochlear fluids are noncompressible, the vibration of the stapes results in the displacement of the noncompressible cochlear fluids along with a compensatory displacement (bulge) of the round window. This round window accommodation to the stapes' input happens almost instantaneously and before the TW is fully propagated. The round window is a highly compliant membrane that easily allows for pressure accommodation (Geisler, 1998). The pressure wave that originates at the oval window travels the entire spiral of the cochlea, transferring the fluid movement from the scala vestibuli to the scala tympani at the helicotrema. The stapes' input to the cochlea creates temporary pressure differences between the scala vestibuli and the scala tympani. This, in turn, causes transverse pressures and vertical displacements along the BM (Buser and Imbert, 1992). Owing to the physical characteristics of the BM and the sensory and supporting cells of the organ of Corti, this fluid bulge moves down the BM, hence the origins of the term *traveling wave* (von Bekesy, 1953, 1960). The specific movement pattern of the BM depends on whether the input from the stapes is a compression wave or a rarefaction wave. In general, compression waves drive the BM downward and rarefaction waves drive the BM upward (von Bekesy, 1960, 1970) (Figures 5.2 and 5.3a).

An important aspect of the TW is the speed at which it travels down the length of the cochlea. The physical characteristics of the BM, the organ of Corti, and the cochlear duct all play a role in the velocity of the TW (Dallos, 1996). Recall that the BM is smaller and stiffer at the basal end, which makes this end more conducive to quick movements (i.e., higher frequencies) than the larger, less stiff tissue at the apical end. As the stiffness gradient decreases down the length of the BM, so does the speed of the TW. Certainly the speed of the TW is much greater at the basal end than at the apical end of the BM. Zwislocki (2002) relates that at the basal-most aspect of the cochlea, the TW velocity is between 45 and 50 m per second and that it slows down to about 1 to 2 m per second at or near the apex. These velocity measurements, however, were based on the original data from von Bekesy (1960), who had derived these measures from cadavers. Subsequent in vivo measurements made by Zwislocki (2002) using the Mongolian gerbil showed the TW velocity to be about twice as fast (e.g., 100 m/second at the base), and computations for "alive" humans (based on mammalian interspecies similarities) were judged to be consistent with the velocities noted for the gerbil (Figure 5.3b). Also, since the stiffness of the BM decreases from the basal to the apical end, the amplitude of the TW increases as it courses along the BM. In fact, the volume displacement at the apical end is more than 10 times what is at the basal end (Zwislocki, 2002) (Figure 5.3c). As the TW begins to travel down the BM, it originates as a uniform nondispersive wave that becomes more dispersive and less uniform as it continues to travel the length of the BM (Lighthill, 1981; Dallos, 1996). This phenomenon has implications related to the sharpness of tuning along the BM and other related functions.

● Figure 5.2

Schematic drawing of the location of the traveling wave on the basilar membrane for various frequencies. Note that the envelopes of the traveling waves are asymmetric in shape and that they progress toward the basal end of the cochlea as the stimulus frequency increases.

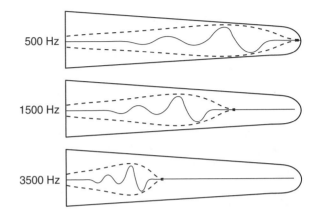

CLINICAL CORRELATE

The speed of the TW at the basal end of the cochlea coupled with the large BM deflections that would be caused by high-intensity stimuli are likely to result in greater damage in this segment of the cochlea as opposed to more apical regions of this structure. This may be why high-frequency hearing losses are much more common than low-frequency deficits in patients with histories of noise exposure. Fast, whip-like motions at the basal end may result in a strain on the hair cells and their stereocilia at the basal end of the cochlea that results in significant compromise of these fine sensory structures. ●

CLINICAL CORRELATE

The greater speed and less dispersive nature of the TW at the basal segment of the cochlea can result in a more synchronous discharge of hair cells and auditory nerve fibers in this portion of the BM than at the apical end (Kiang, 1975). This correlates to better auditory brainstem response (ABR) recordings for high-frequency tone bursts or clicks compared to those noted for low-frequency stimuli. Synchronicity is critical to the ABR and is achieved by stimulation of the basal end of the cochlea. It is well known that clicks and high-frequency stimuli provide better ABR recordings than low-frequency stimuli. ●

● **Figure 5.3**

(a) The effects of compression and rarefaction segments of a sine wave on the basilar membrane. A compression part of the wave results in the stapes moving inward. This results in the round window moving outward to allow the fluid motion to take place. The stapes' inward movement results in a downward movement of the basilar membrane. A rarefaction part of a wave results in the stapes moving outward and the round window moving inward. As a result, the basilar membrane moves upward (modified from Perkins and Kent, 1986, with permission). (b) Cochlear traveling wave velocity computed for humans (from Zwislocki, 2002, with permission). (c) Amplitude of basilar membrane vibration (from Zwislocki, 2002, with permission).

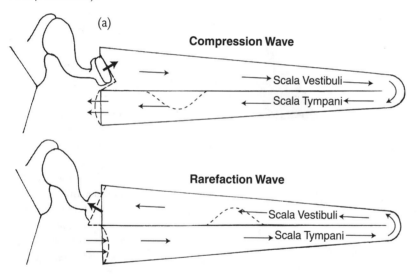

(a)

Compression Wave

Scala Vestibuli
Scala Tympani

Rarefaction Wave

Scala Vestibuli
Scala Tympani

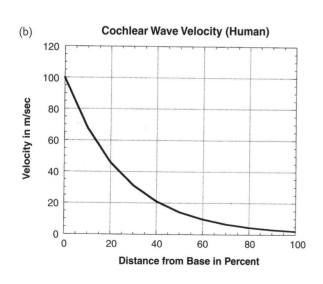

(b)

Cochlear Wave Velocity (Human)

Velocity in m/sec

Distance from Base in Percent

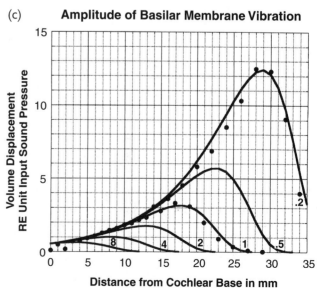

(c) **Amplitude of Basilar Membrane Vibration**

Volume Displacement
RE Unit Input Sound Pressure

Distance from Cochlear Base in mm

● Figure 5.4

The frequency to distance relationship from the stapes to a place along the human basilar membrane.

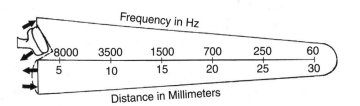

● *Frequency and Intensity Representation*

The stapes' input or displacement is linear and reflects the frequency and the intensity of the stimulus at the oval window. That is, if the sound is a 500-Hz tone that is 75 dB sound pressure level, then the stapes vibrates 500 times per second and causes a displacement at the oval window that would be greater than that for any sound of less than 75 dB SPL (sound pressure level) at the same frequency. The TW must be able to represent the frequency and intensity of the stimulus in some manner, and it does so by the location of maximum displacement of the BM and the amount of the deflection of the BM, respectively. Different frequencies produce TWs that reach their maximum deflections at different places along the cochlear partition (Figure 5.4). High-frequency stimuli cause maximal displacement of the BM in the basal region of the cochlea, whereas low-frequency sounds result in maximal deflection in the apical region of the cochlea. Since the TW moves from the base to the apex, the basal end of the cochlea is stimulated by low-frequency sounds as well as by high-frequency acoustic stimuli (von Bekesy, 1947). When the low-frequency sounds are of relatively high intensity, the TW action causes significant stimulation at the basal end of the cochlea, which is likely responsible for the **upward spread of masking** effect (the masking of a stimulus at one frequency by a stimulus of a lower frequency). The oscillations of the BM, which constitute the TW envelope, increase with the frequency of the stimulus (Figures 5.1 and 5.2). However, it is believed that the displacement location of maximum deflection on the BM is more important physiologically in the representation of frequency than is the velocity of BM oscillations or periodicity (see Geisler, 1998 for review). This is not to say, however, that the oscillation rate (also referred to as temporal coding) does not contribute in some manner to the coding of frequency—it does so at least for some frequencies. Oscillation rate, or frequency periodicity, as it is also called, is likely to play a role in the coding of frequency, particularly for low-frequency sounds. There is evidence from auditory nerve recordings that periodicity cannot faithfully operate at high frequencies because of the refractory period of auditory nerve fibers. However, oscillation rate or periodicity is feasible at lower frequencies, and there may be interactions between place and periodicity information for some frequencies. The role of each of these theories of frequency coding continues to be debated (see Moller, 2000 for additional information).

A variety of physical conditions produce "tonotopicity" in the cochlea, or more specifically along the BM (von Bekesy, 1960, 1970). The TW is a result of the BM moving up and down in a rapid whip-like motion. This rapid motion creates an envelope of activity as the TW travels from the base to the apex of the BM. This whip-like action is faster for the high frequencies than it is for low frequencies and there is greater displacement of the BM for high intensities compared to low intensities. The degree of BM displacement also varies depending on the width and stiffness of the BM. The normal TW gradually builds in amplitude as it moves away from the base of the cochlea, then after reaching its maximum it decays rapidly on

CLINICAL CORRELATE

The upward spread of masking becomes clinically relevant in a number of ways. One of the most common is in hearing aid fittings. If an amplifying device provides too much low-frequency gain, the increased intensity of the low frequencies that is provided by the hearing aid may mask the higher frequencies, and overall hearing performance may suffer. ●

the apical side (Rhode, 1971). This results in an envelope of activity that is markedly asymmetric in shape (Figure 5.2). Similar patterns of BM movement are noted for both air-conducted and bone-conducted signals. Since the BM has 100 times greater stiffness at the base compared to the apex, there is a predictable pattern of physical action; that is, the TW propagation flows from an area of minimal compliance to one of maximum compliance (Buser and Imbert, 1992). Therefore, all things being equal, as the TW moves from base to apex it increases in amplitude. When the TW approaches the resonance point for a particular input frequency, the admittance of the cochlear partition increases and there is enhanced BM movement. This is the point along the BM where the maximum deflection of the TW occurs and it is the primary mechanism by which frequency information is represented within the cochlea.

Resonance in the cochlear partition happens when stiffness and mass limitations are equal in magnitude but opposite in phase (Pickles, 1988). The resonance point takes place at different loci on the BM, depending on the frequency of the stimulus. Inertial forces are greater for high frequencies; thus, these matching forces (stiffness and mass) take place at the stiffer end of the BM (i.e., the base) for higher-frequency sounds, while the mass and stiffness conditions match for low-frequency sounds toward the apical (or less stiff) end of the BM (Pickles, 1988). Beyond the resonance point, the TW dies quickly, as it is moving at a much slower velocity than at the base and more damping is occurring because of the physical characteristics of the BM and the organ of Corti.

Von Bekesy's work, which implicated the TW motion as the basis for frequency selectivity, won him the Nobel Prize in 1961. However, a problem that surrounded this early work was that the frequency tuning of the BM was much too broad to explain fully the psychoacoustic measurement of frequency discrimination (i.e., the frequency discrimination observed behaviorally was much sharper than that which could be predicted by the frequency tuning of the BM). Several factors enter into this observation—especially with the new information now available on cochlear mechanics. Von Bekesy's measurements were conducted on the ears of cadavers, and we now know that the BM's fine-tuning is metabolic dependent (Moller, 2000). Since there is no metabolic activity in cadavers, the resultant BM tuning in these ears was found to be quite broad. Also, many of von Bekesy's measurements of BM movement were taken at high intensities, and it is now known that the best frequency selectivity occurs at low intensities. Finally, as will be discussed in greater detail later, outer hair cell (OHC) motility can influence the tuning potential of the BM. The **cochlear amplifier,** which is mediated by the OHC function, sharpens frequency tuning, especially at low intensities. Briefly, this is accomplished by the OHCs contracting upon upward movement of the BM and expanding upon the downward deflection of the BM. This expansion and contraction of the OHCs adds to the total displacement of the BM. This added BM movement enhances the amplitude of the signal; thus, the term *cochlear amplifier* has been used to describe this function. Because the additional contraction and expansion of the OHCs occurs in a restricted area of the BM, the peak region of deflection is sharper in this area and the frequency tuning is enhanced. This cochlear amplifier works at only low- to mid-intensity ranges and is dependent on metabolic activity for influencing frequency selectivity; hence, von Bekesy's investigations of BM displacement in cadaver ears could not account for these particular types of cochlear processes (see Neely and Kim, 1983 and Geisler, 1998 for review).

The spatial sorting of maximal deflections along the BM leads to **frequency selectivity** and pitch discrimination. That is, the area of maximal deflection on the BM corresponds to the frequency of the stimulus and to the tuning of the hair

● Figure 5.5

(a) The increase in the number of hair cells stimulated as the basilar membrane deflection increases with higher intensities. (b) Basilar membrane displacement associated with intensity increments. Note the amplitude compression, lack of sharpness, and greater displacement at the higher intensities.

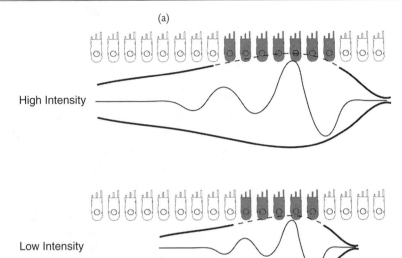

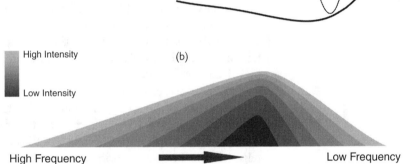

cells (von Bekesy, 1960). Related to the fact that a given hair cell (at suprathreshold levels) responds to frequencies both above and below its characteristic frequency (CF), a single pure tone results in a TW that spreads along the BM (Hudspeth, 2000a,b) (Figure 5.5a). Two tones of different frequencies will have two different areas of maximum deflection. When complex tones or complex signals such as speech are the stimuli being represented on the BM, the maximal deflection points along the BM change quickly over time. This allows the coding of the various frequencies of complex acoustic signals such as speech. The BM pattern of deflection related to the TW is the basis for the stimulation of the cochlear hair cells, which begins the transduction process from vibratory to electrical energy in the cochlea.

To elaborate further upon the function of the BM, the BM action for complex stimuli such as speech provides insight as to how this membrane works. Hudspeth (2000a) provides the following example. If a person hears a vowel sound, that vowel could have three dominate frequency components. A TW is established for each frequency component, and each wave is by first approximation dependent on the waves produced by the other waves. The excursion size of the TW is related to the intensity of the stimulus, and the peak of the excursion is related to the frequency component of the stimulus. Hence, the BW serves as a mechanical frequency analyzer as it distributes energy to the hair cells along the length of the cochlea according to the frequencies that make up the stimulus. This is one of the early steps in the process of encoding the intensity and frequency characteristics of sounds.

• *Nonlinearity*

The tectorial membrane, which comes in contact with the OHCs, bends the cilia as the hair cells "ride" the movement of the BM (see previous chapter). As the intensity of the acoustic stimulus increases, the peak displacement of the BM becomes broader and grows in amplitude, but with considerable compression across the intensity range (Figure 5.5b). This is especially the case at high intensities. Ruggero (1992) made some comparisons for a 3 dB SPL and an 83 dB SPL 9-kHz tone in an animal model. If the BM responses were linear, the 83 dB SPL tone should have yielded a BM deflection that was 10,000 times greater than the deflection that would have occurred for the 3 dB SPL tone, but obviously this does not happen. Instead there were major compression effects that resulted in an amplitude increase of only four times over this intensity range as opposed to the predicted increase of 10,000 times. This compression function within the cochlea serves as a protective mechanism to the organ of Corti. If the BM excursions did increase 10,000 times when increasing intensity from 3 to 83 dB SPL, the result would be severe damage to the cochlea. That is, the deflections would be so great that the BM would hit the bony structures of the cochlea during both negative and positive deflections, causing significant trauma to the BM and the hair cells. In Ruggero's experiments, these compressions that resulted in nonlinearities in the displacement of the BM as a function of intensity were measured at high frequencies.

Because of the anatomy of the mammalian cochlea, it is difficult to measure BM vibrations at the apical end; hence, the data on these effects for low-frequency stimuli are sparse. However, it seems that there is less compression for low frequencies than there is for high frequencies (Rhode and Cooper, 1996). At very low intensities, the BM gets a boost from the cochlear amplifier, resulting in increased BM excursions, although these effects for low-frequency stimuli (i.e., the apical end of the BM) are not nearly as great as those noted for the higher frequencies (represented at the basal end of the BM). At the higher intensities, some compression does take place at the apical end of the BM, but again the extent of these compression effects is not equivalent to those manifested at the high frequencies. Finally, it should be noted that this phenomenon is not limited to the CF (such as with high frequencies), but rather it is present across most of the frequencies surrounding the CF.

The mechanical amplification of low-intensity tones and the compression of BM responses to high-intensity tones can also be demonstrated by comparing BM responses to those of the stapes (Ruggero, 1992; Geisler, 1998). Unlike the BM response, the stapes' displacement for acoustic stimulation is close to linear. Ruggero (1992) demonstrated that the BM response to a weak tone (3 dB SPL at 9 kHz) is much greater than that of the stapes and that as the tonal intensity increases, the BM response compresses while the stapes displacement increases linearly. Therefore, the ratio of stapes displacement to BM displacement drops dramatically as intensity increases. When the animal from which these measurements are made dies, the low-level amplification phenomenon rapidly disappears and the sharpness of the BM response becomes broad. Therefore, it is clear that the enhancement (increased deflection and sharpness of the BM response) of low-intensity stimuli measured at the BM is a result of the action of a biological amplifying system (see next chapter for further discussion).

It is important to realize that the amplification and compression effects, which are recorded at the BM, precede the coding of these vibrations by the auditory nerve. The compression at the BM is critical before the coding of intensity at the auditory nerve since if this mechanism did not occur, the large range of intensities that can be heard could not be handled by the number of auditory nerve fibers available (Moller, 2000).

Based on what has been reviewed in this chapter thus far, it can be concluded that BM excursions increase with increases in intensity of the stimulus. However, the particular manner in which the BM responds to increases in sound intensity is complex (Sellick, Patuzzi, and Johnstone, 1982; Ruggero, 1992; Ruggero, Rich, Recio, Narayan, and Robles, 1997). Nonlinear compression takes place at high intensities, and the area of maximum deflection of the BM becomes larger at higher intensities, reducing frequency selectivity. Also, at high intensities the cochlear amplifier is not active (Figures 5.5a,b and 5.6).

In addition to the physiological actions just mentioned, another BM phenomenon happens at high intensities. It appears that for high intensities represented at the basal end of the BM, there is a shift in maximum deflection of the membrane in the direction of the basal end. This has been shown in small animals (Sellick et al., 1982) and recently in humans based on psychoacoustic findings (Moore, Alcantara, and Glasberg, 2002).

CLINICAL CORRELATE

It is interesting to speculate that when the biological amplifying system and compression systems of the cochlea malfunction, imperfect auditory experiences may result. If the biological amplifier is damaged, then low intensity sounds may not be heard. In addition, frequency selectivity is compromised. On the other hand, if the normal compression of the size of the BM excursions at high intensities does not take place in an appropriate manner, then sounds may be perceived as too loud. Both of these phenomena translate into common clinical symptoms of individuals with hearing disorders. It is possible that when the cochlea is damaged, a resultant dysfunction affects not only the amplification of movement for low-intensity sounds, but also the appropriate compression of the BM movement for high-intensity stimuli. Therefore, symptoms related to less than optimum BM actions could include decreases in both hearing sensitivity and frequency discrimination as well as result in hyperacusis (i.e., increased sensitivity) to relatively intense acoustic stimuli.

● Figure 5.6

A theoretical sketch of basilar membrane displacement for an individual with normal hearing (a) and a person with a severe sensorineural hearing loss (b). The arrows point to the dotted line, which is the point of basilar membrane excursion where the hearing threshold is reached. Also shown are sketches of the resultant behavioral tuning curves for individuals with normal (c) and impaired hearing (d). Note that at (or near) threshold, the peak of the basilar membrane deflection and the associated tuning curve is much sharper for the individual with normal hearing than for the individual with hearing loss. This is because the threshold for the normal hearer occurs at a lower intensity level than for the person with hearing loss. Although both examples are at behavioral thresholds, the greater intensity needed to reach threshold for the person with hearing loss results in a much larger and broader basilar membrane displacement than for the normal hearer.

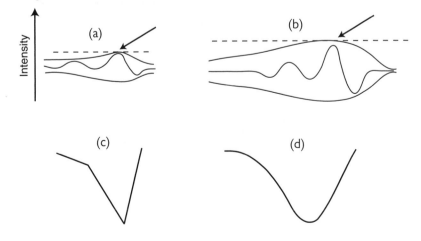

CLINICAL CORRELATE

The mechanical dynamics of the BM are likely to be influenced by disease processes such as endolymphatic hydrops (EH). It is a common theory with some evidence from pathology that EH is associated with increased pressure in the cochlear duct, possibly secondary to increased quantities of endolymph (Horner, 1995). Increased pressure or increased endolymph can affect movement of the BM, resulting in reduced deflection amplitudes. It is also inviting to speculate that increased pressure within the scala media may have more influence at the apical end of the cochlea where the BM is less stiff and more likely to accommodate increased pressure (Figure 5.7a,b,c,d). This increase in pressure at the apical portion of the BM would likely result in a (hydro) mechanically based hearing loss for the low frequencies, consistent with what is often seen in a hydropic hearing loss in its early stages (Tonndorf, 1957). In addition, the increased pressure would likely increase the stiffness of the apical part of the BM. This in turn could result in the TW moving faster at the apical end than would typically be the case. This increased velocity of the TW at the apical end of the cochlea could be translated into shorter latency times for such measures as low-frequency auditory brainstem

● Figure 5.7

(a) An audiogram showing a mild, low-frequency sensorineural hearing loss for the right ear that is typical in the early stages of Meniere's disease (endolymphatic hydrops). (b) An audiogram showing a relatively flat, moderate to severe hearing loss for the right ear, often noted in long-standing Meniere's disease. (c) A sketch showing how endolymphatic hydrops may expand the scala media, distending both Reissner's membrane and the basilar membrane. (d) A sketch showing an 'expansion' of the scala media at the apical end of the cochlea consistent with what may be seen in endolymphatic hydrops. X = left ear, O = right ear, [= right bone conduction,] = left bone conduction, RM = Reissner's membrane, BM = basilar membrane, SV = scala vestibuli, ST = scala tympani, SM = scala media.

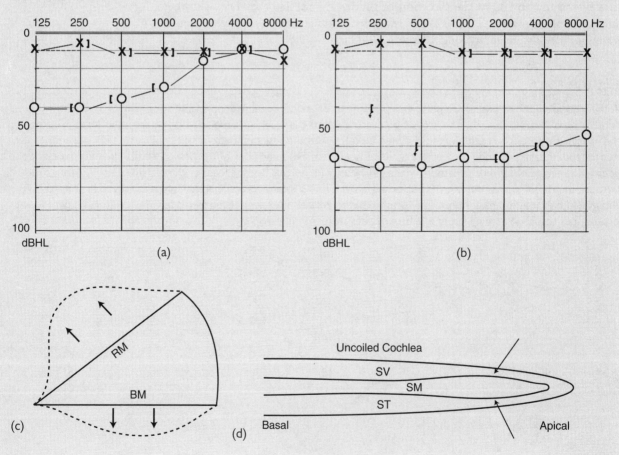

(continued)

responses (ABRs). In the early stages of EH it appears that the hair cells are not damaged to any great extent. Evidence of this is the relatively common finding in EH of hearing sensitivity and speech perception deficits returning to normal values after a meniere's attack. In the later stages of EH, herniations and perforations of the endolymphatic system often evolve and result in biochemical alterations in the cochlea that compromise hearing sensitivity to a greater degree and over a wider range of frequencies than what is typically observed in the early stages of the disease. In addition to greater hearing loss, later stages of EM often result in the hearing not returning to normal after a meniere's episode (Figure 5.7a,b,c,d) (see Schwaber, 1997 for review). ●

HAIR CELL MECHANICS

The hair cells, and especially the **cilia**, have their own mechanical activity. As our technical skills of investigation of cochlear function increase, so does our knowledge of cochlear micromechanics. It seems that more and more critical functions are being attributed to smaller and smaller structures within the cochlea. In hair cell mechanics the tip-links and their ability to open and close ion channels is an area of relatively new and increased interest among hearing scientists. The motility of the OHCs, also dependent on micromechanics, has garnered tremendous interest, mostly because of the advent of otoacoustic emissions (OAEs) and the understanding of the cochlear amplifier (see next chapter). Hence, the area of hair cell mechanics is presently receiving much attention from many researchers. Clearly a review of some of the fundamentals of this exciting area of cochlear physiology is in order.

Upon stimulation, the BM begins to move in either an upward direction toward the scala vestibuli or a downward direction toward the scala tympani, depending on the phase of the stapes movement (Figure 5.3). The direction of this initial movement of the BM is determined by the phase of the acoustic stimulus (i.e., rarefaction or condensation segment of the sound pressure wave) that is reflected in the phase of the stapes' movement. If the acoustic stimulus is a compression or condensation wave, the eardrum is pushed inward, as is the stapes. The inward movement of the stapes causes the TW to deflect the BM downward. Conversely, when the wavefront of the stimulus is a rarefaction, the eardrum and stapes are drawn outward and the BM moves upward. Conventionally, the upper movement of the BM has been considered excitatory, whereas the downward movement has been considered inhibitory (see Moller, 2000 for review). This classic view of compression and rarefaction waves as inhibitory and excitatory has been challenged by a more complex explanation that seems to be dependent on the frequency of the stimulus (Zwislocki and Sokolich, 1973). However, a discussion of these more complex theories is beyond the scope of this chapter. Those interested in a review of these alternative interpretations are directed to Moller (2000).

Let us entertain the classic view of compression and rarefaction stimuli in regard to cochlear mechanics. If a compression wave results in the BM being deflected downward, it will not result in hair cell firing until the rarefaction segment of the wave causes the BM to move upward. On the other hand, a rarefaction stimulus will result in the BM moving upward initially, which causes the hair cell(s) to fire immediately. This means there would be a time difference between hair cell firing with a rarefaction versus a compression stimulus. This time difference is dependent on the frequency of the stimulus and the condition of the cochlea.

CLINICAL CORRELATE

In the clinical application of the ABR (as well as electrocochleography), the use of rarefaction and compression (condensation) clicks can have important implications. It can be demonstrated that a rarefaction click often results in an earlier waveform (usually by 0.1 to 0.2 msec) than does a compression (condensation) click. It also has been suggested that the time difference between waveforms elicited with rarefaction as opposed to compression (condensation) clicks is often exaggerated in patients with meniere's disease (Orchik, Ge, and Shea, 1998). These time differences associated with differences in stimulus parameters (rarefaction and compression stimuli) are important to the proper interpretation of the ABR for clinical use. It is also one of the reasons why one should not change polarity when planning to compare ABR waveforms (except in cases considered to be at risk for meniere's disease). A short difference in latency (0.1 or 0.2. msec), which could be created by changing polarity, could lead to a misinterpretation of latency if one is not cognizant of the latency effects related to different polarities. ●

Let us now take a closer look at what happens in the cochlea, with emphasis on hair cell mechanics when a compression sound wave is the stimulus. A compression wave creates a TW as a result of the stapes moving inward. This causes compression of the perilymph, which results in the scala media being deflected downward, and the BM is also deflected downward. This deflection is carried out with the component parts (BM, tectorial membrane, hair cells, supporting cells) maintaining relative uniformity because the pillar cell complex keeps the BM and scala media in shape. The pillar cell complex's triangular shape permits it to lend support to all the organ of Corti structures during stimulation (see Geisler, 1998).

The pivot point for movement of the BM is at the foot of the inner pillar cell, which is near the tip of the bony spiral lamina. This connection, which serves as a hinge upon which the BM moves up and down, also provides stabilization to the BM during movement. During a compression wave, the OHCs move away from the limbus as the BM rotates downward. The OHCs' cilia, which are attached to the tectorial membrane, move toward the limbus because this membrane is stretched by the deflection of the BM (see Figures 5.8 and 5.9). Although the cilia are relatively stiff, they rotate quite easily at their bases. (The rotation of the cilia at their bases is the primary movement mechanism involved in the OHCs, as opposed to the cilia bending throughout their lengths. This permits the cilia to remain stiff while still moving easily to accommodate fluid and membrane influences.) In downward deflection,

● Figure 5.8

Cilia deflection and basilar membrane movement. (a) A rarefaction stimulus results in an upward movement of the basilar membrane, deflection of cilia away from the limbus, and depolarization (excitation) of the hair cell. (b) Resting state of the basilar membrane. (c) A compression stimulus results in a downward movement of the basilar membrane, deflection of cilia toward the limbus, and a hyperpolarization (inhibition) of the hair cell.

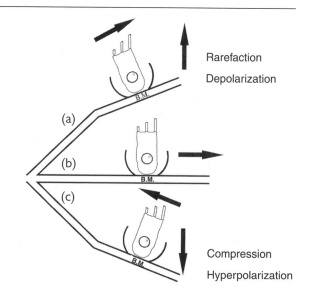

• Figure 5.9

Hair cells that are (a) depolarized, (b) resting, and (c) hyperpolarized and their relative electrical discharge via the auditory nerve. The vertical arrows indicate contraction of the hair cell (during depolarization, with basilar membrane movement upward) and expansion of the cell (during hyperpolarization, with basilar membrane movement downward).

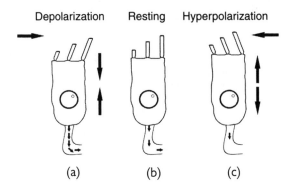

the cilia rotate counterclockwise. The stereocilia motion related to BM movement and tectorial membrane shearing of these cilia is a key step in the transduction process. This mechanical process requires extremely small movement of the hair cell cilia. Dallos (1996) draws an interesting analogy to relate the micro movements of the cilia during the hearing process. He relates that at threshold, the cilia are moved the proportional equivalent of Chicago's Sears Tower moving 5 cm. Put another way, if a cilia were scaled up to be the same height as the Sears Tower, it would move 5 cm at hearing threshold!

The hair cell mechanics of the inner hair cells (IHCs) are different because their cilia are not imbedded in the tectorial membrane—or at least the current thinking is of this opinion. Since the IHCs' cilia do not touch the tectorial membrane, their deflections must be indirect. The most likely scenario is that the fluid in the subtectorial space is pushed away or toward the IHC's cilia. This could be a result of the deflection of the OHCs' cilia pushing fluid toward the IHCs when there is downward movement of the BM. It is also possible that **Hensen's stripe,** an eminence protruding downward from the underside of the tectorial membrane immediately above the IHCs, may play a role in the deflection of the IHCs' stereocilia. More specifically, as the fluid flows in the subtectorial space to the region of the IHC cilia, Hensen's stripe may cause a constriction, adding to the force of the fluid flow against the cilia (Figure 5.10) (see Geisler, 1998, pp. 82).

As mentioned earlier, our understanding of the mechanics of the hair cell has been advanced significantly by recent developments in our understanding of OAEs and the related cochlear amplifier. Brownell, Bader, Bertrand, and de Ribaupierre (1985) demonstrated that OHCs can expand and contract upon electrical stimulation. This expansion and contraction works synergistically with the deflection of the BM (Figure 5.9). That is, the OHC contracts when the BM moves upward and expands when the BM moves downward. This action results in greater deflection and sharpness of BM movement and is referred to as the cochlear, or biological, amplifier (Dallos, 1992). Since the OHC activity is associated with lower-intensity acoustic stimuli, the cochlear amplifier's influence is noted for lower intensities and is probably not active at high intensities. The influence of the OHC expansion and contraction sharpens the point on the BM where there is maximum deflection, resulting in better tuning and frequency selectivity, i.e., at lower intensities. The next chapter, which discusses electromotility and OAEs, will address the function of the cochlear amplifier in more depth.

The next major topic in hair cell mechanics is **tip-links** and **cross-links** (Hudspeth, 1982, 2000a,b). The cilia of the hair cells are arranged in rows of different

● **Figure 5.10**

Hensen's stripe and the junction between the hair cells and tectorial membrane. Arrows show endolymph flow that probably results in stimulation of the cilia of the inner hair cells (modified from Perkins and Kent, 1986, with permission).

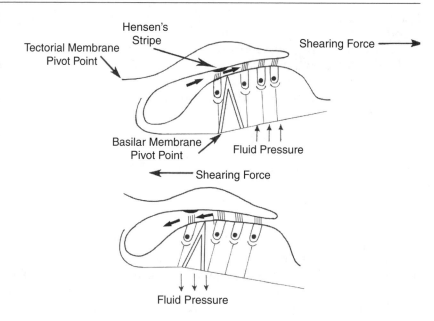

heights. The graded heights of the cilia set up the function of the tip-links. Tip-links are fine strands of an elastic substance that connect to the sides of taller cilia and to the tops of shorter cilia (see Figure 5.11).

There are also cross- or lateral-links that course in various directions connecting neighboring cilia. The cross-links support the cilia and allow the cilia to move in unison (Hudspeth, 1982). The tip-links open up pores in the cilia to allow ion flow through channels whenever the cilia are deflected toward the tallest cilia (excitatory mode). These pores and their associated ion channels are closed when the cilia are deflected away from the tallest cilia (inhibitory mode). Interestingly orthogonal displacement appears to be ineffective and does not result in either excitation or inhibition (see Dallos, 1996; Hudspeth, 2000b). It is believed that tip-links play an important role in the transduction process. When tip-links are destroyed or calcium ions are removed from the external medium, the transduction process of the hair cells is lost (Assad, Shepard, and Corey, 1991; Preyer, Hemmert, Zenner, and Gummer, 1995).

The specific function of the tip-links and cilia is probably best explained by what is known as the trap door theory (Geisler, 1998). If there is a compression wave, the cilia are bent toward the limbus or toward their smaller neighbors. This movement results in the tip-link losing its tension on the so-called trap door, and the trap door closes entirely (hyperpolarization). This means no ion flow into the cells occurs. Conversely, when there is a rarefaction stimulus, the cilia are pushed toward their taller neighbors (away from the limbus). This in turn causes considerable tension on the tip-links, and the trap door is opened to allow ion flow into the cells (depolarization). It has been stated that movements of 100 nm are sufficient to open the ion channels (Fettiplace, Ricci, and Hackney, 2001). Specifically, K+ and Ca+ ions from the endolymph are driven into the cells because of the electrical potential that exists between the positively charged endolymph and the negatively charged cell interior. There is evidence that mechanotransducer rates for such things as ion channel opening and closing speeds may play a role in frequency selectivity. That is, for cells tuned to higher frequencies, these channels open and close faster than for cells that are tuned to low frequencies. It also may be the case that there are more mechanotransducer channels for high-frequency tuned hair bundles than for low-frequency tuned bundles (Fettiplace et al., 2001). Additional information about ion channels and their function will be provided in the following chapter.

SUMMARY

A number of key elements in hair cell mechanics have been introduced in this chapter and will be briefly summarized here. A compression (or condensation) wave results in the hyperpolarization of the cell, which means there is little or no electrical discharge. This happens when the fluid in the cochlea, displaced by the stapes' inward movement, pushes the BM downward. The tectorial membrane is stretched and the cilia are pulled toward the limbus or counterclockwise. The tip-links become slack, which allows the trap doors to close, disallowing any ion flow into the cell. A rarefaction wave results in the opposite function. This type of acoustic wave results in depolarization of the cell, which results in a discharge of electrical impulses. With rarefaction waves, the BM is moved upward because the stapes is moved toward the middle ear and away from the oval window. When this movement pattern occurs, the tectorial membrane that is in contact with the cilia of the OHCs shears the cilia of these cells, and there is a resultant discharge of electrical impulses. The OHCs contract at the peak of the BM deflection and expand at the trough of the downward deflection, resulting in greater BM movement (amplification) and sharpening. This cochlear amplifier works most effectively at low intensities. As intensity increases, the cochlear amplifier plays a lesser role and the cochlear response becomes broader and grows, but with considerable compression—especially at high intensities (Ruggero, 1992).

Cochlear mechanics are affected by changes in the cochlear fluid pressure such as in meniere's disease. This disorder results in increased endolymphatic pressure, with its greatest influence likely at the apical end of the cochlea. This may result in somewhat restricted movement of the BM in this region, which may translate into low-frequency hearing loss—a common finding in meniere's disease.

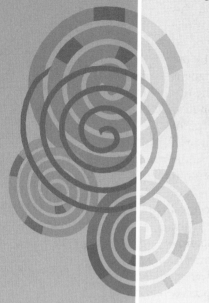

6

Cochlear Physiology II: Mostly Electrophysiology

Contributed by:

Richard J. Salvi, Ph.D., Ann Clock Eddins, Ph.D., and Jian Wang, Ph.D.

Introduction

The preceding chapters have highlighted the basic anatomical features of the inner ear and the pattern of sound-induced mechanical vibration that provides the input to the hair cells, the sensory transducers that convert the sound into a neural response. This chapter will review the electrical events that give rise to hearing. The chapter will focus on (1) the gross cochlear potentials that originate from large groups of cells in the inner ear, (2) the transduction process in the stereocilia bundle and the physiological properties of inner hair cells (IHCs) and outer hair cells (OHCs), (3) the electro-motile response of the OHC body, and (4) spontaneous and sound-evoked otoacoustic emissions generated by the OHCs. To put the electrophysiological processes into perspective, the general organization of the cochlea will be briefly reviewed, with emphasis on the electrochemical nature of the fluid compartments, the morphological features of the stereocilia transduction apparatus, and the motor proteins in the lateral wall of the OHCs.

COCHLEAR ORGANIZATION

Fluid Compartments

The mammalian cochlea is composed of a relatively thin bony shell, or labyrinth, called the otic capsule, which has two openings, the oval and round windows, through which sound energy enters and leaves the cochlea. Inside the bony labyrinth is a membranous labyrinth that consists of three fluid-filled canals that spiral around the central core of the cochlea, referred to as the modiolus. Figure 6.1 shows a cross-section of the cochlea with the three canals: the scala vestibuli, scala tympani, and scala media.

The scala vestibuli begins at the oval window in the base of the cochlea and spirals around the modiolus until it reaches the apex. It is the largest of the canals and is filled with a fluid called perilymph, which is similar in ionic composition to cerebrospinal fluid (i.e., high Na+, low K+). The scala tympani extends from the round window to the apex of the cochlea where it communicates with the scala vestibuli through a small opening called the helicotrema. The scala tympani is also filled with perilymph. Lying between the scala vestibuli and scala tympani is another fluid-filled duct known as

● Figure 6.1

Cross-section of one turn of the cochlea showing the three fluid-filled ducts: scala vestibuli, scala media, and scala tympani (from Geisler, 1998 and Fawcett, 1994).

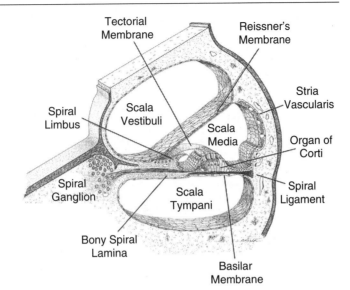

the scala media. The scala media is closed at the apical end of the cochlea but communicates with the vestibular portion of the inner ear at the basal end of the cochlea through the ductus reuniens. The fluid within the scala media is called endolymph and is similar in ion composition to intracellular fluid (i.e., high K^+, low Na^+). The ionic composition of endolymph is such that it gives rise to a positive endocochlear potential that is critical to normal cochlear function.

Cochlear Duct and Organ of Corti

Before discussing the physiological properties of the cochlea, we will review the anatomical structures located within the scala media (Figure 6.2) because they are important for understanding how the cochlea functions. On the modiolar side of the organ of Corti, a bony shelf, referred to as the osseous spiral lamina, extends out from the modiolus and provides structural support to the spiral limbus and supporting cells. Narrow openings in the spiral lamina, called the habenula perforata, provide a passageway for dendrites of the spiral ganglion neurons (type I and type II nerve fibers) to enter the organ of Corti. The spiral limbus, which rests on the top surface of the spiral lamina, provides a point of attachment for Reissner's membrane, which separates the scala tympani from the scala media.

The spiral ligament, spiral prominence, and stria vascularis are located along the lateral wall of the scala media. The spiral prominence is a ridge of tissue that projects into the endolymphatic space and contains capillary loops, fibroblast-like cells similar to those found in the spiral ligament, and dark cells. The spiral ligament, located lateral to the spiral prominence and stria vascularis, is the lateral point of attachment for the basilar membrane. Some spiral ligament cells contain actin and myosin, suggesting that they may apply tension to the basilar membrane (Henson and Henson, 1988). The stria vascularis is a highly vascularized structure with three primary cell layers: marginal cells, intermediate cells, and basal cells. The marginal cells are in direct contact with the endolymphatic space of the scala media and are responsible for secreting K^+ into the endolymph. The cells are joined together by tight junctions, which provide an electrochemical barrier between the endolymph and the intrastrial fluid within the stria vascularis. The basal cells form a

● **Figure 6.2**

The structures within the organ of Corti including the hair cells, supporting cells, tectorial membrane, basilar membrane, Reissner's membrane, and stria vascularis.

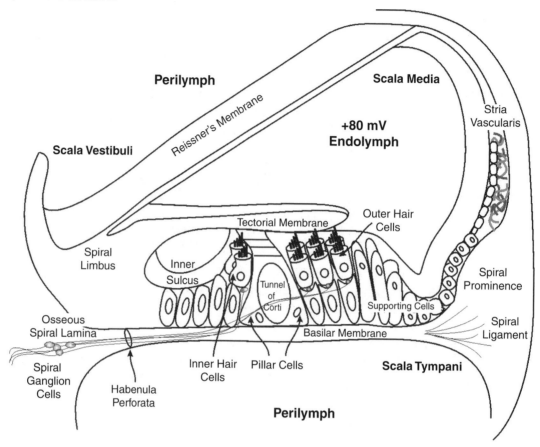

second electrochemical barrier, which communicates by way of gap junctions with intermediate cells on the intrastrial side, and to fibrocytes on the outer spiral ligament side of the stria vascularis (Kikuchi, Kimura, Paul, and Adams, 1995).

The superior boundary of the scala media is formed by Reissner's membrane, which consists of two cell layers. Reissner's membrane extends from the upper edge of the stria vascularis to the medial edge of the spiral limbus. Reissner's membrane is impermeable to large molecules, and there is minimal ATPase in the cells of Reissner's membrane, suggesting that ion transport through the membrane is likely to involve predominantly passive rather than active transport.

The organ of Corti, which contains the sensory cells, rests on the basilar membrane. The basilar membrane, composed of connective and fibrous tissue, stretches radially from the osseous spiral lamina to the spiral ligament. The basilar membrane also extends longitudinally from the base of the cochlea to the apex. The width of the basilar membrane increases from about 150 μm in the base to approximately 450 μm in the apex. The stiffness of the basilar membrane, which influences its mechanical response, decreases from base to apex. The mass and stiffness gradient along the length of the basilar membrane contributes to the overall tonotopic organization of the cochlea.

Sitting on top of the basilar membrane is a collection of supporting cells and sensory cells that make up the organ of Corti. The supporting cells include inner sulcus cells; inner and outer pillar cells; cells of Deiters, Hensen, Claudius, and Boettcher; and outer sulcus cells. The sensory receptor cells include the IHCs and OHCs. Lying just above the sensory and supporting cells is the tectorial membrane, an acellular, fibrous structure that is attached medially at the spiral limbus and extends over the tops of the hair cells. The longest row of OHC stereocilia attach to the underside of the tectorial membrane. The IHC stereocilia, by contrast, appear to be free-standing.

Sensory Hair Cells

● *Gross Features*

The IHCs are flask-shaped and are completely surrounded by supporting cells (Figure 6.3). They contain numerous mitochondria and microtubules. The apex of the cells, made up of a fibrous network of actin, myosin, and fimbrin, form the cuticular plate (Flock, Bretscher, and Weber, 1982; Slepecky and Chamberlain, 1982). Stereocilia, which emerge in rows from the apical surfaces of the IHCs, form a gently curving arc (Figure 6.4). The stereocilia rows are arranged in a staircase pattern: the tallest row of stereocilia faces the lateral wall and shortest faces the modiolus. Approximately 20 type I spiral ganglion neurons make one-to-one synaptic contact at the base of each IHC. Lateral olivocochlear efferent fibers make synaptic contact with the type I afferent fibers that are located beneath the IHCs.

The OHCs are cylindrically shaped; the base of each OHC rests in the cup of a Deiters' cell (Figure 6.3). The phalangeal process of the Deiters' cell extends toward the surface of the organ of Corti where it makes contact with the apical pole of the OHC. Importantly, the lateral wall of the OHC is surrounded almost entirely by fluid, thereby allowing this region to move without interference from its neighbors.

● Figure 6.3

The main morphological features of an IHC and an OHC.

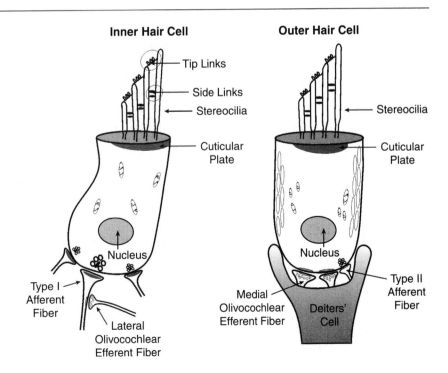

● Figure 6.4

Scanning electron micrograph showing the stereocilia bundles on the three rows of OHCs and the single row of IHCs (courtesy of D. Ding).

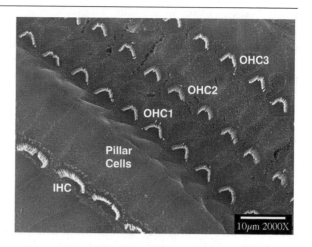

The OHC lateral wall is characterized by lateral **cisternae** made up of smooth endoplasmic reticulum. A cortical lattice adjacent to the cisternae is made up of a series of circumferential filaments that impart radial rigidity but permit longitudinal movement (Holley and Ashmore, 1988). The rows of stereocilia on the OHCs are arranged in a "W" pattern (Figure 6.4); the stereocilia are graduated in height, with the tallest row of stereocilia facing the lateral wall of the cochlea. Medial olivocochlear efferent neurons and type II spiral ganglion neurons synapse on the basal pole of the OHCs.

● *Stereocilia Tip-Links and Side-Links*

The stereocilia maintain a constant thickness along most of their length but taper to a narrow shaft as they enter the cuticular plate; this creates a point where the stereocilia can pivot when they are deflected (Figure 6.3). The cilia are composed of actin filaments, which impart rigidity to the stereocilia. Two types of filaments form lateral cross links within and between the rows of stereocilia. The cross-links hold the stereocilia together, causing the bundle to move in unison when a mechanical force is applied to the bundle. A thin filament, the so-called tip-link, courses from the shaft of one stereocilium to the tip of the shorter stereocilium in the next shorter row. As the stereocilia bundle is deflected in the direction of the tallest row of stereocilia, tension increases in the tip-link; this in turn pulls open the mechanically gated ion channels located near the tip of the cilia (Hudspeth, 1982).

Stria Vascularis: Ion Pumps and Potassium Recycling

The stria vascularis plays a critical role in maintaining the ionic composition of the endolymph and the endocochlear potential. The electrical potential and ionic composition of endolymph is maintained by several different ion transport mechanisms that recycle potassium from the endolymph through the sensory hair cells, the fibrocytes in the spiral ligament, the cells of the stria vascularis, and back into the endolymph. Figure 6.5 illustrates the flow and transport of various ions through the cochlea. When the stereocilia are deflected, K^+ in the endolymph flows through the hair cells into perilymph, through the spiral ligament and stria vascularis, and then back

The flow of potassium ions from the scala media back into the stria vascularis via the basilar membrane and spiral ligament, and via Reissner's membrane.

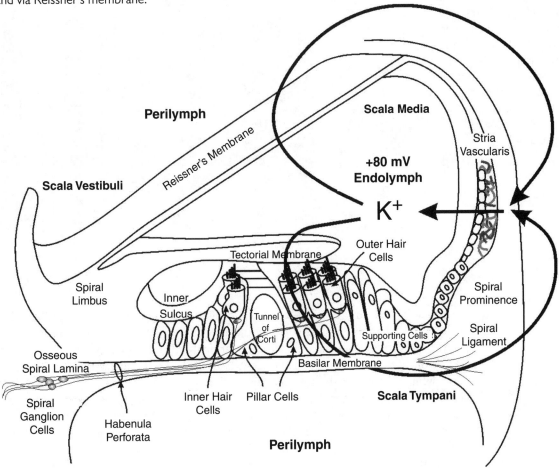

into the endolymph. Ions also flow from the endolymph to the stria vascularis through the outer sulcus cells and through Reissner's membrane (Spicer and Schulte, 1996). A more detailed view of how K^+ is cycled through the spiral ligament and stria vascularis and into the scala media is illustrated in Figure 6.6. Within the stria vascularis, four ion transport mechanisms have been identified for maintaining the high K^+ concentration in the endolymph. The first mechanism involves a selective K^+ channel, located on the apical membrane of the marginal cells, which releases K^+ into the endolymph. The membrane potential across the apical surface of the marginal cells is about 0 to 10 mV, and the activation and deactivation of K^+ is relatively slow (Marcus, Sunose, Liu, Bennett, Shen, Scofield, and Ryan, 1998). If the proteins forming this channel are abnormal, as in certain mutant mice (Casimiro, Knollmann, Ebert, Vary, Greene, Franz, Grinberg, Huang, and Pfeifer, 2001; Lee et al., 2000; Letts, Valenzuela, Dunbar, Zheng, Johnson, and Frankel, 2000), it can impair the flow of K^+ into the endolymph, resulting in a hearing loss. A second transport mechanism involves the electrogenic Na^+/K^+-ATPase pump located in the basolateral membrane of the marginal cells. During one cycle of adenosine tri-phosphate hydrolysis, the marginal cell takes up two K^+ ions, and three Na^+ ions are extruded into the intrastrial fluid. A third mechanism involves the $Na^+/2Cl^-/K^+$ cotransporter that contributes to the uptake

The main ion transport mechanisms in the lateral wall of the cochlea. Four main mechanisms include (1) transport from fibrocytes of the spiral ligament and basal cells of the stria vascularis, (2) transport from intermediate cells to the intrastrial space, (3) transport across the basal surface of marginal cells, and (4) transport across the apical surface of marginal cells into the scala media.

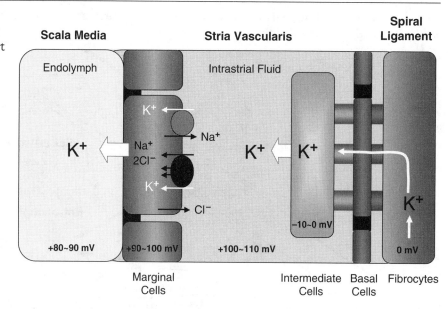

of an additional three K^+ ions from the intrastrial space as well as Na^+ and Cl^-. Finally, a Cl^- channel, also located in the basolateral membrane of marginal cells, contributes to the flow of Cl^- from the marginal cells into the intrastrial space. As a result of these mechanisms, the concentration of K^+ in the intrastrial space is quite low, while that inside the intermediate cells is quite high. Although the marginal cells are responsible for the movement of K^+ from the intrastrial space to the endolymph, it is the large potential difference between the intrastrial fluid and the cytosol of the intermediate cells that is now thought to be responsible for the +80-mV endocochlear potential (Wangemann, 2002a). The +80-mV endocochlear potential and high potassium ion concentration play critical roles in hair cell transduction.

Hair Cell Transduction

● *Receptor Potential*

Sound-induced mechanical vibrations of the cochlear partition are converted into electrical activity through a process referred to as transduction. The mechanically gated transduction channels located near the tip of the stereocilia on OHCs and IHCs are responsible for converting sound into neural activity, as illustrated in Figure 6.7. Movement of the basilar membrane results in radial shear between the tectorial membrane and the apical surface of the organ of Corti. Since the tallest stereocilia on the OHCs are embedded in the tectorial membrane, the radial shear force is coupled directly to the stereocilia. The stereocilia on the IHCs are free-standing; therefore, the stereocilia are deflected by viscous fluid drag of the endolymph. When the bundle is deflected toward the tallest stereocilia, tension is applied to the tip-links, which in turn pulls the mechanically gated channel open. The opening of the channel allows ions in the endolymph to flow into the hair cell, leading to **depolarization.** Because of the high concentration of potassium in the endolymph, the predominant ion that flows into the hair cell is K^+. The opening and closing of the mechanically gated

● Figure 6.7

The connection between the tip-links
and the mechanically gated ion channels.
Deflection of the stereocilia bundle toward
the tallest stereocilium creates tension
on the mechanically gated channel that results
in the opening of the channel, allowing
potassium ions to flow into the hair cell.

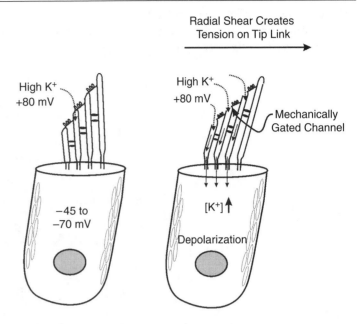

channels generates a transduction current that changes the intracellular potential and produces the receptor potential.

● Davis Battery Theory

The Davis model provides a general framework for understanding how the hair cells are activated by sound-induced mechanical movements of the basilar membrane. As shown in Figure 6.8, the stria vascularis along the lateral wall of the cochlea produces a DC potential of approximately +80 mV in the endolymphatic space. At rest, the inside of the hair cell sits at −70 mV. Thus, the total voltage drop across the apical pole of the hair cell is on the order of 150 mV. The large voltage gradient and the high concentration of potassium in the scala media are the main forces that drive K^+ ions into the hair cells. Davis correctly predicted that sound-induced movement of the basilar membrane modulated a variable resistance located across the apical membrane of the hair cell (Hallpike and Rawdon-Smith, 1937; Davis, 1965). The variable resistance is now recognized as the opening and closing of the mechanically gated ion channels in the stereocilia (Hudspeth, 1982, 1985; Hudspeth and Corey, 1977; Hudspeth and Jacobs, 1979; Roberts, Howard, and Hudspeth, 1988).

● Excitation and Inhibition

Deflection of the stereocilia bundle toward the tallest stereocilia increases the number of transduction channels that are open and results in depolarization of the hair cell (Figure 6.9). Deflection of the stereocilia bundle toward the shortest stereocilia increases the number of transduction channels that are closed and results in hyperpolarization of the hair cell. The receptor potentials generated by IHCs and OHCs play fundamentally different roles in cochlear function. Depolarization of an IHC results in the release of neurotransmitter and excitation of auditory nerve fibers that contact the base of the IHC. Conversely, hyperpolarization of the IHC decreases the release of neurotransmitter from the hair cell and leads to a decreased frequency of firing of auditory nerve fibers. Activation of the OHC leads to a

● Figure 6.8

The main components of the Davis battery model of the cochlea including the stria vascularis as the primary energy source, the basilar membrane, Reissner's membrane, the spiral limbus, and the spiral ligament as sources of fixed resistance and the hair cells as sources of variable resistance.

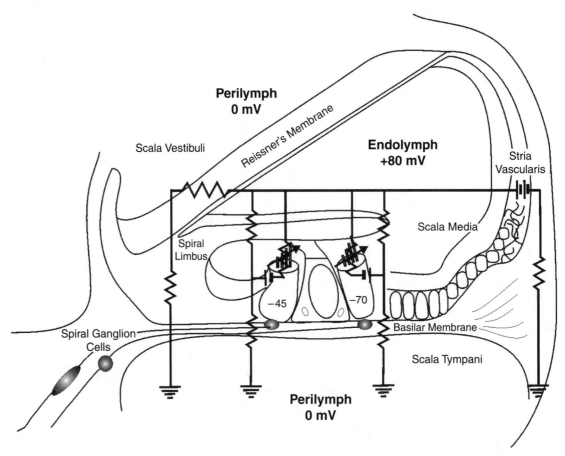

fundamentally different type of response, namely electrically induced motion along the longitudinal axis of the OHC as discussed below. The electromotile response represents a source of frequency-tuned energy that is transmitted back into the cochlea to enhance the sound-induced movements of the basilar membrane.

● Location of Transduction Channels

The mechanically gated **ion channels** are believed to be located near the tips of the stereocilia. Electrophysiological evidence supporting this view comes from experiments in which the stereocilia bundle of hair cells were displaced from their resting position toward the tallest stereocilia and then back to the resting position. During the step-displacement (Figure 6.10), the extracellular voltage was measured at different locations along the side and top of the stereocilia bundle (Hudspeth, 1982). Displacement of the bundle produced a voltage step that increased in size as the electrode was moved from the base toward the tip of the stereocilia bundle. The largest voltage steps occurred when the electrode was located near the tips of the stereocilia in the middle of the bundle. This suggests that the transduction channels are located near the tips of the stereocilia (Russell and Sellick, 1978; Howard, Roberts, and Hudspeth, 1988).

● Figure 6.9

Schematic illustrating how the deflection of the stereocilia bundle depolarizes or hyperpolarizes an IHC. Depolarization leads to the release of neurotransmitter, most likely glutamate, which depolarizes the afferent terminal of the auditory nerve fibers attached to base of the IHC. Depolarization of the afferent terminal leads to an increase in spike rate in auditory nerve fibers. Hyperpolarization of the IHC reduces the spontaneous release of neurotransmitter and causes a decrease in spike rate in the auditory nerve.

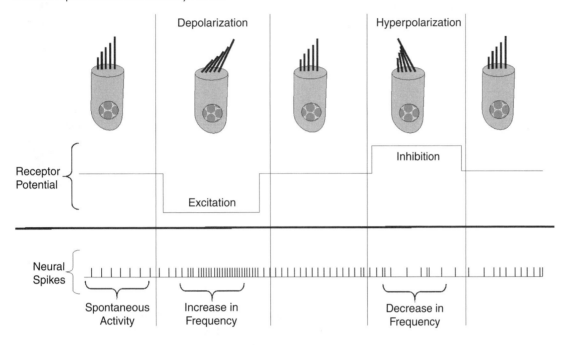

● *Transduction Kinetics*

To faithfully reproduce high-frequency acoustic signals, the kinetics of the transduction channels must be extremely fast. Measurements of the gating current in response to mechanical steps of hair bundle deflection indicate that the response is extremely rapid, consistent with the notion those mechanical links directly gate the channels. The mechanical links, termed "gating springs" (Corey and Hudspeth, 1983; Crawford, Evans, and Fettiplace, 1989), may correspond to the thin tip-links that attach along the side of the taller stereocilia and project to the tip of the shorter, adjacent stereocilia (Figure 6.11) (Pickles, Comis, and Osborne, 1984; Osborne, Comis, and Pickles, 1988; Pickles and Corey, 1992). The mechanically gated channels operate in synchrony because the stereocilia in different rows are coupled together by side links (Figure 6.11). Consequently, if the tallest stereocilia in the bundle is deflected, the entire bundle moves in unison (Pickles et al., 1984; Pickles and Corey, 1992).

Channel Selectivity

To determine which ions passed through the transducer channel, the ionic solution bathing the stereocilia bundle was varied (Corey and Hudspeth, 1979). Sodium, potassium, and other alkali cations

● Figure 6.10

The amplitude of the voltage change detected by an electrode at different locations around the stereocilia bundle as the bundle is displaced toward the tallest stereocilia. Voltage steps are largest when the electrode is placed near the tips of the stereocilia bundle and smallest near the base of the stereocilia (from Hudspeth, 1982, with permission).

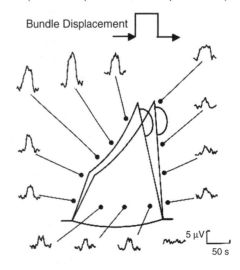

● Figure 6.11

Transmission electron micrograph showing the location of the cross-links (cross-hatched arrow) connecting adjacent stereocilia in the bundle and the tip-link (thin black arrow) that connects the side of the taller stereocilium to the tip of the next shorter stereocilium. Specimen stained with ruthenium red to visual the cell coat on the membrane (white arrow). The mechanically gated channel is presumably located at the tip of the stereocilium in the darkly stained region (courtesy of R. Hamernik).

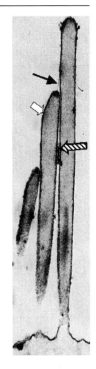

such as lithium pass through the channel with similar permeability while the divalent cation, calcium, was less permeable (Corey and Hudspeth, 1979). Tetramethylammonium, which has a diameter of 0.54 nm, passes through the transduction channel with somewhat lower permeability, suggesting that the diameter of the channel is equal to or slightly greater than this size. Although the mechanically gated channel shows approximately equal permeability to alkali cations, the dominant charge carrier of the transducer current in vivo is potassium because of its extremely high concentration in endolymph.

Studies of nonmammalian hair cells, such as those from the frog, turtle, and chick, have provided the most complete descriptions of the hair cell transduction process (Figure 6.9) (Hudspeth and Jacobs, 1979; Fuchs and Mann, 1985; Hudspeth, 1986). In vertebrate hair cells, the influx of K^+ initiates depolarization of the cell, which then leads to the opening of Ca^{2+} channels in the basolateral membrane (Lewis and Hudspeth, 1983). The influx of Ca^{2+} leads to the activation of Ca^{2+}-activated K^+ channels, allowing the outward flow of K^+, which repolarizes the hair cell. Increased intracellular Ca^{2+} promotes the release of neurotransmitters from the base of the hair cell.

● *Neurotransmitters*

It is generally accepted that the IHCs are the main sensory cells involved in transduction, whereas OHCs are considered to be modulators of transduction through mechanical processes. As such, one primary role of the IHCs is to release a neurotransmitter that diffuses across the synaptic cleft, activates receptors on the postsynaptic membrane of afferent nerve fibers, and depolarizes the fibers enough to generate action potentials. There is sufficient evidence to indicate that the afferent excitatory transmitter released by IHCs is the amino acid, **glutamate**. It is still uncertain what afferent transmitter(s) is released by OHCs. The major inhibitory neurotransmitter in the organ of Corti that is released by medial efferent neurons is acetylcholine (Ach). Other efferent neurotransmitters believed to be present in the inner ear include dopamine (lateral efferent neurons), gamma aminobutyric acid (GABA), substance P, enkephalins, and dynorphins (Altschuler, Hoffman, and Wenthold, 1986; Fex and Altschuler, 1986; Eybalin, 1993; Eybalin, Charachon, and Renard, 1993). The release and uptake of these neurotransmitters is responsible for initiating and modulating the physiologic response of auditory nerve fibers and hair cells and the eventual transmission of electrical signals from the cochlea to the central auditory pathway.

GROSS COCHLEAR POTENTIALS

Endocochlear Potential

Much of our current understanding of cochlear function is based on intracellular and extracellular measures of electrical activity generated in the cochlea. The voltage gradients in different fluid-filled compartments can be assessed by passing an electrode from the scala tympani through the organ of Corti and into the scala media (Figure 6.12). As noted above, a large +80-mV **endocochlear potential**

● **Figure 6.12**

The upper portion of figure shows the penetration of a microelectrode from the scala tympani, through the organ or Corti, into the scala media and finally into the scala vestibuli. Letters indicate the location of the electrode: (a) scala tympani, (b) organ of Corti, (c) OHC or IHC, (d) scala media, and (e) scala vestiibuli. (From Salvi, McFadden, and Wang, 2000, with permission).

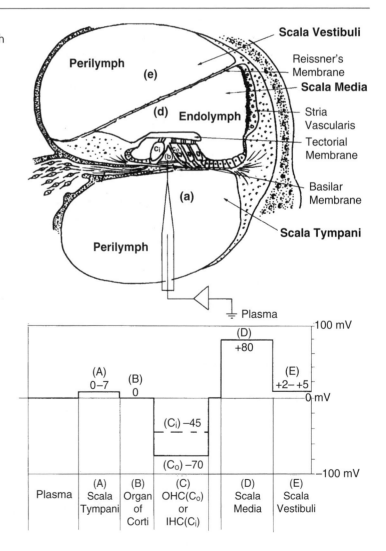

is recorded when the electrode is in the scala media. The endocochlear potential is the main driving force that is responsible for moving positively charged ions through the transduction channels of the hair cell stereocilia. Evidence from normal and impaired cochleae has demonstrated that the endocochlear potential is generated by active metabolic processes in cells within the stria vascularis. Specifically, the endocochlear potential is thought to be a product of the high K^+ concentration inside the intermediate cells relative to the stria and the low K^+ concentration in the intrastrial fluid space outside of those cells (Wangemann, 2002a,b). The important role of intermediate cells in the generation of the endocochlear potential has been demonstrated in a number of ways. For example, mutant mice that lack intermediate cells lack an endocochlear potential (Carlisle, Steel, and Forge, 1990; Cable, Barkway, and Steel, 1992; Cable, Huszar, Jaenisch, and Steel, 1994; Schulte and Steel, 1994). The endocochlear potential is also reduced in experimental animals treated with drugs that block the KCNJ10 K^+ channel, localized to the intermediate cells, or knockout mice lacking the gene that codes for the KCNJ10 K^+ channel (Ando and Takeuchi, 1999; Marcus, Wu, Wangemann, and Kofuji, 2002; Rozengurt, Lopez, Chiu, Kofuji, Lester, and Neusch, 2003).

Cochlear Microphonic Potential

When an acoustic stimulus is presented, it evokes a change in the electrical current flowing through the hair cells. The three sound-evoked cochlear potentials are the **cochlear microphonic (CM),** the **summating potential (SP)**, and the **compound action potential (CAP)** (Figure 6.13). These three potentials can be measured in the fluid-filled spaces of the cochlea, or at locations outside, but near, the cochlea (e.g., round window, cochlear promontory).

The CM represents the vector summation of the individual responses from a large number of hair cells distributed along the basilar membrane. The CM is an alternating current (AC) whose frequency response mimics that of the stimulus. Wever and Bray (1930) were the first to demonstrate that acoustic signals could be transduced into electrical signals that mirrored the stimulus waveform, much like a microphone. Because these original recordings were made from an electrode placed on the auditory nerve, the CM was originally assumed to represent electrical potentials produced by the auditory nerve. Destruction of the auditory nerve, however, has no effect on CM amplitude (Zheng, Ding, McFadden, and Henderson, 1997).

● **Figure 6.13**

The gross evoked potentials recorded from the cochlea. The compound action potential (CAP) consists of two negative deflections (N1, N2) and occurs at the onset of the signal. The cochlear microphonic (CM) is an AC response that mimics the waveform of the tonal signal, and the summating potential (SP) is a DC response that follows the envelope of the signal.

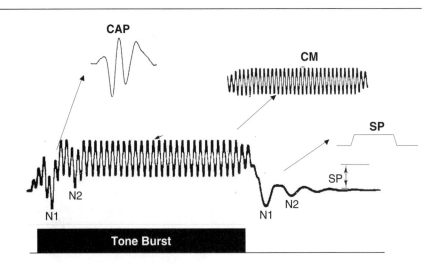

Moreover, when an electrode is passed through the hair cells of the organ of Corti into scala media, the CM increases in amplitude and reverses polarity (Tasaki, Davis, and Eldredge, 1954). It is now recognized that the CM is a reflection of receptor currents flowing through the hair cells (Dallos, Billone, Durrant, Wang, and Raynor, 1972; Dallos and Cheatham, 1976). The CM is predominantly generated by the OHCs, consistent with the fact that there are roughly three times as many OHCs as IHCs; however, the IHCs also make a small contribution to the generation of the CM.

Figure 6.14 illustrates the relationship between the logarithm of CM amplitude and dB of signal intensity recorded in the base of a normal cochlea. For a given stimulus frequency, the CM amplitude increases linearly as intensity increases from low to moderate levels but then it saturates and often decreases at higher levels (Dallos, 1973). The nonlinear nature of the CM input/output function may be due in part to the nonlinear mechanical response of the cochlea. The spatial distribution of the CM along the length of the cochlear duct also reflects the basilar membrane vibration pattern. Figure 6.15 shows the magnitude of the CM as a function of frequency in the basal turn (T1), middle turn (T2), and apical turn (T3) of the cochlea. Low-frequency stimuli are capable of generating a CM response in all three turns, consistent with the basilar membrane vibration pattern. In contrast, high-frequency stimuli generate a CM response only in the basal end of the cochlea, consistent with the fact that high-frequency stimuli activate the basal but not the apical or middle turns of the cochlea.

● **Figure 6.14**

The logarithm of CM amplitude as a function of stimulus intensity. The response amplitude grows linearly over low to moderate level signals but saturates at high levels.

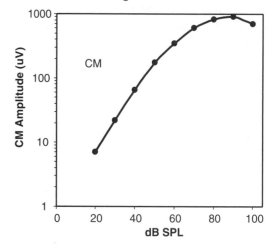

Summating Potential

As shown in Figure 6.13, acoustic stimuli also evoke a DC shift in the extracellular response that is referred to as the SP; the response generally follows the envelope of

● **Figure 6.15**

CM amplitude as a function of stimulus frequency for recordings made in apical turn 3 (T3), middle turn 2 (T2), and basal turn 1 (T1) of the cochlea. The CM recorded from basal turn 1 is smaller in amplitude but can be measured in response to a broad range of frequencies. The CM recorded from apical turn 3 is larger in amplitude but is measured only in response to a range of low frequencies.

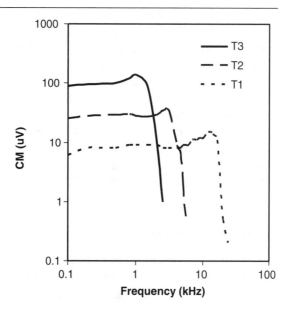

● **Figure 6.16**

CM amplitude and SP amplitude as a function of frequency obtained from differential electrode recording techniques using electrodes in the scala tympani (ST) and scala vestibuli (SV). The CM is a broadly tuned response that drops off rapidly above 1 kHz. The SP is more narrowly tuned, with a negative polarity near CF, but reverses polarity as the signal moves above or below CF (~0.5 to 1 kHz).

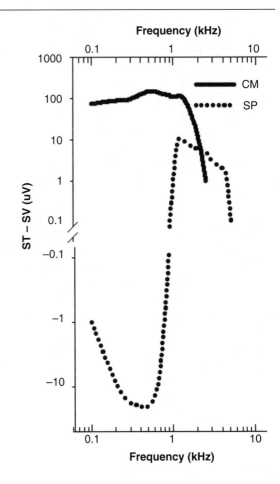

the stimulus. Like the CM, the SP can be measured from electrodes placed inside the cochlea or from locations outside the cochlear, such as the round window, cochlear promontory, or ear canal. The polarity and the magnitude of the SP are affected by the parameters of the evoking stimulus as well as the recording location. When the SP is recorded from an electrode in the scala media or differentially between electrodes in the scala tympani and scala vestibuli (Figure 6.16), the polarity of the SP is negative at the characteristic frequency (CF) of the recording site but reverses polarity in response to lower or higher frequencies (Dallos, 1973). The CM frequency response curve, on the other hand, is quite broad. Accordingly, the SP provides a better estimate of the frequency tuning of the basilar membrane than does the CM.

The source of the SP is not entirely clear. However, recent lesion studies indicate that selective destruction of all the IHCs substantially decreases the SP (Figure 6.17). SP amplitude is further reduced by the additional loss of OHCs (Zheng et al., 1997; Durrant, Wang, Ding, and Salvi, 1998). These data suggest that while both IHCs and OHCs contribute to the generation of the SP, the IHCs make the dominant contribution at low and moderate intensities.

Compound Action Potential

The **compound action potential (CAP)** originates from the spiral ganglion neurons that give rise to the auditory nerve's physiological response. Similar to the CM and SP, the CAP can be measured from an electrode placed in or near the cochlea.

● **Figure 6.17**

The SP input/output function obtained from normal animals, animals with selective IHC loss, and animals with IHC loss plus OHC loss. Ordinate plotted on logarithmic scale. IHC loss has the greatest effect on SP amplitude at low to moderate signal levels, whereas the addition of OHC loss contributes to greater reduction for higher-level signals.

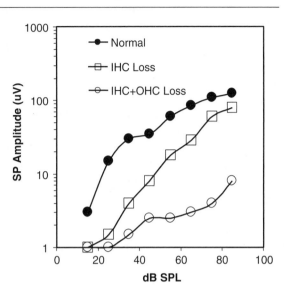

The CAP is an onset response that arises from the synchronous response of a group of auditory nerve fibers. The CAP waveform illustrated in Figure 6.18a consists of two prominent negative peaks; N1 occurs with a latency of approximately 1.0 ms and N2, at about 2.0 ms in response to moderate-to-high-level stimuli. Like the CM and SP, the CAP is a graded potential whose amplitude increases with increasing signal level as shown in the intensity series in Figure 6.18b. In addition to changes in amplitude, the latency of the peaks decreases systematically with increasing intensity.

The threshold of the CAP is the lowest stimulus level at which a reliable CAP response can be detected visually. In most cases, the CAP threshold is 10 to 20 dB above the behavioral threshold in experimental animals (Dallos, 1975) as well as in humans (Eggermont and Odenthal, 1974). Because of this close correlation, the CAP is a valuable clinical tool that can be used to estimate changes in hearing threshold

● **Figure 6.18**

(a) CAP recording showing the N1 and N2 peaks. (b) CAP intensity series showing the increase in CAP amplitude and the decrease in N1 and N2 latency with increasing sound intensity.

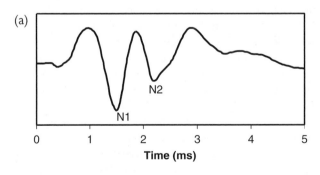

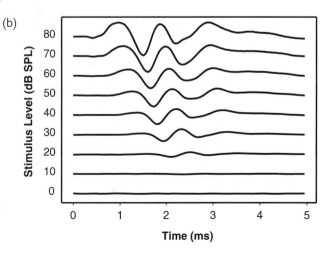

● **Figure 6.19**

CAP input/output functions in normal animals and animals with partial IHC loss or OHC loss. IHC loss produces little change in CAP threshold but decreases amplitude at moderate to high levels. OHC loss produces a large shift in threshold but only a small reduction in amplitude at high levels.

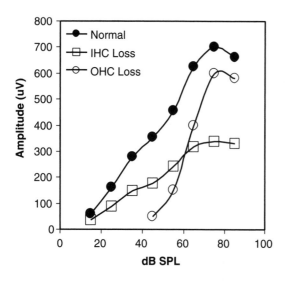

following cochlear damage. Figure 6.19 is a schematic of the CAP input/output functions from control animals and from experimental animals with selective damage to IHCs or OHCs. IHC loss reduces the amplitude of the CAP by a constant proportion, leading to a decrease in the slope of the input/output function. There is only a small change in CAP threshold (Trautwein, Hofstetter, Wang, Salvi, and Nostrant, 1996; Wang, Powers, Hofstetter, Trautwein, Ding, and Salvi, 1997). Selective destruction of the OHCs, on the other hand, causes a shift in the CAP threshold, but once the threshold is exceeded, the CAP amplitude increases rapidly so that there is only a modest reduction in amplitude at high intensities (Ozdamar and Dallos, 1976).

Clinically, the stimulus-evoked cochlear potentials recorded with either ear canal or transtympanic electrodes can play an important role in diagnosing such disorders as meniere's disease and auditory neuropathy. Meniere's disease, for example, is a progressive inner ear disorder with symptoms such as vertigo, tinnitus, and fluctuating sensorineural hearing loss. Although the pathophysiology is not entirely understood, a well-documented sign of meniere's disease is an abnormally large SP/AP amplitude ratio in response to click stimuli, as well as an enhanced SP amplitude to tone burst stimuli (Ferraro, Blackwell, Mediavilla, and Thedinger, 1994a; Ferraro, Thedinger, Mediavilla, and Blackwell, 1994b).

CLINICAL CORRELATE

Electrocochleography (Ecog) is a way in which the CM, SP, and AP can all be recorded (see Durrant and Ferraro, 1999 for review). This procedure has been and is used clinically. In the normal human auditory system, the CM is the earliest and smallest electrical response. This is followed in time by the SP and then the AP, which is larger in amplitude than the SP (Figure 6.20a).

The Ecog can be recorded in three main ways: (1) by placing an electrode in the ear canal (tiptrode), (2) by positioning the electrode on the tympanic membrane (TM electrode), or (3) by inserting a needle through the TM to the promontory (transtympanic electrode). Obviously, the closer the electrode is to the cochlea, the larger the response will be. However, the morphology remains quite similar regardless of recording site. Although the morphology remains consistent across recording sites, the smaller Ecog responses are more likely to be affected by noise, which may seriously affect their identification.

When a canal electrode is used, it is relatively easy to also record the auditory brainstem response (ABR)

(Figure 6.20b). An ABR cannot be observed with a transtympanic recording because the Ecog response is so large that the display gain on the instrument must be decreased to the point that the ABR tracing is too small to be seen.

Both clicks and tones are used as stimuli for Ecog. Clicks are recorded as two or three negative and positive deflections before the SP, and the SP often appears as a shoulder of the AP or wave I (of the ABR). Using a tone burst, the CM looks like the stimulus, whereas the SP consists of a baseline shift (usually negative) on which the CM is superimposed. At times the CM can be confused with the AP. Use of an alternating polarity click can help identify the AP, as this recording procedure cancels the CM waveform, leaving only the SP and AP (Figure 6.20c).

Currently, the main clinical use of Ecog is helping in the diagnosis of meniere's disease. It is also used in differentiating cochlear from retrocochlear problems, estimating hearing threshold, and enhancing wave I of the ABR when needed. The diagnosis of meniere's disease

(continued)

● Figure 6.20

(a) An example of a transtympanic ECog that has been smoothed to show the components. In this example the SP/AP ratio is about 40%. (b) An ABR recording made on a patient with a tympanic membrane electrode. This permitted the ABR to be recorded but also greatly enhanced the amplitude of the summating and action potential. In this example the SP/AP ratio is about 20% for the top tracing and almost 30% for the bottom tracing. (c) A transtympanic ECog from a patient with meniere's symptoms. The SP/AP ratio is slightly over 50% for each tracing. All the recordings were made with an insert phone signal delivery system and hence a 0.9 msec delay. CM = cochlear microphonic, SP = summating potential, AP = action potential (or wave I) (courtesy of Frank Musiek, University of Connecticut).

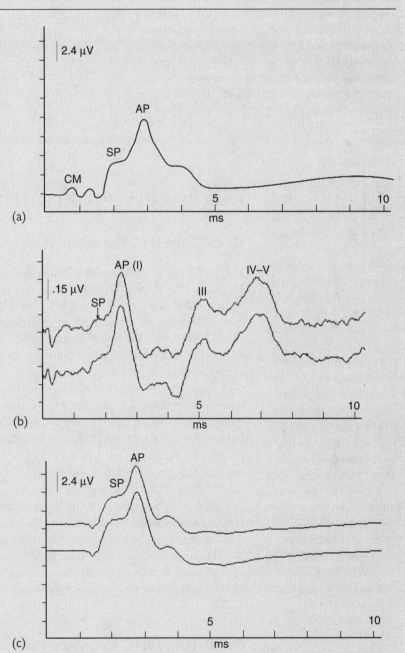

is often made when the SP is enlarged—yielding an SP/AP ratio that is abnormal (Figure 6.20c,d). The criteria for abnormality are not universally agreed upon, with some advocating SP/AP of 0.4 or greater, whereas others use 0.5 or greater. The sensitivity of Ecog for meniere's disease is marginal. This could be related to the less than clear categorization of meniere's disease as well as to the time when the patient with meniere's disease is tested. If the patient is asymptomatic at the time of testing, the SP/AP would likely be normal; however, if the patient is symptomatic, it is likely the SP/AP ratio would be abnormal (Ferraro, Arenburg, and Hassanein, 1985). In this case, specificity of the Ecog is high.

(continued)

In differentiating cochlear from retrocochlear involvement, especially in the diagnosis of auditory neuropathy, recording the CM is most helpful. In auditory neuropathy, the CM should be present (indicating an intact OHC) and the AP absent (see Chapter 7). The Ecog can be used to estimate hearing threshold, but with the popularity of ABR and OAEs, it is not often used in this capacity.

Wave I amplitude of the ABR can be enhanced by using Ecog recordings. This can help in the interpretation of the ABR for diagnostic purposes when wave I is either absent or unclear. The identification of wave I allows the use of interwave interval measurements, which would not be possible if wave I cannot be identified within the ABR waveform recorded. ●

CLINICAL CORRELATE

Auditory neuropathy, which is a relatively newly defined disorder with an uncertain pathophysiology, also presents with a range of unique symptoms that can include moderate hearing loss and severely impaired speech understanding. Interestingly, one of the diagnostic indicators of auditory neuropathy is the presence of a normal CM, suggesting normal OHC function, and an abnormal or absent CAP and ABR, suggesting pathology associated with the neural elements originating in the cochlea (El-Badry, 2003; Starr, Picton, Sininger, Hood, and Berlin, 1996). ●

HAIR CELL RECEPTOR POTENTIALS

Basal Turn IHC Receptor Potential

Using sharp microelectrodes with tip diameters less than 1 μm, it is possible to penetrate the IHCs or OHCs and record their responses (Russell and Sellick, 1977; Sellick and Russell, 1978). In quiet, the IHC resting membrane potential is typically in the range of −40 to 50 mV, while the OHC resting potential is generally around −70 mV (Cody and Russell, 1987). Figure 6.21 shows the typical response of an IHC as a function of stimulus frequency. The 300-Hz tone burst produces a predominantly AC response that depolarizes and hyperpolarizes around the resting potential. The AC response to low-frequency tones is asymmetrical, with the depolarizing phase being significantly larger than the hyperpolarizing phase. The asymmetry results in an AC response that rides upon a DC depolarization. As the frequency rises above 1000 Hz, the amplitude of the AC response declines and it is greatly attenuated above 3 to 4 kHz. The decline in the AC response with increasing frequency is due to the capacitance of the cell's membrane that forms a low-pass filter that attenuates the high frequencies.

The AC component of the receptor potential resembles the CM recorded in the extracellular fluid; however, the CM response can be recorded at much higher frequencies than the intracellular AC response. The intracellular DC component of the IHC resembles the SP; however, a major difference between the two is that the SP can shift from positive to negative polarity, whereas the DC intracellular response is predominantly depolarizing.

Basal Turn OHC Receptor Potential

AC and DC responses can also be recorded from OHCs; however, the responses tend to be smaller than in IHCs (Cody and Russell, 1992). In addition, the electrophysiological properties of OHCs appear to vary from base to apex of the cochlea. Figure 6.22 compares the responses of an OHC to an IHC in the base of the cochlea. The stimulus was either a 600-Hz tone burst at 68 dB SPL (sound pressure level) (top row) or an 18,000-Hz tone burst at 78 dB SPL (bottom row). Both the IHC and OHC produce an AC response to the 600-Hz tone; however, the OHC response is smaller and predominantly hyperpolarizing (Figure 6.22a), whereas the IHC response is predominantly depolarizing (Figure 6.22b). The characteristics of the OHC's AC response are level dependent. AC responses are symmetrical

● Figure 6.21

Intracellular response from an IHC in the base of the cochlea in response to an 80 dB SPL tone. Frequency varied from 300 to 5000 Hz (frequency shown on right side of each trace). AC and DC components are labeled in the 2000-Hz trace. The dashed line on the left side of the 300-Hz trace shows the resting potential. Note that the response to the 300-Hz tone is asymmetric, with a larger response in the depolarizing than hyperpolarizing direction. AC and DC responses are evident from the 300-Hz trace to the 2000-Hz trace. Note that AC response is nearly absent in the 5000-Hz trace (from Palmer and Russell, 1986, with permission).

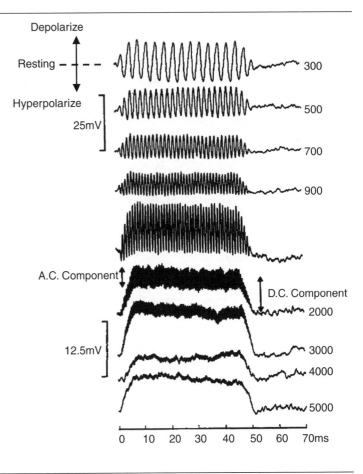

● Figure 6.22

Responses of an IHC and an OHC in the base of the cochlea to a low-frequency tone (upper row) and a high-frequency tone (lower row). The IHC response (a) to a low-frequency tone is highly asymmetric in the depolarizing direction, whereas the OHC response (b) is asymmetric in the hyperpolarizing direction. The IHC response (c) to a high-frequency stimulus shows large depolarizing response, whereas the OHC shows little or no DC response (d) (modified from Cody and Russell, 1992, with permission).

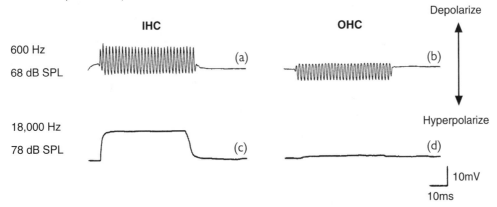

at low levels, predominantly hyperpolarizing at moderate levels (68 dB SPL, Figure 6.22b), and depolarizing at high levels. OHCs and IHCs produce little or no AC response to the 18,000-Hz tone (Figure 6.22c,d). However, the IHC produces a large DC depolarization response (Figure 6.22c), whereas the OHC produces only a small depolarization (Figure 6.22d).

Apical Turn IHCs and OHCs

The responses of IHCs and OHCs in the apex of the cochlea are illustrated in Figure 6.23. The panel on the left shows the amplitude of the AC and DC receptor potential from an IHC and those on the right show the AC and DC responses from an OHC. At moderate stimulus intensities, both the IHC and OHC show maximum responses around 800 to 900 Hz; however, the responses drop off rapidly at frequencies above and below the best frequency (BF), resulting in a sharply tuned response. The tuning bandwidths are similar for OHCs and IHCs.

The DC receptor potential from apical turn OHCs differs from basal turn OHCs in two respects. First, at low to moderate intensities, apical turn OHCs show a pronounced depolarization around BF and a hyperpolarizing response below BF (Figure 6.23, right panel); the hyperpolarizing response below BF does not occur in basal turn OHCs (Figure 6.22d). Second, apical turn OHCs show a pronounced DC depolarizing response at BF, unlike basal turn OHCs, which produce a weak depolarizing response at high intensities.

Hair Cell Tuning

What is the relationship between the tuning of IHCs and OHCs, and how does hair cell tuning compare with mechanical tuning of the basilar membrane? Figure 6.24 shows the tuning curves for an IHC and an OHC in the base of the cochlea. The

● Figure 6.23

AC and DC receptor potential from an IHC (left) and OHC (right) in the apical turn of the cochlea (from Dallos, 1986, with permission).

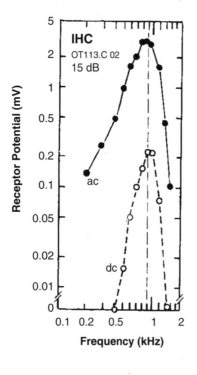
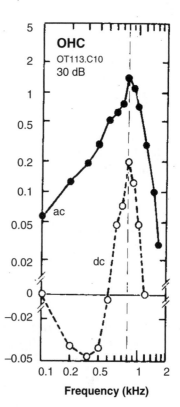

● Figure 6.24

IHC and OHC receptor potential tuning curves are similar and closely resemble the basilar membrane tuning curves (from Cody and Russell, 1987, with permission).

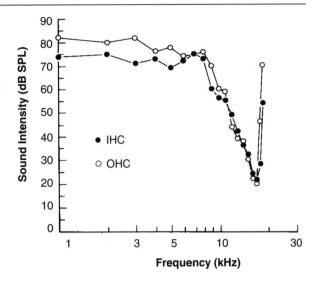

tuning curves represent the sound pressure level needed to produce a criterion, low-level AC response, or DC response (Cody and Russell, 1987). The IHC and OHC tuning curves both have a low threshold, a narrowly tuned tip near the best frequency, and a high-threshold, broadly tuned, low-frequency tail. These responses closely resemble the basilar membrane mechanical vibration patterns (Sellick, Patuzzi, and Johnstone, 1982), suggesting that the hair cell response is closely linked to the mechanical response.

Hair Cell Input/Output Functions

The basilar membrane input/output function is highly nonlinear at CF, but linear above and below CF (Sellick et al., 1982). The same type of nonlinearity is present in the input/output functions of the IHC and OHC receptor potentials near CF. Figure 6.25 shows the AC input/output functions for (a) an IHC and (b) OHC; the AC response of the OHC has been corrected for the cell's membrane capacitance. The dashed line in the top panel of Figure 6.25 has a slope of 1 when the receptor potential amplitude is plotted on a logarithmic scale. The input/output function at CF (~17 kHz) and slightly above and below CF increases linearly at low intensities, but at higher intensities the slope decreases, that is, a compressive nonlinearity (Cody and Russell, 1987). By contrast, the input/output functions far above or below CF are approximately linear. Thus, the compressive nonlinearity is mainly present around CF.

Efferent Stimulation

The axon terminals of the efferent neurons in the crossed olivocochlear bundle (COCB) synapse on OHCs. Electrical stimulation of the COCB increases the amplitude of the CM potential and decreases the amplitude of the CAP (Gifford and Guinan, 1987), which is generated by the type I auditory nerve fibers that contact the IHCs (Trautwein et al., 1996; Wang et al., 1997). COCB stimulation decreases the amplitude of the IHC's AC and DC receptor potentials evoked by stimuli near CF but has little or no effect on the receptor potentials elicited by frequencies

● **Figure 6.25**

(a) IHC and (b) OHC AC receptor potential input/output functions. OHC responses compensated for membrane capacitance. Dashed line in (a) represents the linear slope (from Cody and Russell, 1987, modified with permission).

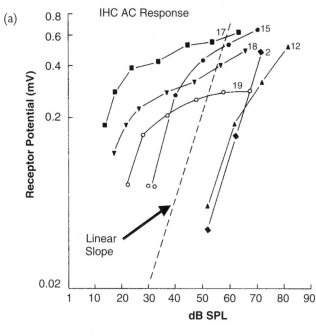

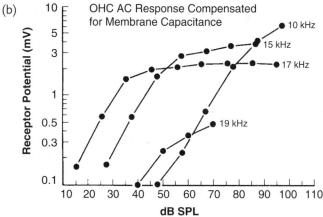

remote from CF (Brown and Nuttall, 1984). The IHC's AC and DC receptor potential tuning curves demonstrate a similar loss of sensitivity near the CF during COCB stimulation (Figure 6.26). The loss in sensitivity near the tuning curve tip is equivalent to a 9–24-dB decrease in sound intensity. The effects of COCB stimulation on the IHC response are presumably mediated indirectly through the OHCs, which attenuate the mechanical input to IHCs near the CF. This interpretation is consistent with results showing that COCB stimulation reduces basilar membrane motion around the CF (Murugasu and Russell, 1996), presumably by modulating the electromotile response of OHCs.

OHC Function

The mammalian inner ear contains roughly three times as many OHCs as IHCs, but only 5 to 10% of the auditory nerve fibers synapse on OHCs; the remaining 90 to 95% synapse on IHCs. Type I auditory nerve fibers that synapse on IHCs produce an AP in response to sound stimulation (Liberman, 1982a,b), whereas type II fibers that contact OHCs do not appear to produce discharges to sound (Robertson, 1984). If the OHC type II complex does not transmit sound-evoked information to the brain, then what do the OHCs do?

Selective hair cell lesion studies have provided some important clues regarding the functional role of IHCs and OHCs. Selective destruction of OHCs results in an elevation of psychophysical and physiological thresholds of up to 40 to 60 dB and a significant widening of tuning curves (Ryan and Dallos, 1975; Dallos and Harris, 1978; Ryan, Dallos, and McGee, 1979). Changes similar to these are seen in IHC and OHC receptor potential tuning curves following acute acoustic trauma (Figure 6.27) (Cody and Russell, 1992). The OHC and IHC AC receptor potential tuning curves (left side) and DC receptor potential tuning curves (right side) have a low-threshold, narrowly tuned tip near 20 kHz before the traumatizing exposure. After a 15-second exposure to a 12.5-kHz traumatizing tone, the IHC AC and DC receptor potential tuning curves show elevated thresholds around CF, but little change in sensitivity in the low-frequency tail of the tuning curve. Changes similar to this also occur in the OHC AC receptor potential tuning curve. The OHC DC receptor potential tuning curve shows less change after acoustic trauma; this is most likely due to the high sound levels required to generate OHC tuning curves. Changes in tuning similar to this have been observed in basilar membrane mechanical tuning curves (Sellick et al., 1982; Russell, Richardson, and Cody, 1986). The loss of the nonlinear response, increase in threshold, and widening of the tuning curve appear to be closely linked to the deterioration in the mechanical input to the IHCs.

These results suggest that there is a division of labor whereby the OHCs enhance the sensitivity and tuning around the CF; the enhanced response near CF is then relayed to the IHCs, which are responsible for transmitting the information to the central auditory system. The physiological processes that improve the sensitivity and tuning of the inner ear are often referred to as the "cochlear amplifier." The amplifier is thought to involve metabolically active processes (e.g., the EP and hair cell resting potentials). Cochlear pathologies that damage the active process result in the loss of sensitivity and tuning.

The cochlear amplifier did not have a strong empirical foundation until the discovery of two fundamental auditory phenomena: otoacoustic emissions and the OHC's electromotile response. Otoacoustic emissions, discovered by Kemp in the late 1970s (Kemp, 1978) and predicted by an astronomer (Gold, 1948) in the late 1940s, are sounds emitted from the inner ear either spontaneously or in response to acoustic or electric stimulation. The second major finding was the discovery of electrically evoked OHC motion along the longitudinal axis (Brownell, Bader, Bertrand, and de Ribaupierre, 1985). The electromotile response suggests that the active source of mechanical energy in the cochlea resides in the OHCs.

● **Figure 6.26**

Electrical stimulation of the crossed olivocochlear bundle (COCB) elevates the narrowly tuned low-threshold tip of IHC receptor potential tuning curves. Recovered shows normal IHC tuning curve (from Brown, Nuttall, and Masta, 1983, with permission).

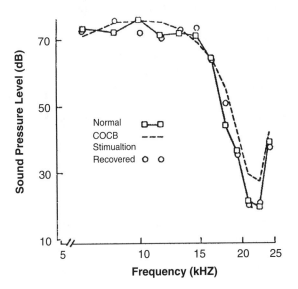

● Figure 6.27

OHC (top row) and IHC (bottom row) AC (left column) and DC (right column) tuning curves measured before and after acoustic overstimulation. Tuning curves show an elevation of threshold near the low threshold tip with the exception of the OHC's DC response, which does not, presumably because its high threshold was high initially (from Cody and Russell, 1992, with permission).

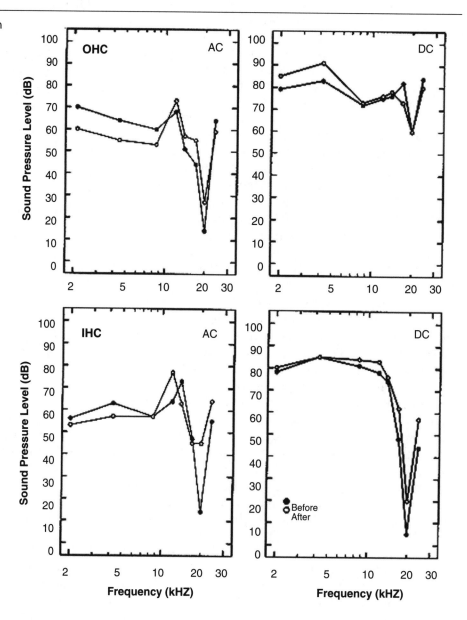

ELECTROMOTILITY

Electromotility refers to the longitudinal motion of OHCs in response to changes in transmembrane voltage (Brownell et al., 1985). To measure the electromotile response, OHCs are removed from the organ of Corti and placed under a microscope equipped with a photodiode to measure hair cell movements. The OHC membrane potential can be altered by placing the basal end of an OHC (Figure 6.28) in a large bore micropipette and changing the voltage in the pipette with respect to the external bath solution (Ashmore and Brownell, 1986; Dallos and Evans, 1995). As shown by the line in Figure 6.28, DC depolarization results in shortening of the OHC, whereas hyperpolarization leads to elongation. When an OHC is stimulated with a sinusoidal signal, the length of the OHC follows the stimulus in

● Figure 6.28

Photomicrograph of a gerbil OHC with the base of the OHC inserted in a glass micropipette, which is used to deliver electrical stimulation to the hair cell. DC depolarization (top panel) causes contraction of the OHC. The solid line shows OHC length in the contracted state. Hyperpolarization (bottom panel) shows an OHC elongation. The long solid line shows an OHC in contracted state; the short solid line near the cuticular plate of the OHC shows the increase in cell length relative to contraction (Photomicrographs courtesy of Z.Z. He).

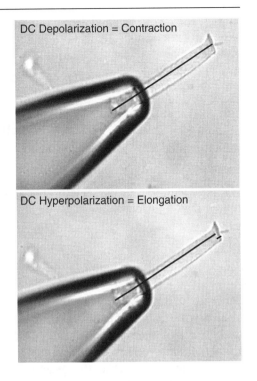

DC Depolarization = Contraction

DC Hyperpolarization = Elongation

a cycle-by-cycle manner. However, the OHC response is asymmetric such that contraction is substantially greater than elongation (Figure 6.29). Because of the asymmetry, the AC length change is superimposed upon on an overall decrease in OHC length. In guinea pigs, the AC electromotile response extends out to 79 kHz, a value exceeding the upper range of hearing (Frank, Hemmert, and Gummer, 1999). The high-frequency cutoff of the AC electromotile response is greater for short OHCs in the base than for long OHCs in the apex. The overall length change for hair cells in the apex is on the order of $+/-2$ microns, or 4% of OHC length (Ashmore, 1987).

The electromotile response is thought to play a role in reverse transduction; that is, acoustical stimulation changes the transmembrane voltage of OHCs, which in turn causes the OHC to send mechanical energy back into the cochlea to help overcome the viscous fluid damping and enhance the vibration of the cochlear

● Figure 6.29

OHC electromotile response of gerbil OHC to AC stimulation. Vertical arrows show shortening (up) and lengthening (down) of the OHC. AC voltage applied to the microchambers shown in bottom trace (from He et al., 2003, modified with permission).

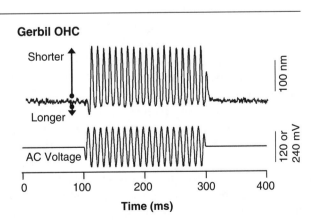

Gerbil OHC

Shorter

Longer

100 nm

AC Voltage

120 or 240 mV

Time (ms)

● **Figure 6.30**

Basilar membrane velocity response in response to acoustic stimulation (solid line) and electrical stimulation delivered to the round window (dashed line) (from Nuttall and Ren, 1995, with permission).

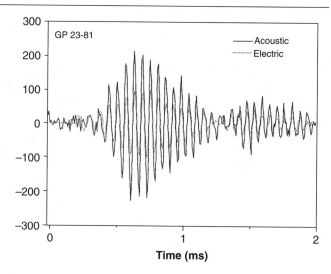

partition. Electromotility has been studied in situ using the excised temporal bone preparation. By changing the membrane potential of an OHC using a patch clamp electrode, movements can be induced in neighboring cells of the organ of Corti (Mammano, Kros, and Ashmore, 1995). Similarly, when electrical current is passed across an isolated segment of the organ of Corti, electrically evoked changes in OHC length induce place-specific vibrations of the basilar membrane (Mammano and Ashmore, 1993). Finally, injection of electrical current into the intact cochlea, which would be expected to elicit changes in OHC length, results in basilar membrane motion (Nuttall and Ren, 1995; Xue, Mountain, and Hubbard, 1995b). Sinusoidal current delivered to the scala media induced basilar membrane movement equivalent to that produced by a 60-dB SPL sound. Brief current pulses produced damped oscillations of the basilar membrane similar to the vibrations caused by an acoustic click (Figure 6.30).

Electromotility Motor and Prestin

The OHC lateral wall is composed of three distinct layers: the subsurface cisternae (SSC), the cortical lattice (CL), and the plasma membrane (PM) (Figure 6.31). The outermost PM layer contains numerous heterogeneous, intramembranous protein particles with an estimated density of $6000/\mu m^2$ (Forge, 1991). The PM is characterized by numerous wrinkles that would permit the cell to elongate and shorten (Oghalai, Patel, Nakagawa, and Brownell, 1998). The SSC, which forms the innermost layer, is composed of multiple sheets of flattened membranes (Saito, 1983). The CL, which lies between the SSC and PM, is made up of cross-linked actin and spectrin filaments that form a lattice of circumferential filaments, the so-called cytoskeletal spring (Holley, Kalinec, and Kachar, 1992). The CL is anchored to the PM by connecting pillars.

The molecular motor responsible for OHC electromotility is thought to reside in the dense network of proteins in the PM. Using subtractive hybridization polymerase chain reaction of cDNA from OHCs and IHCs, a gene, prestin, was identified that codes for the motor protein, **prestin** (Zheng, Shen, He, Long, Madison, and Dallos, 2000). The cDNA for prestin is only expressed in OHCs, not in IHCs or cells from other organs. When prestin was transfected into kidney cells, the cells

● Figure 6.31

The plasma membrane (PM), cortical lattice (CL) and subsurface cisternae (SSC) of the OHC lateral wall. Actin and spectrin cytoskeleton is coupled to the plasma membrane by connecting pillars. The plasma membrane contains a high density of protein particles (from Zheng et al., 2000, with permission).

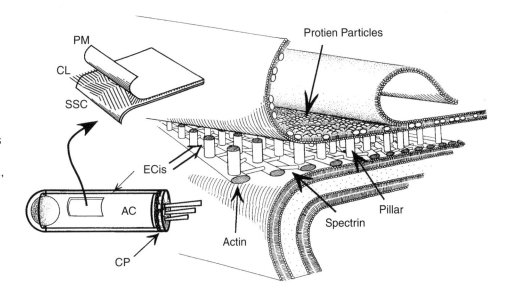

expressed a nonlinear capacitance to voltage steps, a signature of OHC electro-motility. The prestin-transfected kidney cells also changed length in response to voltage steps (Figure 6.32). Prestin is a member of the gene family coding for anion transporter–related proteins, known as the solute carrier family (SLC) 26 (Dallos and Fakler, 2002). Unlike other members of the SLC26 family, prestin does not transport anions across the membrane but instead imparts electromotility and non-linear capacitance to the membrane.

Prestin is thought to consist of two elements, a voltage sensor that detects the change in transmembrane voltage and an actuator molecule that undergoes a con-formational change that leads to the electromotile response (Oliver et al., 2001; Dallos and Fakler, 2002). Experimental evidence indicates that prestin uses an ex-trinsic sensor; the sensor is an anion, Cl⁻, in the cytoplasm. In response to voltage change, the anion binds to a site on prestin. Membrane hyperpolarization causes the anion to translocate toward the extracellular side of the membrane, causing the

● Figure 6.32

Electromotile response from cultured human kidney cells transfected with the gene for prestin. The top two traces are from prestin-transfected cells, the third trace is from the control cell, and the bottom trace shows the electrical stimulus in microvolts. Length change is expressed in nanometers (nm) (from Zheng et al., 2000, modified with permission).

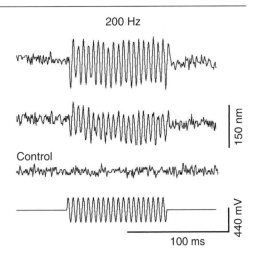

prestin molecule to elongate; depolarization shifts the location of the anion toward the cytoplasmic side, causing the prestin molecule to shorten.

The preceding results indicate that the OHC can elongate and contract at high rates in response to changes in transmembrane voltage and cause the basilar membrane to move. Such movements would create pressure fluctuations in the fluid-filled cochlea that would be coupled back to the stapes and tympanic membrane.

OTOACOUSTIC EMISSIONS

Types of Otoacoustic Emissions

Consistent with the concept of active amplification in the cochlea is the finding of otoacoustic emissions—sounds generated in the inner ear by OHCs that propagate in the reverse direction back into the external ear canal. Otoacoustic emissions come in three main "flavors." Spontaneous otoacoustic emissions (SOAEs), as implied by the name, occur in the absence of external sound stimulation. Sound-evoked otoacoustic emissions fall into two main groups: transient evoked otoacoustic emissions (TEOAEs) and distortion-product otoacoustic emissions (DPOAEs). Finally, electrically evoked otoacoustic emissions (EEOAEs) are elicited by injecting current into the inner ear. Because of their noninvasive nature and ease of measurement, TEOAEs and DPOAEs are used extensively in clinical settings to assess the functional integrity of the inner ear, specifically the OHCs and stria vascularis.

TEOAEs

Because otoacoustic emissions are low-level sounds, typically less than 30 dB SPL, they need to be recorded under low-noise conditions using a sensitive microphone coupled to a signal averager or spectrum analyzer. To measure TEOAEs, a probe assembly containing an earphone and a sensitive microphone is inserted in the ear. A foam or rubber cuff surrounding the tip of the probe occludes the ear canal, thereby reducing background noise (Figure 6.33a). A click or a short-duration tone burst (<3 ms) is presented to the ear and the sound pressure is measured over time. To improve the signal-to-noise ratio, the stimulus is presented several hundred to a thousand times and the sound pressure picked up by the microphone in the ear canal is signal averaged for 10 to 20 ms following the stimulus. Figure 6.34 shows a TEOAE measured with a click stimulus (81 dB pSPL). The pressure-time waveform of the click stimulus is shown in Figure 6.34a; note that the amplitude is scaled in Pascals (Pa) and the time window is 5 ms. Figure 6.34b shows the pressure-time waveform sampled for 25 ms following stimulus onset. Note that the amplitude is scaled in mPa (a scale 1000 smaller than that for the stimulus in the upper left) to enhance the low-amplitude TEOAE waveform. The acoustic stimulus that would normally occur in the first few milliseconds has been suppressed in the middle panel in order to visualize the low-amplitude TEOAE. Panel B shows two traces, A and B, which represent the averaged TEOAE waveforms collected on every other stimulus presentation. Traces A and B are nearly identical, indicating that the TEOAE is highly reproducible in this ear. The TEOAE, which consists of a series of oscillations, begins several ms after the onset of the click, rises to its peak

● Figure 6.33

Schematic showing equipment needed to measure (a) TEOAE and (b) DPOAE. Output of a low-noise, sensitive microphone is generally sent to a computer for signal averaging or spectral analysis. Two sound sources are used for DPOAE measurements, whereas a single sound source is used for measurement of TEOAEs (modified from Lonsbury-Martin, Whitehead, and Martin, 1991, with permission).

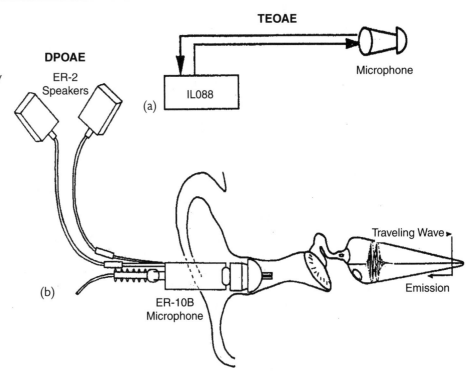

● Figure 6.34

TEOAE obtained from adult, using a click stimulus. (a) Waveform of click stimulus in ear canal. (b) TEOAE waveform with stimulus artifact suppressed 0 to 2 ms. (c) Spectrum of stimulus (solid line), TEOAE from panel B (dark area), and background noise (shaded area).

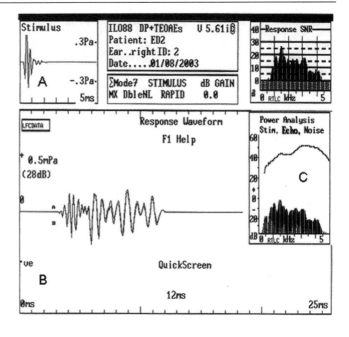

amplitude around 3 to 10 ms, and then gradually decays away. The time between peaks in the TEOAE waveform is shortest near the beginning of the waveform, indicating high-frequency content, and gradually increases toward the end of the waveform, indicating low-frequency content. This indicates that the TEOAE energy spectrum is dispersed over time, with high-frequency energy emerging from the cochlea first, followed by lower frequencies. This is consistent with basilar membrane mechanics, which predicts a shorter latency for high frequencies than for low frequencies. The onset latency of the TEOAE, which contains high-frequency energy, is approximately 3.5 ms. The latency is believed to reflect the time it takes for the stimulus to travel to the region of the cochlea, where it is transduced and the emission is generated, plus the time it takes for the signal to propagate in the reverse direction back to the microphone in the external ear canal (Norton and Neely, 1987; Neely, Norton, Gorga, and Jesteadt, 1988). The low-frequency components of the signal must travel to and return from more apical locations of the cochlea; hence, they have longer latencies and appear much later in the TEOAE response.

Figure 6.34c shows the spectrum of the stimulus (upper line), the spectrum of the TEOAE (dark black area), and the spectrum of the background noise (gray area). The click produces a broadband signal, with a peak around 4 kHz, which stimulates much of the cochlea. Note that the upper frequency range of the TEOAE response is around 5 to 6 kHz. The spectrum of the TEOAE in panel C is substantially greater than the noise between 1 and 4 kHz but begins to drop off at higher frequencies. Because the upper frequency range of the TEOAE response is around 5 to 6 kHz, TEOAEs have limited utility at very high frequencies.

Click-evoked TEOAEs are highly reproducible within a given ear; however, the TEOAE waveform varies noticeably from one individual to the next. TEOAE amplitude tends to increase with stimulus level at low intensities; however, the response is nonlinear and saturates at moderate to high stimulus levels. TEOAEs can also be elicited by narrow-band stimuli such as tone bursts (Kemp, 1978; Probst, Coats, Martin, and Lonsbury-Martin, 1986). Tone burst–evoked TEOAEs have spectral peaks with a maximum near the frequency of the stimulus. In addition, the latency of tone burst–evoked TEOAEs increases as the frequency decreases, consistent with the mechanical properties of the basilar membrane.

TEOAE amplitude can be suppressed by presenting a broadband noise stimulus in the contralateral ear; however, the maximum suppression is on the order of 2 to 3 dB. Contralaterally induced TEOAE suppression is most likely mediated through the olivocochlear efferent system, since the suppression effect can be abolished by drugs known to block neurotransmission of efferent neurons that synapse on OHCs (Kujawa, Glattke, Fallon, and Bobbin, 1992; Kujawa, Glattke, Fallon, and Bobbin, 1993).

In listeners with sensorineural hearing loss, which involves damage to the OHCs (e.g., acoustic trauma or aminoglycoside antibiotics) or stria vascularis (e.g., diuretics such as furosemide), the TEOAE response is reduced or absent (Marshall and Heller, 1998; Anderson and Kemp, 1979; Stavroulaki, Apostolopoulos, Dinopoulou, Vossinakis, Tsakanikos, and Douniadakis, 1999; Withnell, Yates, and Kirk, 2000). TEOAEs are greatly reduced or absent in listeners with thresholds greater than 40 dB hearing level (HL) (Bray and Kemp, 1987; Prieve, Gorga, Schmidt, Neely, Peters, Schultes, and Jesteadt, 1993). Because TEOAEs can be recorded within a matter of minutes, are sensitive to cochlear pathology, and do not require a response from the subject, they are now commonly used to screen for hearing loss in newborns (Aidan, Avan, and Bonfils, 1999).

DPOAEs

When the ear is stimulated with two tones of similar frequency and amplitude, new tones, referred to as intermodulation distortion tones, can be recorded in the ear canal in addition to the original stimuli (Kemp, 1979). The most prominent distortion products occur at $2f_1$-f_2, the cubic distortion product, and f_2-f_1. The equipment used to measure DPOAEs is schematized in Figure 6.33b. A low-noise microphone is used to record the signals in the ear canal, and the output of the microphone is evaluated with a spectrum analyzer to determine the spectral content of the signal. To minimize intermodulation distortion produced by the equipment, two separate earphones are used to generate pure tones at primary frequencies of f_1 and f_2, where f_1 is the lower frequency and f_2 is the higher frequency, and sound levels of L_1 and L_2. To enhance the production of DPOAEs, the f_2/f_1 ratio is normally set to 1.1 to 1.3, and the amplitudes of the primary tones are set to the same level ($L_1 = L_2$) or with L_1 set approximately +10 dB above L_2 (Whitehead, McCoy, Lonsbury-Martin, and Martin, 1995). Figure 6.34a shows the spectrum of the acoustic signal measured in a human ear canal with $f_1 = 1636$, $f_2 = 2002$, and L1 = L2 = 67 dB SPL. In addition to the two primary tones generated by the earphones, a prominent 2f1-f2 distortion product, generated by the ear, can be seen at 1270 Hz at 8 dB SPL, well above the surrounding noise floor. In this example, the distortion product is approximately 60 dB below the level of the primary tones.

A convenient and clinically useful method of assessing DPOAEs is to sweep a pair of primary tones, locked in a fixed frequency ratio, from low to high frequency while holding the level of the two primary tones constant. DPOAE amplitude is typically plotted as a function of the f2 frequency or the geometric mean frequency of the primaries $((f1*f2)^{0.5})$. The resulting graph, shown in Figure 6.35b, is referred to as a DPgram. The Xs in Figure 6.34b show the data for an individual

● **Figure 6.35**

DPOAE from an adult. Primary tones: f1 = 1636 Hz, L1 = 67 dB SPL, f2 = 2002 Hz, L2 = 67 dB SPL (a) Spectrum of the acoustic signal recorded in the ear canal shows the two primary tones plus the cubic difference tone, 2f1-f2, with a level of 7.7 dB SPL. (b) DPgram obtained by sweeping the two primary tones with an f2/f1 ratio of 1.224 from low to high frequencies at a constant level of 67 dB SPL. Crosses show amplitude of 2f1-f2; shaded area shows mean (+/−1 SD) from control group.

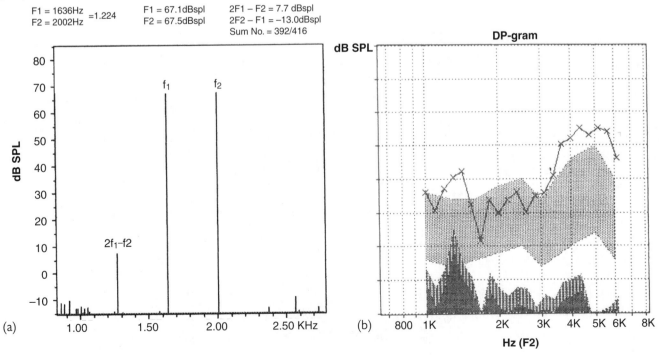

subject, and the lightly shaded area shows the range of normal values (+/−1 SD around the mean). The dark, shaded area near the bottom shows the noise floor. The DPOAE amplitude ranges from 5 to 10 dB below 3 kHz, but then increases to around 18 dB from 4 to 6 kHz. DPOAEs can be measured out to higher frequencies than TEOAEs, and thus DPOAEs are more useful for assessing high-frequency hearing loss than TEOAEs.

An alternative method of assessing DPOAEs is to measure the amplitude as a function of stimulus level while holding the primary tone frequencies constant. Once the noise floor is exceeded, DPOAE amplitude increases with stimulus level, but the response typically saturates above 75 dB SPL. The so-called DPOAE threshold is often specified as the sound intensity that produces a DPOAE that exceeds the surrounding noise floor by 3 to 6 dB.

Hair cell lesion studies in rodents have helped confirm that the OHCs are the generators of the DPOAEs (Brown, McDowell, and Forge, 1989; Trautwein et al., 1996; Hofstetter, Ding, Powers, and Salvi, 1997). Selective destruction of IHCs has no effect on DPOAE amplitude; DPOAE amplitude is only depressed in ears with OHC lesions. At high frequencies, DPOAE amplitudes decrease approximately 4 dB for every 10% loss of OHCs in chinchillas. Furthermore, the frequency-specific loss of DPOAE amplitude is closely linked to the location of damage along the cochlear partition.

SOAEs

SOAEs are tonal signals, usually of low level (<10 dB SPL), but sometimes as high as 40 to 50 dB SPL, that can be recorded in the ear canal with the aid of a low-noise microphone and narrow-band spectrum analyzer. Figure 6.36 shows an SOAE in a human subject; the frequency of the SOAE is near 1 kHz and the SPL is approximately −15 dB SPL. The prevalence of SOAEs has been reported to be as high as 72% in normal hearing human subjects (Penner, Glotzbach, and Huang, 1993;

● Figure 6.36

SOAE from an adult. Spectrum analysis of microphone output shows a distinct peak of approximately −8 dB SPL near 980 Hz.

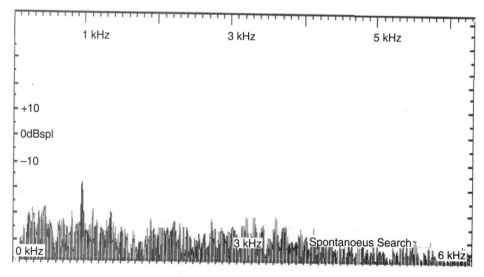

Talmadge, Long, Murphy, and Tubis, 1993). In humans, SOAEs typically occur between 1 and 2 kHz, and women are almost twice as likely as men to have SOAEs. Multiple SOAEs can be recorded in the same ear, and subjects frequently have SOAEs in both ears. SOAEs can be suppressed by external tones near the frequency of the SOAE. A suppression-tuning curve can be obtained by varying the level and frequency of the suppressor needed to suppress the SOAE by a fixed amount (e.g., 3 dB). Suppression tuning curves are shaped much like single auditory nerve fiber or psychophysical tuning curves (Ruggero, Rich, and Freyman, 1983; Ruggero, Kramek, and Rich, 1984; Powers, Salvi, Wang, Spongr, and Qiu, 1995). SOAEs are generally abolished by cochlear damage involving OHCs (Long and Tubis, 1988; Norton, Mott, and Champlin, 1989).

EEOAEs

EEOAEs, while not used clinically, provide an important link between OHC electromotility and otoacoustic emissions (Mountain and Hubbard, 1989; Xue, Mountain, and Hubbard, 1995a; Reyes, Ding, Sun, and Salvi, 2001). Injection of AC current into the scala media or scala tympani, which induces basilar membrane motion (Figure 6.29), would be expected to produce a pressure fluctuation in the cochlear fluids that propagates in the reverse direction into the ear canal (Nuttall and Ren, 1995; Xue et al., 1995a,b). Figure 6.37 shows the spectrum of the EEOAE recorded in the ear canal of a chinchilla when sinusoidal current (220 μA peak–peak) was injected into the cochlea from an electrode placed on the round window membrane (Reyes et al., 2001). As the stimulus was swept from low to high frequency, the amplitude of the EEOAE was recorded at the stimulus frequency. The AC current

● **Figure 6.37**

EEOAE from a chinchilla. An electrode on the round window was used to deliver sinusoidal current (220 µA p-p). The frequency of the AC signal varied from low to high frequency. The amplitude of the acoustic signal in the ear canal was measured at the stimulus frequency.

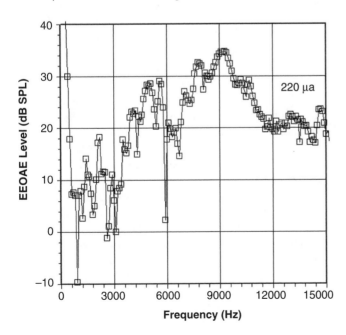

produced a robust EEOAE over a wide frequency range. The peak in the amplitude spectrum (35 dB SPL) was near 9 kHz; this frequency corresponds closely to the characteristic frequency of the basilar membrane associated with the site of stimulation. Destruction of the IHCs had little effect on EEOAE amplitude, whereas OHC loss caused a significant reduction in EEOAE amplitude, confirming that EEOAEs are generated by the OHCs.

Prestin, DPOAEs, and Threshold

A growing body of evidence suggests that OHC electromotility is responsible for the production of otoacoustic emissions, but is the motor protein, prestin, essential for the production of emissions? To test this hypothesis, mutant mice were generated that lacked the gene for prestin (Liberman, Gao, He, Wu, Jia, and Zuo, 2002). OHCs and IHCs in homozygous mutant mice ($-/-$), which lack both copies of the prestin gene, were morphologically normal; however, electrical stimulation failed to induce an electromotile response in isolated OHCs. In addition, DPOAEs were absent or greatly reduced in homozygous mutant mice, and their auditory brainstem response (ABR) thresholds were elevated by 40 dB or more. In heterozygous mice ($+/-$), lacking one copy of the prestin gene, OHC electromotility was only slightly reduced and DPOAEs and ABR thresholds showed minimal change. These results provide convincing evidence that the motor protein, prestin, is needed to maintain normal auditory sensitivity and otoacoustic emissions.

CLINICAL CORRELATE

During the past 50 years, considerable progress has been made in understanding the biological source(s) of many of the physiological signals generated in the inner ear. Because of advances in the basic sciences, clinicians now have powerful tools at their disposal to assess the functional status of different structures in the inner ear. TEOAEs and DPOAEs are perhaps the most important new tools in the clinical armamentarium; measurements can be obtained rapidly and easily using noninvasive measures. Assuming the middle ear is intact, abnormal DPOAEs or TEOAEs would most likely indicate damage to the OHCs or, alternatively, the stria vascularis, which provides a significant proportion of the driving voltage across the apical pole of the OHC. Distinguishing between OHC damage and strial dysfunction is problematic in humans because of the lack of noninvasive methods for assessing endocochelar potential voltage. Noninvasive techniques to assess endocochelar potential in humans would represent an important clinical breakthrough, one that could prove useful in distinguishing between strial versus sensory presbycusis (Schuknecht, 1974).

Cochlear hearing loss: One of the most common forms of hearing loss is attributed primarily to OHC damage. Since OAE measures were first introduced into the clinical test battery, a number of studies have demonstrated a high correlation between the pure-tone frequencies at which a hearing loss is observed and the frequency region where OAE response amplitudes are reduced or absent (Probst, Lonsbury-Martin, Martin, and Coats, 1987; Harris, 1990; Probst, Lonsbury-Martin, and Martin, 1991). This is illustrated in Figure 6.38a, which shows an audiogram of a 71-year-old male with a slightly asymmetric sloping, high-frequency hearing loss. The DPOAEs recorded for this individual are shown in Figure 6.38b,c for the left and right ears, respectively, where the DPOAE amplitude is represented by the solid line and the noise floor by the shaded region. Although the DPOAE amplitude measures appear to reflect a similar asymmetry to that observed in the pure-tone thresholds, caution is warranted in attempting to use OAE data to predict pure-tone thresholds. Studies of individuals with normal middle ear and cochlear function have demonstrated that while test–retest reliability of OAE amplitudes produces relatively small within-subject variability ($\sim$4 dB), the between-subject variability can be as much as 30 dB (re: noise floor) (Gorga, Neely, Bergman, Beauchaine, Kaminski, Peters, and

(continued)

● Figure 6.38

A patient with a cochlear hearing loss showing (a) the audiogram and (b,c) the left and right ear DPOAEs.

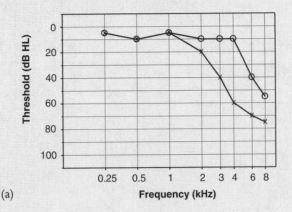

(a)

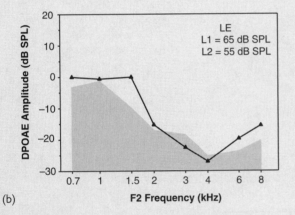

(b)

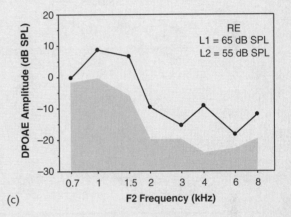

(c)

Jesteadt, 1993; Gorga, Stover, Neely, and Montoya, 1996; Marshall and Heller, 1996; Robinette, 2003). Further, when cochlear hearing loss is present and exceeds about 30 to 40 dB HL at a particular frequency, the probability of obtaining a measurable emission in that frequency region is less than 50% (Probst et al., 1987; Harris and Probst, 1997). Clinically, OAE amplitude measures appear to be most useful as a tool for monitoring cochlear and/or middle ear function within individuals and they likely reflect changes in OHC and/or strial function.

Auditory neuropathy: Clinicians occasionally encounter patients who present with confusing signs and symptoms. A good example of this would be patients with auditory neuropathy who have unusual auditory performance characteristics (see also Chapter 7 for more on auditory neuropathy). Auditory neuropathy patients have fairly normal OAEs and hearing thresholds that are normal to mildly impaired (Starr et al.,

1996). Figure 6.39a shows the audiogram of an auditory neuropathy patient who was evaluated in our clinic at 14 years of age. Hearing thresholds in quiet were measured with pure-tone stimuli as well as narrow-band noise stimuli and found to be less than 20 dB HL in both ears. Interestingly, the patient reported that it was easier to hear the narrow-band noise stimuli than the pure tones. Speech discrimination was extremely poor, except when the patient was given visual cues. The patient also found it difficult to distinguish speech stimuli from noise stimuli. Surprisingly, despite having normal pure-tone thresholds, the patient's speech production and voice quality were similar to those of patients with profound hearing loss.

To assess the condition of the OHCs, DPOAE testing was carried out on this patient (F2/F1 = 1.21, L1 = L2 = 75 dB SPL). The DPgram in Figure 6.38b revealed fairly robust DPOAEs except for a large dip near 6 kHz. The large, reliable DPOAEs suggest that

(continued)

● **Figure 6.39**

A patient with presumed auditory neuropathy. (a) Pure-tone thresholds. (b) Distortion product otoacoustic emissions for the right ear. (c) Auditory brainstem response, (d) middle latency response, and (e) late potential response for the right ear.

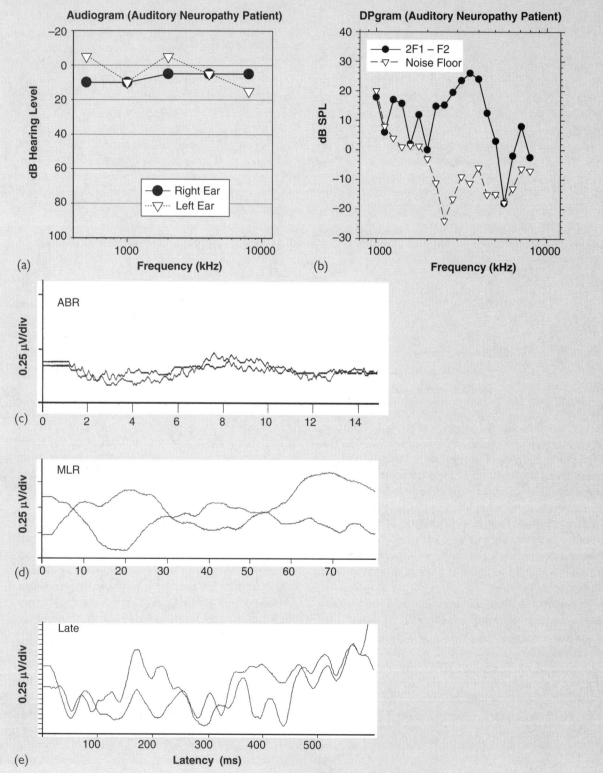

the OHCs and the stria vascularis, which generates the EP, must be fairly normal in this individual.

Additional testing was carried out to assess the condition of the more central auditory structures. The ipsilateral and contralateral acoustic reflexes were evaluated and found to be absent in both ears. Masking-level difference (MLD) testing was performed and found to be abnormal, consistent with poor speech discrimination scores and lack of acoustic reflexes. Several electrophysiological tests were conducted to identify possible sources of neural activity in the peripheral or central auditory pathway. Auditory brainstem response (ABR) testing was performed with condensation or rarefaction click stimuli presented at 80 dB nHL. Wave I, the first peak in the ABR, presumably reflects the summed neural output of type I neurons that make exclusive contact with IHCs. Later peaks in the ABR are thought to reflect the response of successively higher auditory relay centers from the cochlear nucleus up to the lateral lemniscus. As shown in Figure 6.39c, wave I of the ABR was absent along with later peaks in the ABR response. The lack of a wave I response suggests that little neural activity is being transmitted by the type I neurons because of damage to either the IHCs, the type I neurons, or the synapse connecting these two structures. To confirm that little neural activity was being transmitted to the central auditory system, further evoked potential testing was carried out to assess the middle latency response (MLR) and the late cortical evoked potential. Stimuli used to elicit the MLR or late cortical responses were 1000 Hz tone bursts presented at 70 dB nHL to the left or right ear. The MLR (Figure 6.39d) and late cortical response (Figure 6.39e) were absent in this patient (Figure 6.39b,c), consistent with the absence of the ABR.

Other investigators have used electrocochleography to perform a more in-depth assessment of cochlear function in auditory neuropathy patients (Arslan, Santarelli, Sparacino, and Sella, 2000; Starr, Sininger, Nguyen, Michalewski, Oba, and Abdala, 2001; Santarelli, and Arslan, 2002). As noted above, the CM can be used to assess the status of the OHCs, the SP can be used to assess the OHCs and IHCs, and the CAP can be used to assess the condition of type I neurons in the auditory nerve. In some auditory neuropathy patients, the CM and SP are relatively normal, but the CAP is absent or reduced in amplitude and broader than normal. Results such as these suggest that either the type I auditory nerve fibers are damaged or the neural transmission between the IHCs and type I neurons is impaired (Santarelli and Arslan, 2002). In cases where the SP is greatly reduced or absent, it would be reasonable to conclude that the hearing deficits are the result of IHC damage as well as possible damage to type I auditory neurons. It is clear from the preceding example that accurate interpretation of clinical results rests on a solid scientific understanding of cochlear anatomy and the origins of the various physiological responses in the inner ear. ●

Acknowledgments: The authors are supported in part by grants from NIH 1P01DC03600 and NSF IBN9996379.

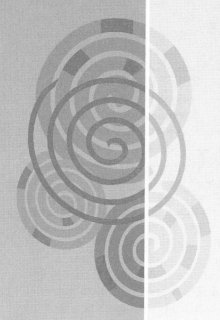

7

Structure and Function of the Auditory Nerve

Introduction

The **auditory nerve** (AN) connects the cochlea with the brainstem. Functionally, it relays information about the intensity, frequency, and timing of a sound after the cochlea has completed the initial processing of the incoming stimulus. The AN is part of the eighth cranial nerve, which also includes vestibular nerve tracts as well as AN fibers. As mentioned in the section on the temporal bone, the AN courses from the cochlea through a small canal in the temporal bone known as the **internal auditory meatus (IAM)** before it reaches the brainstem. The AN is partially myelinated (proximal to the habenula perforata) and its cell bodies are located in the spiral ganglion. Impulses representing the auditory information that were analyzed and coded in the cochlea are preserved in the AN and then passed on to the cochlear nucleus in the brainstem. The AN's fibers are **tonotopically** arranged and have some specificity in terms of intensity gradients. Since the AN is reasonably accessible for study in both animals and humans, its structure and function have been the subject of in-depth investigations for many years.

From a historical perspective, the AN has a long history of scientific investigation. In this regard, Folloppia is given credit for first describing the AN in the 1500s (see Moller, 2000). In the 1930s and 1940s, some outstanding work was done on the structure and function of the AN by Guild and Rasmussen (see Moller, 2000). One of the major discoveries of AN anatomy was reported in a number of papers by Spoendlin in the late 1960s and early 1970s (Spoendlin, 1969, 1972). Spoendlin described the AN's connections to the inner (IHC) and outer hair cells (OHC) and categorized AN fibers into two basic types. About the same time William and Howard House, two otologic surgeons, were developing new approaches to acoustic neuroma surgery. In developing these new surgical approaches, these two surgeons also learned much about the structure of the human AN and its blood supply (see House, Luetje, and Doyle, 1997). In the 1980s, Aage Moller performed physiologic recordings directly from the AN of humans during neurosurgery (Moller, 1983). His observations led to new knowledge about the structure and function of the AN and brainstem nuclei. This work became especially important, as it drew attention to notable differences between the ANs of animals and humans. Investigations into the anatomy and physiologic properties of the AN continue to the present day.

The AN can be viewed as an **auditory bottleneck**. This is because all of the auditory information being transmitted from the cochlea to the higher auditory centers in the brain must travel through the AN fibers. In the cochlea, activity is spread throughout the structure before it converges in the AN. Once the auditory impulses leave the AN, they again become dispersed in the many tracts of the brainstem and beyond. This concept was attributed to James Jerger and it has important clinical consequences. In particular, if the bottleneck region in the AN is damaged, there is considerable compromise of functions at and beyond this region. This is why in some patients that what appears to be slight damage to or compromise of the structure of the AN actually results in a major dysfunction of the auditory system and a related hearing loss.

ANATOMY OF THE AUDITORY NERVE

The AN in the adult human ranges in length from approximately 22 to 26 mm (Moller, 2000). It is usually slightly longer in men than in women, most likely because men's heads tend to be slightly larger than women's. Most measurements of the AN begin at the point where all of the fibers from the cochlea converge in the modiolus and end at the point where the AN connects to the cochlear nucleus in the pons. In actuality, however, the AN fibers connect to the hair cells at the terminal buttons before they course through the habenula perforata (openings in the spiral lamina) to form the spiral ganglion and then enter the IAM (Figure 7.1). At the brainstem level, there is a root entry zone of AN fibers that projects into the area between the anterior and posterior ventral cochlear nucleus (see next chapter for additional information). Therefore, AN fibers probably have a slightly longer route than is typically measured.

Most of the anatomical and physiological studies performed on the AN have been conducted on cats. Although much has been learned from these animal studies, certainly the anatomy of cats is much different than that of humans. For example, in cats the AN is only 0.8 mm long, but has 50,000 nerve fibers (Lang, 1981, 1991). Hence, it is difficult to estimate how applicable information derived from studies of animal auditory nerves is to our understanding of the structure and function of the AN in humans. The AN has both afferent and efferent fibers, with the preponderance of fibers being afferent. In this chapter, only the afferent AN fibers will be discussed. The efferent fibers of the AN will be discussed in Chapter 15, which will address the efferent system within the AN and the central auditory nervous system (CANS).

In general, the course of the AN as it proceeds from the cochlea to the cochlear nucleus in the brainstem is relatively predictable. Although the nerve twists as it leaves the cochlea (as do most cranial nerves as they course to the brain), it follows a reasonably straight course. As the AN approaches the brainstem, it often takes a slightly posterior course before it connects to the first major nucleus in the auditory brainstem, that is, the cochlear nucleus. As alluded to earlier, the AN travels through a bony channel, the IAM. Within the IAM, the AN occupies a location that is beneath the facial nerve and to the side of the vestibular nerves that also course through the IAM on their way to the brainstem (Figure 7.2). Because the AN twists as it courses through the IAM, the location of

● **F i g u r e 7 . 1**

The auditory nerve connections from the spiral ganglion to an inner hair cell.

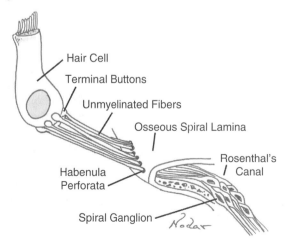

Hair Cell

Terminal Buttons

Unmyelinated Fibers

Osseous Spiral Lamina

Rosenthal's Canal

Habenula Perforata

Spiral Ganglion

● **Figure 7.2**

The internal auditory meatus at its opening (porus acousticus) where the auditory, vestibular, and facial nerve fibers exit and proceed to the brainstem.

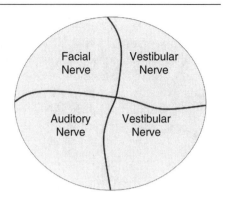

the AN relative to the other nerve fibers in the IAM changes slightly as it travels medially; that is, the AN rotates clockwise as it approaches the brainstem (see Moller, 2000).

Specifically, the afferent course of the AN involves a number of important structures that play a critical role in hearing. The fibers of the AN originate at the base of the cochlear hair cells at the **terminal buttons** where the AN contacts the bottoms of the hair cells. These are fragile connections and they may be a weak link in the system in terms of their susceptibility to trauma during surgical procedures involving the AN (Robinette, 1992). The AN fibers that connect to the OHCs course through the tunnel of Corti before they course along with the fibers from the IHCs toward, and then through, the **habenula perforata**. The habenula perforata is a bony structure of the osseous spiral lamina that has small openings through which the AN fibers pass (Gelfand, 1998). The ganglion cells of the AN converge in a slightly enlarged area known as **Rosenthal's canal** and then the fibers collect in a smaller area to form the trunk of the modiolus as the nerve proceeds into and through the IAM. The auditory, facial, and vestibular nerves course through the IAM and they all twist slightly, rotating clockwise, as they approach the brainstem (Moller, 2000). The AN fibers are unmyelinated in the region between their endings on the hair cells and the habenula perforata but may become **myelinated (Schwann cells)** as they pass through the IAM (there are some differences in myelination in regard to different types of AN fibers, which will be discussed later). As the fibers approach the brainstem, the myelin changes to more of an **oligdendrocyte myelin**. This myelin is similar to that found in the brain, and as such, is often referred to as central myelin (Moller, 2000). As they leave the IAM, the auditory, facial, and vestibular nerves course through a recess called the cerebellopontine angle (CPA) to enter the brainstem at the lateral, posterior pontomedullary junction and then provide input in an area between the dorsal and posterior ventral cochlear nucleus (root entry zone) (Figure 7.3).

The anatomy of the innervation of the IHCs and the OHCs by the AN reveals two distinct types of fibers as described by Spoendlin (1972). The type I fibers, sometimes referred to as radial fibers, make up 90 to 95% of all of the AN fibers, whereas type II fibers, at times referred to as spiral or longitudinal fibers, constitute only 5 to 10% of the total number of AN fibers. The type I fibers largely innervate the IHCs, and each IHC receives innervation from a number of individual type I fibers, as there are many more type I nerve fibers than there are IHCs. Because of this relative difference in the numbers and the orientation of the IHCs within the cochlea, the type I fibers, when viewed running from cochlea, give a radial appearance. The

● Figure 7.3

View of the base of the human brain. The seventh and eighth cranial nerves (1) are shown exiting the internal auditory meatus into the region of the cerebellopontine angle (CPA) and connecting to the lateral pons (2). Also shown are the basilar artery (3) and the cerebellum (4).

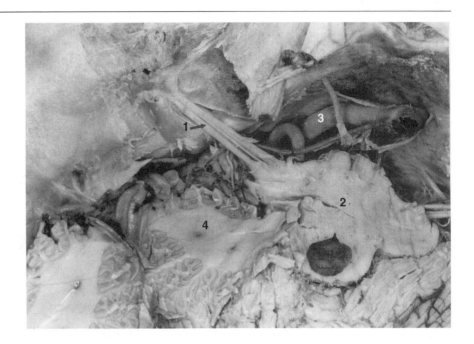

type II fibers innervate primarily the OHCs. Since there are many more OHCs than type II nerve fibers, these fibers tend to distribute across a number of OHCs and make connections with multiple OHCs. Because these fibers connect to more than one OHC, many of them run in longitudinal fashion—practically perpendicular to the type I fibers (Figures 7.4 and 7.5).

This rather unique distribution of AN fibers with a heavy orientation toward IHCs is consistent with the greater "physiological workload" of the IHCs as discussed in previous chapters. The type II fiber connections to the OHCs are rather complex (see Spoendlin, 1972 and Yost, 2000 for reviews). In the basal portion of the cochlea, these fibers connect primarily to the outer row of OHCs. As the innervation pattern moves toward the apical end of the cochlea, the middle and then the innermost rows of OHCs become the main connection regions. Besides the differential innervation patterns of the different hair cells, there are a number of biological differences between type I and type II fibers—probably related to the different functional tasks that each of these fiber types must accomplish. It should be realized that type I fibers are the ones that most AN researchers study because of their accessibility, size, and number. Most of what is known about the AN and its function is based on the investigation of type I fibers. Type II fibers are more difficult to locate in the AN core. In fact, some researchers believe type II fibers may not make effective connections to the brainstem, and if they do they are likely responsible for very little neural activity (Spoendlin, 1983; see also Gelfand, 1998 and Yost, 2000 for reviews). On the other hand, some researchers have studied type II fibers and believe that they play a definite role in AN physiology (Hurd, Hutson, and Morest, 1999; Moller, 2000; Yost, 2000). We subscribe to the latter view of type II neuron function.

Some anatomic differences between the type I and type II fibers are clear. Although the overall size of auditory fibers is about 2.5 μm in diameter, the type I fibers are consistently larger than the type II

● Figure 7.4

Type I and II auditory nerve fibers connecting to inner and outer hair cells (IHCs, OHCs).

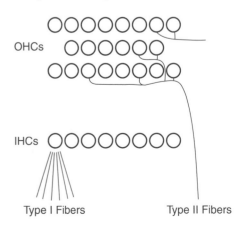

● **Figure 7.5**

(a) Photomicrograph of an auditory nerve showing radial (running up and down) and longitudinal (crosswise) fibers.
(b) An exposed organ of Corti and auditory nerve fibers. The arrows show a transition area where the nerve fibers (dark) become depleted owing to damage to the inner hair cells in the same region (courtesy of Marilyn Pinheiro).

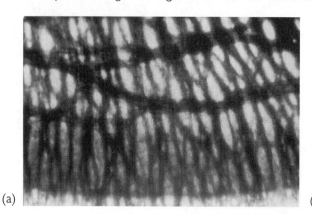

(a)

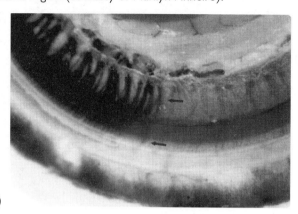

(b)

fibers. This difference in diameter is mostly attributable to the greater amount of myelin on type I axons. Many of the type II neurons have either little myelin or are without myelin altogether (Hurd et al., 1999; Yost, 2000). Interestingly, neither type I nor type II fibers have vesiculated endings (see Yost, 2000).

The innervation density of myelinated AN fibers varies greatly along the length of the cochlea. At the most basal and apical ends there are about 400 fibers per millimeter; however, in the 1- to 2-kHz region, innervation density is nearly 1400 fibers per millimeter. This means there are about three or four nerve fibers per IHC at the apex and base of the cochlea and about 15 per IHC in the 1-kHz region. The most heavy concentration of unmyelinated nerve fibers is found at the basal turn. These fibers (i.e., the unmyelinated fibers) are much smaller in diameter and many fewer in number than are the myelinated fibers (Spoendlin and Schrott, 1989).

The tonotopic organization of the AN has been studied extensively (for reviews, see Kim and Parham, 1997; Moller, 2000; and Yost, 2000). The low-frequency AN fibers connect to the hair cells at the apical end of the cochlea and occupy the central area, or core, of the AN (Figure 7.6). As the fibers arise from the more basal aspects of the cochlea, they progress to higher characteristic frequencies. As a result, the highest frequencies are represented on the circumference of the AN, with lower frequencies being represented by fibers in the center, or core, of the nerve. (This description is easy to remember, but may be slightly oversimplified. Spoendlin and Schrott [1989] have shown that the tonotopic arrangement of the AN is similar to that of the spiral organization of the cochlea. The most basal aspect, or hook area, of the cochlea is represented in a segment of the AN that courses inferior to the inferior vestibular nerve [Figure 7.6b,c]). Hence, in general, damage to the outside of the AN results in a high-frequency hearing loss, while damage to the middle core of the nerve yields a loss of low-frequency hearing. The relative arrangement of high- and low-frequency fibers within the AN is maintained throughout the IAM, although the fibers twist as they enter the brainstem. Since the cochlea is a concave-like structure (i.e., snail-shaped), with the apex in the middle, it appears that the low-frequency fibers may be slightly longer than the high-frequency fibers, which would mean that the high-frequency fibers have a slightly shorter route to the brainstem.

● Figure 7.6

(a) The auditory nerve fibers and their tonotopic array (note the slight twist of the auditory nerve fibers as they leave the cochlea and proceed to the brainstem). (b) Cross-section of auditory nerve fibers, with the "H" indicating the hook area or extreme basal aspect of the cochlea. (c) The arrows indicate the approximate tonotopic course of auditory nerve fibers from high to low frequencies in this cross-section of the auditory nerve.

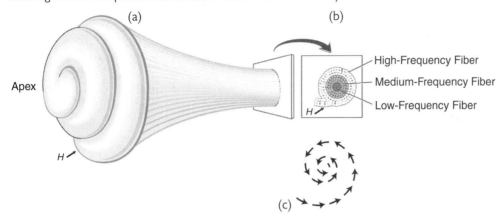

CLINICAL CORRELATE

Before discussing the physiology of the AN, it seems timely to discuss some of the many clinical correlates of the AN. The main clinical disorder of the AN is a serious one—the **acoustic tumor** (see House et al., 1997 for review). The acoustic tumor is really (at least 90% of the time), a **vestibular schwannoma**. That is, these tumors most often arise from the vestibular nerve(s) in the IAM and encroach upon the AN. These tumors are benign but serious because they lie in close proximity to the brainstem and in many situations may grow medially into the CPA and pontomedullary junction of the brainstem (Lustig and Jackler, 1997). Because most tumors affecting the AN approach the outside of the nerve first, the high-frequency fibers are initially compromised, resulting in a high-frequency sensorineural hearing loss. This is why in approximately 75% of acoustic tumors, high-frequency hearing loss is one of the first symptoms (Johnson, 1977).

Tinnitus is also a common symptom related to acoustic tumors. Reports indicate that over 80% of the individuals with this disorder present with tinnitus. This may be from pressure exerted on the AN or from a lack of an adequate blood supply to the cochlea. Tumors that originate in the IAM can grow and exert pressure on the auditory, vestibular, and facial nerves before they erode the bone of the IAM or grow into the CPA, where there is considerably more space to

accommodate the tumor. Some tumors may originate near or in the CPA and may affect the nerves in the IAM minimally (Johnson, 1977; House and Luetje, 1979). Meningiomas, another type of tumor, can grow into the CPA and mimic a true vestibular schwannoma.

Eighth nerve tumors in the IAM can disrupt the AN by slowing or even stopping the impulses that travel along the axon. Slowing of the impulses can delay or desynchronize the auditory brainstem response (ABR), which results in abnormal findings on this test. The ABR is abnormal in about 90% of acoustic tumors (see Selters and Brackmann, 1977 and Durrant and Ferraro, 1999 for reviews). This or similar pathophysiology can result in poor speech recognition abilities and elevated or absent acoustic reflexes. Although acoustic tumors are the most significant disorder of the AN, vascular and viral lesions can also result in dysfunction of the AN (Moller, 2000) (see Figure 7.7).

The best audiological procedure for the detection of acoustic tumors is the ABR. The ABR is usually abnormal because of increased latency between waves I and III or between waves I and V (i.e., the wave I–III and the I–V interwave intervals, respectively). However, often because of the presence of a hearing loss, these waves may not be obtainable, and in these cases a comparison of the latencies between wave V for the left and right ears, referred to as the interaural latency

(continued)

● **Figure 7.7**

Diagnostic test results for a middle-aged patient
with a left-sided acoustic neuroma. (a) Pure
tone and speech audiometry. (b) Distortion
product otoacoustic emissions, right and
left ears, with L1 and L2 = 70 dB SPL.
(c) Auditory brainstem response results using
a low rate, 80 dB nHL click, and 100 to 3000 Hz
filter band. (d) Radiology showing a large
CPA lesion.

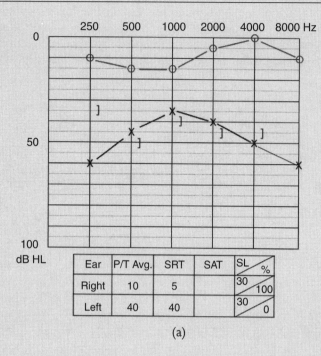

Ear	P/T Avg.	SRT	SAT	SL %
Right	10	5		30 / 100
Left	40	40		30 / 0

(a)

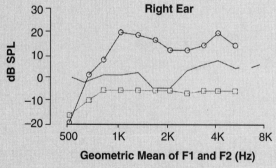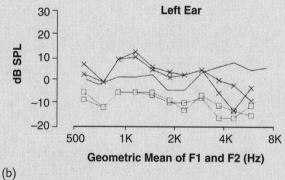

(b)

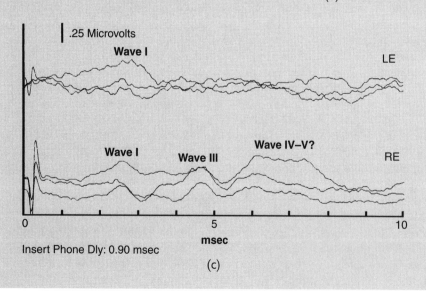

Insert Phone Dly: 0.90 msec

(c)

(continued)

Figure 7.7

(Continued)

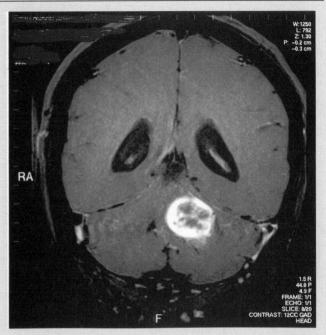

(d)

difference (ILD), is valuable. In cases where hearing is good, it is often possible to obtain a wave I because the tumors are generally located medially to the region of the AN that generates wave I (Musiek, McCormick, and Hurley, 1996).

Large tumors of the CPA often result in abnormal ABRs being obtained from the ear opposite the lesion. In these instances, the ABR generally shows an extended III–V interwave interval in the "unaffected" ear. This is probably the result of the brainstem being compressed and displaced by the large tumor, yielding "brainstem" findings on the ABR (Musiek and Kibbe, 1986). There has

been some concern about the ABR test procedure missing small (<1 cm) intracanicular tumors (Chandrasekhar, Brackmann, and Devgan, 1995). People with these small tumors usually have few symptoms and relatively good hearing. To counter the concerns about the ABR missing small tumors, a new technique called the "stacked ABR" has been introduced. Preliminary reports indicate that this new form of ABR may be more sensitive to small tumors than the traditional ABR procedure (Don, Masuda, Nelson, and Brackmann, 1997). However, it is too early to know if this ABR procedure will be adopted for routine clinical use. ●

CLINICAL CORRELATE

Auditory neuropathy (also termed **auditory dyssynchrony**) has become a popular term recently (see Starr, Sininger, and Pratt, 2000). This term has led to some confusion in that auditory neuropathy infers that the AN is the site of the disorder, which should be the case if the term is applied appropriately. However, it seems that in many instances where patients have been given this diagnosis, auditory neuropathy may not be

the underlying etiology or the condition may coexist with another disorder. The audiological indicators of auditory dyssynchrony are poor ABRs, presence of a cochlear microphonic, abnormal acoustic reflexes, abnormal masking level differences (MLDs), poor speech recognition scores, normal otoacoustic emissions (OAEs), and highly variable pure-tone thresholds (Starr et al., 2000). These audiological findings, however, can

(continued)

● **Figure 7.8**

Test results for a young adult with a diagnosis of auditory neuropathy bilaterally. This patient suffered bilateral facial nerve palsy of unknown etiology. Approximately 1 month after the facial nerve involvement (facial function eventually recovered) the patient noted decreased hearing, which progressed rapidly over the next few weeks to the point where conversational speech could not be understood. Despite various medical interventions, this patient's hearing did not improve. Radiological exams including computed tomography and magnetic resonance imaging were normal. (a) The pure tone thresholds revealed an unusual low-frequency sensorineural hearing loss bilaterally. Speech recognition scores were very poor for the left ear and fair for the right ear (lower left on audiogram). Ipsilateral and contralateral acoustic reflexes were absent bilaterally for frequencies 500, 1000, and 2000 Hz. Tympanograms were normal bilaterally (b, c). Transient otoacoustic emissions were essentially normal bilaterally. (d) The auditory brainstem response was absent for both ears.

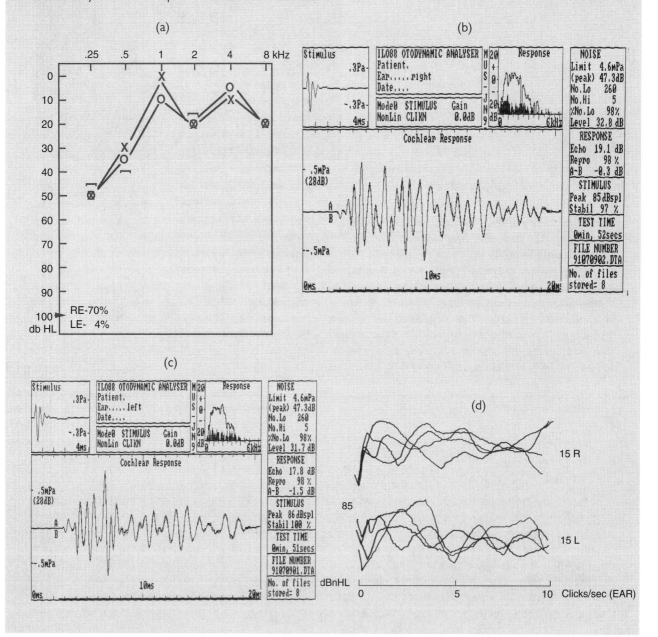

(continued)

also result from abnormalities of the inner hair cells, (low) brainstem pathology or dysfunction, and other AN disorders (Starr, Picton, Sininger, Hood, and Berlin, 1996). Therefore, the diagnosis of auditory neuropathy (dyssynchrony) needs to be carefully pursued while entertaining the possibility of true CANS disorders, such as low brainstem pathology, as well as peripheral disorders such as IHC damage. It may be more appropriate to not make the diagnosis of auditory neuropathy unless the ABR is totally absent. The finding of an absent ABR should occur in concert with clinical findings of absent or abnormal acoustic reflexes and normal OAEs, and if MLD and speech recognition scores can be obtained (older children and adults), these measures should also be abnormal. Careful analysis of test findings and knowledge of auditory pathology is critical to making this diagnosis.

For example, a condition that often is misdiagnosed as auditory neuropathy is that of **hyperbilirubinemia** (or kernicterus in the pathological condition). High bilirubin levels affect the nuclei within the CANS, with the cochlear nucleus especially involved in humans. The AN is not a primary site of this disorder, yet many cases of hyperbilirubinemia are reported as auditory dyssynchrony or neuropathy. There is evidence of the AN being involved in animals with hyperbilirubinemia, but not necessarily in isolation (Nehlig and Vert, 1997) (Figure 7.8).

We share many of the views published by Rapin and Gravel (2003) in regard to auditory neuropathy. These authors relate the following: the term *auditory neuropathy* should be limited to pathology that involves the spiral ganglion cells or axons and their related functions. This condition is an infrequent disorder—likely far less frequent than what is being reported in the literature. The term *auditory neuropathy* should not be used for disorders affecting the brainstem, higher auditory structures, or inner hair cells. It also should not be used for disorders of mixed or uncertain locations in the auditory system. Loose usage of the term only leads to confusion and may compromise proper management of infants and other patients who present with auditory disorders that on the surface may appear to be auditory neuropathy but are in fact related to some other underlying etiology. ●

The anatomy of the AN can be affected by a lack of input from the cochlea, such as in cases of considerable sensorineural hearing loss. In a study of cats, Niparko (1999) demonstrated that induced sensorineural loss altered the fine structure of the AN. Specifically, a subpopulation of AN fibers showed changes in the nerve endings (end bulbs), with smaller terminal swelling and more dendritic branching being noted. Smaller AN nerve dimensions have also been reported in humans who had severe hearing loss (Maxwell, Mason, and O'Donoghue, 1999; Furuta, Ogura, Higano, Takahashi, and Kawase, 2000). Another recent study showed that the IAM in patients with congenital hearing loss was significantly smaller than the IAM in a control group when both groups were evaluated by computed tomography (Fatterpekar, Mukherji, Alley, Lin, and Castillo, 2000). Although the results from the latter study may not be the direct result of lack of input from the cochlea, they do show how the AN or IAM could be affected embryologically. Clearly the collective findings of these reports demonstrate that appropriate presurgical considerations should be entertained before intervention is undertaken for specialized surgical procedures (e.g., cochlear implantation) where the structure and function of the AN are important for success.

PHYSIOLOGY OF THE AUDITORY NERVE

Fundamental Considerations

It should be understood that most of our knowledge about the function of the AN is a result of measurements and recordings from type I fibers. Little is known about type II fibers because they are difficult to locate and to record from with any degree of accuracy. Near- and far-field recordings have been made from the fibers of the AN in animals and humans. The key topics in the function of the AN (as is the case with other auditory structures) center around the frequency, intensity, and temporal coding of acoustic stimuli within this structure. Information on how various AN fibers fire and what constitutes their unique response properties is also of import. Frequency, intensity, and temporal coding is the manner through which approximately 30,000 AN fibers preserve the responses to sound in the cochlea and pass them on to the brainstem for more analysis and processing. Patterns of electrical impulses set up an information stream that is utilized throughout the CANS. Information from these patterns of nerve impulses are studied from single unit recordings and from procedures where hundreds or thousands of fibers firing at similar and sometimes not so similar times are measured (e.g., ABR). Single nerve unit recordings often include firing rates measured over the time period for which the acoustic stimulus is applied. When this type of information is plotted, it provides an "envelope of activity" called a **poststimulus time histogram (PSTH)**. When recordings are made from the AN that reflect large numbers of fibers firing synchronously (i.e., a number of action potentials) at nearly the same time, an **evoked potential** (EP) can be recorded. EPs can be recorded from near- or far-field approaches. Poststimulatory time histograms and EPs will be discussed in greater detail in the following sections of this chapter. A variety of other recordings are used in auditory neurophysiology, with most of them specific to acquiring information about the frequency, intensity, or temporal coding of information within the AN.

The threshold (related to hearing) of the AN is determined by an increase in activity or firing rate above its spontaneous rate that is coincident with the presentation of an acoustic stimulus. This increase above the spontaneous rate is related to the sensitivity of the nerve and to two cochlear functions. These cochlear functions are basilar membrane (BM) displacement and velocity (Ruggero, Narayan, Temchin, and Recio, 2000). The displacement of the BM and the velocity of this displacement determine the threshold for AN fibers.

Frequency Coding of Tones

Perhaps a good starting point in discussing frequency coding of the AN is to mention the term **characteristic frequency** (CF). Auditory nerve fibers each respond best to a particular frequency. This frequency is termed the CF and is usually determined by the frequency for which a given AN fiber's threshold is the lowest. For example, if an AN fiber was stimulated by a variety of tones of various frequencies, the frequency that yielded the lowest threshold would be the CF. It should be understood that this particular nerve fiber responds to tones of other frequencies, but these frequencies have to be presented at higher intensity levels for the neuron to respond. Generally, the further away in frequency from the CF the stimulating tone is, the greater the intensity level required for the fiber to fire or respond. If the intensity level for a threshold response of an AN fiber is plotted for different frequencies, a **tuning curve** (TC) is the result (Figure 7.9). Different fibers may have differing TCs, while some may have very similar TCs (see Pickles, 1988; Gelfand, 1998; and Moller, 2000 for reviews).

Fibers that have low CFs usually have broad TCs, while nerve fibers that have high CFs have TCs that are quite asymmetric with steep high-frequency sides and less steep low-frequency sides (Liberman and Mulroy, 1982; Moller, 2000). It should be remembered that TCs are usually plotted on a log scale for frequency.

● Figure 7.9

(a) Sharp and (b) broad tuning curves (TCs) similar to those that might be seen if recorded from the auditory nerve. The sharp TC is generally associated with high characteristic frequencies, whereas the broader TC is associated with low characteristic frequencies (or in some cases damage to the cochlea or auditory nerve itself). The sharpness of a TC is related by its Q10 value. This value is derived by measuring the bandwidth at 10 dB (indicated by the solid arrow) from the peak (shown by the dotted arrow) and dividing it into the center frequency. The higher the Q10 number, the sharper the TC. For example, if the TC in (a) was at 1000 Hz and its bandwidth was 150 Hz, the Q10 value would be 6.67. If the TC in (b) also had a center frequency of 1000 Hz but its bandwidth was greater, say 200 Hz, then the Q10 would be 5.0—a lower number, meaning that this TC is broader than the TC in (a) (Gelfand, 1998, pp. 150–151).

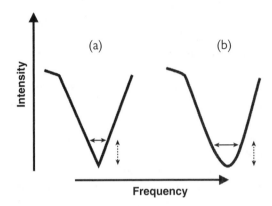

Using this kind of scale, TCs at high frequencies are going to look narrow and sharp compared to those noted for low frequencies. Because of this fact and because a variety of TCs can be recorded from the AN (as well as all of the CANS), there needs to be a way to measure and classify the sharpness or broadness of the TC. This has been accomplished by a ratio measurement that denotes the sharpness of a TC, that is, the Q10 ratio. The Q refers to the ratio of the CF to the bandwidth of the TC, and the 10 to the location within the TC where the ratio measurement is taken. It has been standard practice to measure 10 dB down from the peak amplitude to derive an indication of the sharpness of the TC; hence, the use of Q10 (Gelfand, 1998; Pickles, 1988) (Figure 7.9). A cochlear frequency map can be constructed by plotting the CFs of AN fibers from the basal-most to apical-most part of the BM (Liberman, 1982). When this is done, there is a uniform progression for AN fibers from high to low CFs.

The sharpness of an AN's TC is dependent on the health of the OHCs. Damage to the OHCs raises the threshold of the TC and rounds the tip of the TC (see Harrison, 1981, 2001).

Frequency is coded in two ways. One way has to do with the location along the BM where maximal displacement of the membrane occurs (after von Bekesy). This provides for the AN fiber(s) to be connected to hair cells at a particular place on the BM, and the particular place represents a unique range of frequencies. The basal area of the BM represents high-frequency sounds, while lower frequencies are coded in the apical portion of this membrane. The other mode of coding is more of a temporal coding related to the firing rate of the AN and its phase-locking ability. These two coding processes may work in parallel to provide an accurate coding of frequency (Evans, 1978).

The place coding (sometimes referred to as place-rate coding) mechanism indicates that AN fibers at a particular spatial location along the BM provide maximum firing at that point. Frequency selectivity is controlled by the fact that each afferent AN fiber (or fibers) is connected to only one IHC. This means small vibrations on the BM in the area of a hair cell can result in a differential firing response between this cell and adjacent cells, resulting in finely tuned frequency coding within the cochlea and its associated AN fiber or fibers (Evans, 1978; Kim and Parham, 1997; Moller, 2000). This frequency selectivity is secondary to BM tuning that is related to the biological amplifier that provides sharpening of the response (see previous chapter). This is also related to the CF of the AN fiber.

Temporal frequency coding is not well understood. This kind of frequency coding probably works in parallel with place-rate coding. Key to temporal coding for frequency is the phenomenon of phase-locking. Phase-locking is the time locking of neural discharges to the acoustic waveform (see Hind, 1972; Kim and Parham, 1997; Moller, 2000). The phase-locking of the AN to the acoustic waveform generally involves a particular place on the waveform, such as the compression or rarefaction phase of the signal (see Figure 7.10).

One of the key questions surrounding phase-locking related to coding frequency is whether the nerve fibers can fire rapidly enough to represent each stimulus waveform—even at high frequencies. The answer to this question is dependent on several factors. First is the ability of the neuron to fire rapidly. AN fibers have higher discharge rates than more rostral structures in the auditory pathway; therefore, at the AN level, phase-locking is more prominent than it is in most other regions of the CANS (Eggermont, 1993; Moller, 2000). As Moller and others have reported, there is evidence of some AN fibers phase-locking for tones up to almost 5000 Hz (Johnson, 1978). However, there is fairly good agreement that most AN fibers can only fire at a maximum rate of about 800 times per second (Pickles, 1988).

● **Figure 7.10**

Two sine waves. The arrows on both sine waves show where on the wave the neuron may phase-lock. The upper sine wave represents a low-frequency signal where the auditory nerve locks on every cycle. The lower sine wave is of a higher frequency, and the nerve fiber can only lock onto every other cycle, but a second nerve fiber locks onto the cycles missed by the first so that the summation of the firings of fibers one and two (the total response) captures the frequency of the high-frequency sine wave. This is could be viewed as a representation of the classic volley principle.

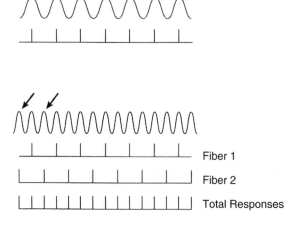

Therefore, for high-frequency sounds it is unlikely that many (if any) AN fibers fire for every cycle of the stimulus. It has been observed that for frequencies above 1000 Hz, phase-locking of AN fibers definitely takes place but deteriorates markedly, with only some fibers responding in this manner (Hind, 1972; Johnson, 1978).

In the case of high-frequency sounds, the AN fibers may fire on every second, third, or fourth cycle of the sound stimulus, while other AN fibers are recruited to lock onto the cycles that are not locked onto by the initial fiber(s). In this manner frequency coding is maintained at the high frequencies (Johnson, 1978). This concept of temporal coding at the high frequencies is related to the well-known **volley principle** of hearing. Simply stated, the volley principle is when a single nerve fiber reaches it frequency limit (firing rate) and another nerve fiber is recruited into action. These two fibers, firing alternately, increase the response rate markedly. Once the second fiber reaches it limit, another fiber is recruited, and so on. Therefore, although one AN fiber may not be able to phase-lock on every cycle of the acoustic stimulus, multiple nerve fibers, if the timing is appropriate, can do so (up to 4000 to 5000 Hz) (see Moller, 2000 and Hanekom and Kruger, 2001 for reviews). Therefore, on an individual basis, AN fibers have more of a limitation for frequency coding than do multiple AN fibers working together. Moreover, the temporal coding process combined with place coding for frequency at the AN level provides a capable basis for the perception of a wide range of frequencies.

Frequency discrimination at the AN level can be potentially expressed by the CF of each nerve fiber (related to place), as well as the firing rate of the fiber. Therefore, the physiologic perception of a frequency change or difference can be related to slight differences in the CFs and firing rates of AN fibers involved in the coding of the acoustic stimuli. That is, both the place and rate code contribute to frequency discrimination, as has been demonstrated by Kim and Parham (1991).

Frequency Coding of Complex Sounds

The frequency coding of complex sounds utilizes the same mechanisms that are applied to pure tones as long as these complex stimuli have periodic or quasiperiodic elements (see Moller, 2000 for in-depth review). Both place and temporal coding of frequency are evident for complex sound stimuli such as speech. For example, consider vowel formats. From a place coding perspective, the BM (and hair cells) can provide selectivity of each of the formats by providing a major deflection at the frequency location of each format. In other words, there would be three areas of maximum deflection along the BM, corresponding to the vowel formats. It then stands to reason that each vowel format has a different set of AN fibers that are phase-locked onto the periodicity of the vowel format.

Two-Tone Inhibition

A phenomenon related to the coding of complex stimuli at the AN level is **two-tone inhibition,** or as it is sometimes called, **two-tone suppression**. This phenomenon is probably a factor in many instances of multiple and complex stimuli actions at the AN level. The following commentary is based on only a few accounts of the many studies performed on this phenomenon (Sachs and Kiang, 1968; Gelfand, 1998; Moller, 2000). For two-tone inhibition to take place, two tones must be presented at the same time. When the two tones are presented, interaction between the tones can take place. This interaction is such that a response from an AN fiber to one tone can be inhibited by the presentation of a second tone if the second tone is within a certain frequency range of the first tone. This range of frequencies represents an inhibitory area of frequencies. These inhibitory areas are usually located on each side of the AN fiber's response area. The extent of a fiber's response area and how it changes in the presence of a second tone has been studied extensively but will not be covered here. The two-tone inhibition phenomenon is well demonstrated at the AN level but probably reflects a true cochlear or preneural action rather than an AN-mediated response (see Gelfand, 1998 for discussion).

The Effect of Intensity on Frequency Coding

Frequency tuning at the AN is dependent on the frequency tuning of the BM and the intensity of the stimulus (de Boer, 1983; Moller, 1983, 2000). At low and moderate intensities, the TCs of the BM and the AN are sharp and similar in form. As the intensity of the stimulus approaches high levels, the sharpness of AN tuning curves tends to be compromised. The broad tuning of the AN at high intensities reflects the less specific tuning at the BM. Moreover, the poorer tuning at the high intensities suggests that the OHCs (cochlear amplifier) do not play as much of a role in fine tuning the cochlear response at higher intensities as they do at lower intensities; hence, less sharpening of the response is seen (see previous chapter). The behavioral correlate to this is that frequency selectivity is not as good at high intensities as it is at low intensities (see Sellick, Ptuzzi, and Johnstone, 1982 and Yost, 2000 for reviews).

The widening of the AN's TCs can also be created by physiological damage to either the OHCs (which affects the biological amplifier) or the AN fibers themselves. Hence, frequency discrimination can be compromised by either cochlear damage or AN damage (Thompson and Abel, 1992; Moller, 2000). This same phenomenon of widened areas of frequency selectivity also negatively impacts the processing of individual speech segments, resulting in poorer speech recognition and discrimination abilities.

Intensity Coding

In this section several aspects of the physiology of how the AN behaves over the wide range of intensities will be discussed. One of the first aspects of intensity coding is the **spontaneous firing rate** of the AN. Kim and Parham (1991) showed a variety of spontaneous rates (SRs) in the AN fibers of the cat (see also Kim and Parham, 1997). A large portion of AN fibers have SRs that are less than 10 per second, but some fibers have SRs of about 100 per second. Liberman (1978) divided AN fibers into three categories on the basis of firing rates (spikes per second): low (0 to 0.5), medium (0.5 to 18), and high (> 18). It is informative to observe how AN fibers with various SRs react to tonal stimuli at different frequencies and intensities (see Kim and Parham, 1997 for review). Plotting discharge rates for a 1000-Hz tone, Kim and Parham (1991) showed a more specific response (from fibers firing in the 1-kHz area) for lower-intensity sounds than for high-intensity sounds for both low- and high-SR fibers. However, the low-SR fibers demonstrated more frequency-specific responses than did the high-SR fibers at both low and high intensities. In this same study Kim and Parham used a 5000-Hz tone stimulus to show a more robust response for high-SR fibers compared to-low SR fibers for low intensities (30 dB sound pressure level). At a mid-intensity level, low- and high-SR fibers showed similar responses for firing rate and frequency specificity, whereas at high-intensity levels the high-SR fibers began to show some nonlinearities, but the low-SR fibers did not. Additional aspects of this study indicated that high-SR fibers responded better for low intensities than did the low-SR fibers. Further, in regard to (fiber) threshold measures (across CFs) it appeared that high-SR fibers had a lower threshold than low-SR fibers.

CLINICAL CORRELATE

It is interesting to entertain the idea of auditory deprivation in regard to spontaneous firing rates of the AN and neurons at higher centers within the CANS. The common thinking is that if a neuron (or groups of neurons) is not stimulated, it will become nonfunctional. Obviously the clinician is concerned that hearing loss in the auditory periphery may preclude stimulation of the neurons in the AN or in the higher centers of the auditory system. For example, reports have documented how speech recognition scores from individuals with long-standing hearing loss improve after the use of amplification, thus implicating the importance of stimulation on the optimal functioning of the auditory system (Silman, Gelfand, and Silverman, 1984). On the other hand, electrophysiological studies on children with long-standing otitis media have revealed delayed latencies on the ABR years after the middle ear condition has resolved. This was presumably related to the deprivation effects caused by the hearing loss associated with the otitis media (Gunnarson and Finitzo, 1991). However, if there is spontaneous activity of neurons without stimulation (Evans, 1972), then it would appear that these neurons should stay viable. That is, the metabolism of the nerve cell should still be working in terms of keeping the cell healthy even in the face of no direct stimulation; hence, no degeneration or deterioration of function should be noted. This thinking could be applied to not only the AN, but also to brainstem neurons and possibility auditory subcortex and cortical fibers.

Obviously many questions enter into this issue of deprivation and the spontaneous activity of neurons.

One major question is whether the neuron that is deprived of acoustic input will lose the response properties that allow it to code the stimulus—even though it may retain its spontaneous activity. For example, perhaps the neuron loses its full dynamic range for intensity. Another question is that perhaps spontaneous activity doesn't guarantee that the nerve cell is viable for stimulation. Is spontaneous activity only present in an intact system? It appears that the spontaneous activity of a nerve fiber deprived of input will be reduced (see Harrison, 2001 for discussion). Therefore, there are some effects of a damaged system or deprivation on neurons of the AN and the CANS. These effects are complex and may vary as to the nature of the deprivation (damage to the nerve or cochlea versus sound deprivation in the environment, the age of the individual experiencing the deprivation, the duration of the deprivation, etc.). We do know that nerve fiber atrophy is linked to lack of auditory input. Therefore, clinically it is of great importance to be sure that auditory deprivation does not occur. Although it appears that spontaneous nerve activity may be present in cases of reduced input, associated metabolic changes will, in time, cause atrophy of these fibers. Total lack of input, such as in ablation of the cochlea, would stop neurotransmission and likely stop spontaneous activity in the AN (Harrison, 2001). However, even this situation is not totally clear. There has been some discussion that even in cases of ablation (of the cochlea) there may still be some spontaneous activity in the AN, although current evidence is definitely against this view (see Geisler, 1998 for discussion). ●

It is well known that the intensity range of human hearing is approximately 110 to 120 dB. This is a large range of intensities, especially when one considers that the relationship between sound pressure level and firing rate of the AN fiber(s) is close to linear (Hudspeth, 2000). Therefore, at high intensities the AN fibers become saturated. Fibers with high SRs may have response thresholds that are in the neighborhood of 0 dB SPL at their CFs. This kind of AN fiber often saturates at moderate intensities (around 40 dB SPL). There are, however, other AN fibers that

● **Figure 7.11**

Examples of low-intensity (high spontaneous rate) and high-intensity (low spontaneous rate) auditory nerve fiber firing rates by level contours (see text). The low-intensity fiber begins to respond at low intensities (at or near threshold) and reaches saturation at around 40 dB SPL. The high-intensity fiber initiates responses at the mid-intensity range and continues to respond at high levels. Hence, between these two auditory nerve neurons a wide intensity range is coded.

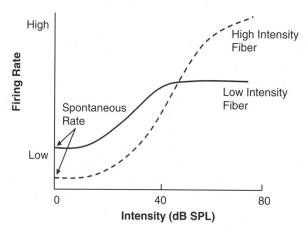

have lower SRs, much higher thresholds, and the ability to provide graded responses for intensities up to 100 dB or greater (Liberman, 1978; Hudspeth, 2000). These high- and low-intensity fibers can set up an orchestrated manner of coding intensities over a large range. As the low-intensity neurons respond at low intensities and saturate at moderate intensities, the high-intensity fibers begin to respond at moderate intensities and do not saturate until the high intensities are reached. This arrangement not only allows the coding of intensity over a wide dynamic range, but also provides a basis for differential intensity coding (Palmer and Evans, 1982) (see Figure 7.11).

Firing Pattern and Adaptation

The AN fibers have a relatively distinct firing pattern as shown by their PSTHs. For normal fibers, there is a strong response at the beginning of the stimulus, followed by an attenuation of the response for a period of time, and then a response plateau over the adaptation period. During the adaptation period there is a slight decrease in firing over time. When the stimulus is turned off, there is a transitory period before the complete cessation of activity occurs (Kiang, Watanabe, Thomas, and Clark, 1965). The envelope of activity is often referred to as a primary-like PSTH (see Figure 7.12).

Adaptation of the AN's is a phenomenon that has received much interest from both the basic and clinical science communities. Adaptation is defined as the decrease in the amplitude of the AN action potential (AP) over time (during stimulus presentation) without a coincident change in the stimulus characteristics. As reviewed by Huss and Moore (2003), there is greater adaptation for high-frequency sounds than low-frequency sounds. Also, there is more signal decay or adaptation in individuals with hearing loss that is greater than 50 dB hearing level (HL) than for those with normal hearing or only mild degrees of hearing loss. After the termination of the acoustic stimulus, recovery from adaptation usually requires only a few seconds (see Keidel, Kallert, and Korth, 1983). Adaptation is a neural activity rather than a sensory response. This is demonstrated by the fact that during adaptation of the AN the CM does not change (Keidel et al., 1983). As shown in Figure 7.12, adaptation is reflected as a decrease in the height of a PSTH, that is, a decrease in the firing rate over time while the stimulus does not change (Moller, 1983). Nerve fibers from various loci in the auditory system have different adaptation rates. The AN fibers are considered to have little to a moderate degree of adaptation (Moller, 1983). However, the longer the continuous stimulation of the auditory system persists without a change in the stimulus characteristics, the greater the adaptation of the AN. The amount of adaptation is measured by noting the amount of change in the response characteristics over time. This concept has transitioned in the clinical domain of audiology with a procedure known as the tone decay test.

Evoked Potentials and the Auditory Nerve

The electrical potentials that are generated by the AN (and other areas of the auditory system) can be measured near or far field. Near-field recordings are obtained with the recording electrode on or very near the structure. Far-field recordings are obtained with the electrodes away from the

● **Figure 7.12**

Poststimulatory time histogram (PSTH) from an auditory nerve fiber to a tone burst. These are often referred to as primary-like responses. (A) The initial strong, abrupt, response to the wave front of the signal followed by quick attenuation. (B) The plateau part of the neural response followed by a transition phase to no activity.

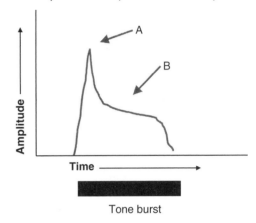

Tone burst

factors influenced the sensitivity of the tone decay test, such as size of the lesion, the method used, the degree of hearing loss, the age of the patient, and so on. Although the test was aimed at AN dysfunction, brainstem and cochlea pathologies also occasionally resulted in excessive decay—although infrequently. In the late 1970s and early 1980s the tone decay test was essentially replaced by the auditory brainstem response (ABR) test, which clearly had a better sensitivity and specificity for detecting acoustic tumors.

The underlying mechanism for tone decay is not clearly understood. It is fairly well accepted that abnormal adaptation is related to the inability of neural elements (auditory nerve) to fire continuously. Perhaps the most popular theory that attempted to explain the physiological mechanism underlying clinical tone decay was suggested by Davis (1962). Davis argued that tone decay could be explained by the Wedensky principle of peripheral nerve function. In essence, this principle related that if a nerve is damaged, the initial impulses will be conducted without problems, and even subsequent impulses will pass along the nerve as long as they are separated by enough time. However, if the impulses are continuous (as from a sustained stimulus), the nerve fiber will not recover sufficiently to respond to the stimulus, and as a result, will not carry the stimulus effectively. With a sustained stimulus, more and more fibers will fail until the system is incapable of maintaining a sufficient response to the stimulus to trigger perception of the stimulus. ●

generating structure. A popular example of a far-field recording is the contemporary clinical ABR, where the electrodes are attached to the scalp, but the EPs are generated by the AN and brainstem nuclei.

In regard to near-field recordings, there are monopolar and bipolar recordings. Monopolar recordings of the AN are conducted with one needle electrode placed directly on the AN (Figure 7.13). Bipolar recordings require an electrode with two tips, with one tip placed more peripherally than the other (Figure 7.13). The bipolar recordings require more area than the monopolar recordings and are difficult to obtain from small animals or whenever the recording field is small for any reason. Bipolar recordings are not only more difficult to obtain in many cases, but they also can be more challenging to interpret (Moller, 2000).

Monopolar recordings of the AN yield a triphasic waveform as described by Moller (2000). This triphasic waveform is propagated by a depolarization that moves along the nerve (Figure 7.14). As this depolarization approaches the area of the electrode site, a positive deflection occurs. As the response moves directly under the needle electrode, a negative deflection occurs, and as the depolarization passes this site, a somewhat weaker positive deflection ensues.

● **Figure 7.13**

Examples of electrode tips from monopolar (top) and bipolar electrodes (bottom) used in measuring responses from the auditory nerve during intraoperative monitoring.

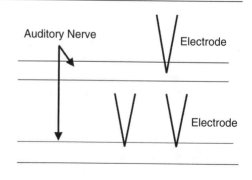

● Figure 7.14

A triphasic waveform that is commonly seen in monopolar recordings from the auditory nerve. When depolarization occurs in the region of the electrode, a positive deflection (A) results. As the depolarization moves under the electrode site a negative deflection (B) occurs, which is then followed by a shallow positive deflection (C) as the depolarization moves away.

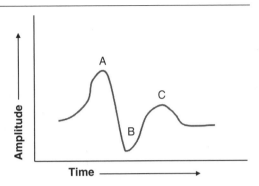

CLINICAL CORRELATE

A number of important clinical applications for EPs are derived from the AN both near- and far-field. Near-field recordings are used during neurosurgical procedures on humans to monitor the activity of the AN in an attempt to preserve hearing. Even with the removal of an acoustic tumor, hearing can often be saved. In other surgical procedures, such as a vestibular nerve section, it is important not to damage the AN. In both of these surgical situations, the monitoring of the neural response either near- or far-field plays a critical role (Moller, Jho, and Jannetta, 1994).

Another near-field, but not direct, recording of the AN includes recordings from the round window or promontory. Clinically, this is done in a procedure that is referred to as transtympanic electrocochleography (Ecog). A needle electrode is passed through the tympanic membrane to the promontory or near the round window of the cochlea. This allows enhanced recordings of the action potential (AP) of the AN but also permits the recording of the cochlear microphonic (CM) and the summating potential (SP). This Ecog technique is often clinically used in the diagnosis of endolymphatic hydrops (meniere's disease). The key measurement in patients with suspected hydrops is the SP/AP ratio. To compute the ratio, the amplitude of the SP is compared to the amplitude of the AN AP. In normal situations the SP is less than 50% of the amplitude of the AN AP. When the SP is greater than the AP,

it is consistent with a hydropic condition (see also previous chapter).

Electrocochleographic responses can also be recorded with electrodes placed on the eardrum (usually a cotton ball or sponge placed on the end of a wire) or deep in the ear canal (tiptrode). These latter two methods are clinically useable but do not provide the large or distinct recordings of the transtympanic approach (see Durrant and Ferraro, 1999).

The APs of the AN can also be recorded by the far-field method. In this situation, the APs recorded are waves I and II of the ABR. As Moller (1983) has demonstrated, waves I and II of the ABR are generated by the distal and proximal portions of the AN in humans.

The presence of wave II is not as consistent a finding as is the presence of wave I—even in normals, so it must be used with caution clinically (Musiek et al., 1996). However, when wave II is present at normal latencies, it is a good indicator that the AN is functioning. However, if wave II is absent, little can be said about the AN function since this wave is often not observed in normal individuals. Most acoustic tumors occur medial to the generator site of wave I. Therefore, unless there is considerable hearing loss, wave I can and should be observed in patients with acoustic tumors. Electrocochleographic methods can also be used to enhance readability of a small or absent wave I noted in ABR testing. ●

Latency–Intensity Functions

Whether recording AN potentials near- or far-field, there is an intensity effect on the latency of the AP. As the intensity of the stimulus increases, the latency of wave I

● **Figure 7.15**

An intensity–latency function for wave I (auditory nerve) of the ABR derived from the responses of an adult human.

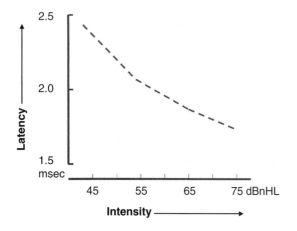

decreases. In the middle intensity range (about 40 to 75 dB nHL) a 10-dB increment results in approximately a 0.3 to 0.4 msec decrease in latency in the normal system (Figure 7.15). At low and high intensities the effect is not the same as the intensity–latency relationships become more nonlinear. The change in latency of the AN's EP is, of course, related primarily to the cochlear traveling wave time and not the response characteristics of the AN itself.

Ngan and May (2001) relate that there are high linear correlations between ABR thresholds and the thresholds for the most sensitive AN neurons. These investigators showed that the most sensitive AN fibers' thresholds were approximately 25 dB better than the ABR thresholds obtained from cats with normal hearing. However, for cats with hearing loss, the ABR and most sensitive AN fibers' thresholds were essentially equivalent. However, even though some differences were noted in the threshold measures for the most sensitive AN fibers and the ABR results between the two groups, there was a consistent linear relationship observed between these two measures when the results were analyzed across all of the animals in each group. In other words, those animals in each group with the "best" thresholds for the most sensitive AN fibers also had the "best" thresholds for the ABR measure, and as the thresholds of the AN fibers increased within a group, so did the threshold measures obtained for the ABR test.

Conduction Velocity of the Auditory Nerve

The conduction velocity of AN fibers can relate important information. Conduction velocity is related to the amount of myelin covering the axon; hence, the larger the diameter of the nerve, the more myelin. Moller and colleagues (Moller, Colletti, and Fiorino, 1994) have recorded neural conduction times in humans during neurosurgery to determine the velocity of impulses traveling down the AN. This measurement involved placing two electrodes 1 mm apart on an exposed part of the AN. Each electrode recorded an AP, and the time between the peaks of the two APs was measured and the velocity computed. The conduction velocity of the AN in humans was found to be about 20 m per second. In cats, the conduction velocity of the AN was slightly slower (11.6 m/sec) (Nguyen, Javel, and Levine, 1999).

Neurotransmitters

Relatively early work suggested that the key neurotransmitters of the AN are likely to be glutamate and aspartate. Wenthold (1978) performed several experiments to indicate that these excitatory neurotransmitters are active in the AN and have receptors in the cochlear nucleus. Perhaps the most striking was the decrease in glutamate and aspartate in the cochlear nucleus after cutting the AN. More recent data supports Wenthold's early work (see Romand and Avan, 1997 for review).

SUMMARY

The AN transmits acoustic information in the form of neural impulses from the cochlea to the brainstem. The AN is part of the eighth cranial nerve and is often referred to as a bottleneck in the auditory pathway because essentially all acoustic information passes through its neurons on the way to the brain. The AN fibers connect to the hair cells, course through the habenula perforata, form the modiolus, and proceed through the IAM to the lateral aspect of the pons. There are type I and type II fibers, with the type I connecting to IHCs and type II to the OHCs. Type I fibers make up about 90% of the total number of AN fibers. The AN trunk has high-frequency fibers on the outside, and low frequencies are present in the middle or core of the nerve. The tuning curves of the AN are sharp for high frequencies and broad for low frequencies. It has been shown that damage to the OHCs translates into broad tuning curves at the AN.

The AN fibers have a wide range of spontaneous firing rates. In general, AN fibers with low SRs respond better to moderate- and high-intensity sounds, whereas fibers with high SRs respond best to low-intensity or threshold-level sounds. Continuing with this idea, there are AN fibers that best respond to low intensities and saturate at moderate-intensity levels and others that only begin to respond at moderately high intensities and saturate at high levels. This allows a large dynamic range for coding intensity. Most AN fibers can time lock onto relatively high frequencies, which indicates good temporal coding. Two-tone inhibition can be well demonstrated at the AN, and adaptation studies have been extensive for the AN. Excessive adaptation to continuous acoustic stimulation has been linked to pathology at this site.

The AN contributes to waves I and II of the ABR and has been directly studied in humans during neurosurgical procedures. The AP from the AN follows a reasonably predictable latency–intensity function for low- to high-intensity stimuli. Acoustic tumors as well as auditory neuropathy (dyssynchrony) are two well-known disorders of the AN. Both can result in major compromise of hearing abilities and both can be well delineated by using contemporary diagnostic methods in audiology.

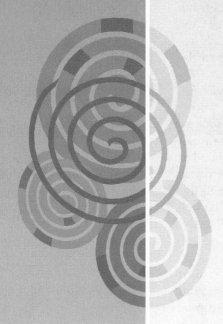

8

The First Central Auditory Structure: The Cochlear Nucleus

Introduction

The auditory nerve (AN), which was discussed in the previous chapter, is the final anatomical structure in the auditory periphery. The fibers of the AN project from the auditory periphery and connect to the first structure within the portion of the auditory system that is referred to as the central auditory nervous system (CANS). The initial and caudal-most neural complex of the CANS is the **cochlear nucleus** complex (CN). The CN is one of the most studied structures of the CANS both in animals and humans. In animals, the investigation of the CN represented a logical extension of the study of auditory function from the periphery of the afferent system to the central mechanisms. The CN was also reasonable to approach anatomically in the animal model. In humans, the recent development of cochlear implants with electrodes that are imbedded in the CN has resulted in additional advances in the understanding of the anatomy and physiology of the CN in man. In addition, surgical removal of acoustic tumors and other mass lesions of the cerebellopontine angle (CPA) have triggered the study of the CN and its surrounding area in humans. In this chapter the human model will be utilized as much as possible, but as will be the case in the rest of this book, reference to animal data will be made when necessary to establish a fundamental foundation for the understanding of the functional aspects of a particular CANS structure.

The CN is a structure that has many functional similarities to the AN. It must preserve the neural coding of auditory information that was performed initially in the AN, while at the same time enhancing or augmenting the processing of that signal at this level. The CN also sets the stage for processing of the neural representations of the acoustic signal at higher levels within the auditory system. Its precise and complex input to other auditory structures in the brainstem is critical if one is to hear and process accurately what is present in one's acoustic environment.

ANATOMY OF THE COCHLEAR NUCLEUS

General Aspects

The CN in humans is covered posteriorly by the cerebellum. In order to observe the CN, the cerebellum must be removed, which requires the sectioning of the greater cerebellar peduncles. Once these peduncles are cut and

● Figure 8.1

Posterior view of the human brainstem. 1 = area of the cochlear nucleus (dorsal portion) directly below the greater cerebellar peduncle, which has been sectioned (also shown laterally are the remnants of the eighth cranial nerve), 2 = fourth ventricle, 3 = inferior colliculus, 4 = superior colliculus, 5 = brachium of the inferior colliculus, 6 = medial geniculate, 7 = thalamus (pulvinar).

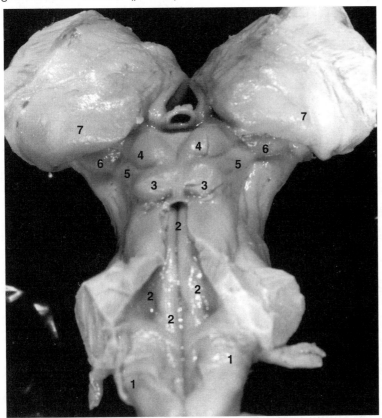

● Figure 8.2

Posterior view of the left half of the human brainstem. The right arrow is pointing to the area of the vestibular nuclei, which is seen in the lateral aspect of the fourth ventricle (IV). The left arrow is pointing to the dorsal cochlear nucleus.

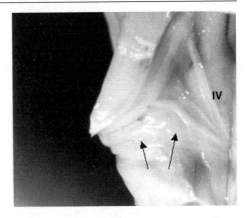

the cerebellum is removed, the CN can be viewed by looking at the postero-lateral aspect of the brainstem immediately beneath the sectioned peduncles (Figures 8.1, 8.2, and 8.3).

The location of the CN in humans is further defined by small tubercles that define the specific region within the brainstem at the level of the ponto-medullary junction where this structure is situated. The CN has three major subdivisions: the

● Figure 8.3

Two views of the upper medulla and pons focusing on the cochlear nucleus. (a) Right dorso-lateral view; (b) right ventro-lateral view. VIIIn = eighth nerve (entering the brainstem at the ponto-medullary junction), DCN = dorsal cochlear nucleus, VCN = ventral cochlear nucleus, icp = inferior cerebellar peduncle, mcp = middle cerebellar peduncle, scp = superior cerebellar peduncle, ms = medullary stria, ol = oliva, p = pons, vIV = fourth ventricle, Vn = fifth cranial nerve, IXn = ninth cranial nerve, vn = vestibular nuclei, d = dorsal, c = caudal, r = rostral, v = ventral (from Terr and Edgerton, 1985, with permission).

(a)

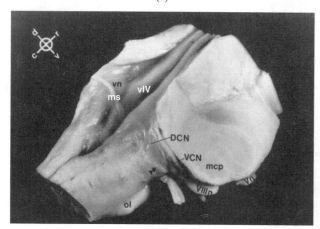

(b)

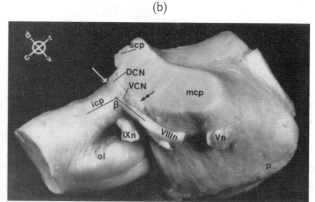

dorsal (DCN), the **posterior ventral** (PVCN), and the **anterior ventral** (AVCN) sections. Viewing the posterior (dorsal) aspect of the human brainstem, the DCN can be observed. A lateral view is required to observe the PVCN and AVCN (Musiek and Baran, 1986; Moller, 2000).

The CN courses along the margin of the postero-lateral aspect of the brainstem, immediately rostral to the ponto-medullary junction (Figure 8.3). The **fourth ventricle** is a large recess that is roughly diamond shaped in the middle of the brainstem, which is easily recognized from a posterior view. The lateral recess of the fourth ventricle at the level of the CN is bordered by the medial aspect of the DCN. The fourth ventricle is sandwiched between the anterior cerebellum and the posterior brainstem.

CLINICAL CORRELATE

Because of the anatomical relationship between the fourth ventricle and the CN (especially the DCN), hydrocephalus occurring here can affect hearing function. Expansion of the fourth ventricle secondary to hydrocephalus can compress the CN as well as the dorsal acoustic stria and possibly the intermediate acoustic stria, both of which course ventrally to the fourth ventricle. The close anatomical relationship among the fourth ventricle and these CN structures may be the reason why hydrocephalus and mass lesions of the fourth ventricle often result in abnormal auditory brainstem responses (ABRs) as well as depressed results for other tests of auditory function that are relevant to this anatomical area (Kraus, Ozdamar, Heydemann, Stein, and Reed, 1984; Donnelly, 1992). In a study of 40 patients with hydrocephalus, Donnelly (1992) found that 88% of the patients had abnormal ABR results—with 25% of the subjects demonstrating no readable ABRs. Hydrocephalus not only can influence the latencies of the ABR waves, but it can also elevate the estimated audiometric thresholds assessed via ABRs. As is the case in other neurologic abnormalities of the brainstem, the ABR procedure may not provide a valid estimate of hearing sensitivity in cases with compromise of the CANS because of the lack of integrity of the neural structures (in this case, the CN) that generate the ABR. However, the procedure, although not always reliable for assessing threshold or hearing sensitivity, is highly reliable for assessing neurologic compromise at this level of the CANS. The pathological mechanisms that may underlie abnormal ABRs in hydrocephalus include increased intracranial pressure, ischemia, and morphological abnormalities that occur secondarily to the build-up of excessive spinal fluid (Donnelly, 1992). ●

● **Figure 8.4**

Transverse section of the cochlear nucleus of the chinchilla. DCN = dorsal cochlear nucleus, PVCN = posterior ventral cochlear nucleus, AVCN = anterior ventral cochlear nucleus (dorsal-most aspect), D = dorsal, L = lateral (courtesy of Tony Sahley).

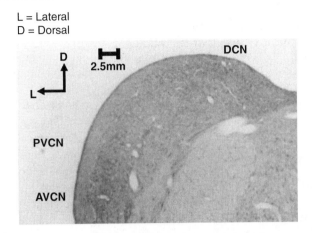

L = Lateral
D = Dorsal

In humans the CN is about 3 mm in length in the rostral to caudal plane, 10 mm in length in the medial to lateral plane, and 8 mm in length in the ventral to lateral plane. These dimensions are considerably larger than those noted in the cat, which measure about 4 mm in all three planes (Moore, 1987; Klose and Sollmann, 2000). This size difference reminds one that there are human–animal differences that must be kept in mind if animal models are used to predict or study similar structures in humans (Figure 8.4).

Inputs to the Cochlear Nucleus

The AN courses laterally to medially as it leaves the cochlea and heads toward the CN in the brainstem, where it enters a region situated between the pons and the medulla. Immediately after entering the lower brainstem, the AN bifurcates into two major fiber bundles, which then connect to various portions of the CN. One branch of the bifurcated bundle travels to the anterior portion of the CN in a region referred to as the AVCN, while fibers from the second branch travel more posteriorly, and they synapse and pass on to the PVCN along their course to the dorsal cochlear nucleus (DCN) (Figure 8.5).

● **Figure 8.5**

Transverse view of the cochlear nucleus showing the auditory nerve entry and its three main branches.

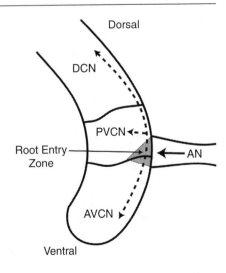

CLINICAL CORRELATE

The root entry zone creates some potential difficulty in differentiating peripheral from central involvement, at least on a clinical basis. The root entry zone is actually a peripheral nerve, but it is located within a central structure—the CN. Therefore, it seems likely that if the CN is damaged in the area of the root entry zone, the AN could also be damaged. It is difficult to say if this type of fine differential between the central and peripheral auditory systems would make a difference clinically; however, this concept should be kept in mind as one might speculate that in cases of **hyperbilirubinemia**, which is known to damage the CN but probably not the AN in humans (Dublin, 1976), the AN could be damaged at the root entry zone because of retrograde degeneration secondary to the insult to the CN. This speculation needs to be studied further to determine if the AN is involved in cases of hyperbilirubinemia, and if so, what are the specific mechanisms involved. The possibility of secondary damage to the AN in the root entry zone is an interesting and highly plausible theory—one that is deserving of investigative attention. Many individuals with histories of hyperbilirubinemia have auditory deficits that are frequently diganosed as auditory neuropathy (this diagnosis implies a peripheral basis for the hearing deficits). Currently, however, the term *auditory neuropathy* is often applied to a variety of hearing disorders, many of which involve or may involve central sites and mechanisms. A more restricted use of the term should be adapted by clincians, reserving it for cases where only the AN or spiral ganglion cells are compromised (see Rapin and Gravel, 2003). ●

There is **a root entry zone** where the AN fibers project relatively deeply into the CN. In small animals this corresponds to the area bordered by the PVCN and AVCN (Roullier, 1997).

Two types of AN fibers (type I and II fibers) project to the CN. The AN fibers project to all parts of the CN in an organized manner. The type I fibers, originating from the inner hair cells, make up approximately 90% of all AN fibers that project to the CN. These fibers are generally well myelinated (Romand and Avan, 1997) (see previous chapter). The type II fibers are thin, mostly unmyelinated fibers, which account for about 10% of the AN fibers. These fibers have connections that are probably of significant importance (Hurd, Hutson, and Morest, 1999). In chinchillas, these fine type II fibers project to the edge of granule cell regions of the CN as well as to small cell clusters and synaptic nests of stellate cells in the CN (Benson and Brown, 2004; Hurd et al., 1999). In smaller animals, the type I and II fibers run a simliar course projecting to various regions of the CN (Brown, Berglund, Kiang, and Ryugo, 1988).

There are also intrinsic connections in the CN, indicating that a tight neural communication network exists within this structure. These connections were described by Lorente de No in 1976 and include connections coursing from the VCN to the DCN, as well as from the DCN to the VCN. Ostapoff, Morest, and Parham (1999) showed that most of the cells projecting from the AVCN to the DCN are stellate and giant cells, which are two of the many cell types found in the CN. The fiber bundle that connects the AVCN and DCN has been termed the ventro-tubercular tract. This pathway is gaining in its anatomical significance as an important structure for communication between the ventral (VCN) and dorsal segments (DCN) of the CN.

Cell Types

The CN has a number of different cell types (Pfeiffer, 1966). The work by Osen (1969) has shown that different cell types have distinct locations within the CN (see Cant, 1992 for review). The spherical bushy cells are located in the anterior portion of the AVCN, while globular bushy and multipolar (stellate) cells are located in the posterior part of this segment of the VCN. In the PVCN one can find multipolar, granular (small cells), giant, and octopus cells, whereas in the DCN, small, giant, granular, and pyramidal (fusiform) cells can be found (Figure 8.6).

● **Figure 8.6**

Transverse view of the cochlear nucleus
showing the approximate location
of the various cell types.

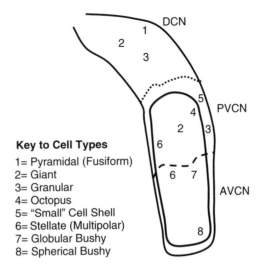

Key to Cell Types
1= Pyramidal (Fusiform)
2= Giant
3= Granular
4= Octopus
5= "Small" Cell Shell
6= Stellate (Multipolar)
7= Globular Bushy
8= Spherical Bushy

PHYSIOLOGY OF THE COCHLEAR NUCLEUS

Acoustic Responses of Cell Types

The early work by Pfeiffer (1966) and Osen (1969), as well as more recent reviews
by Roullier (1997) and Rhode (1991), have articulated the differential temporal response patterns associated with the various cell types in the CN. The different cell
types in the CN provide different types of output patterns known as **poststimulus
time histograms** (PSTHs), which provide the input to higher auditory structures
in the brainstem. These differences in the PSTHs associated with the various cell
types are presumed to be related to differences in the structures or functions of the
different cell types, which through their synaptic connections with AN fibers modify the input of these fibers in important and differential ways. This means, at least
in some sense, that there is a repackaging of the auditory (neural) information at
this level of the auditory system—a situation that suggests that the acoustic stimulus is defined in a slightly different way at the CN than it is at the AN level. The AN
fibers have one firing pattern, but when these fibers input to the various cells in the
CN, multiple firing patterns emerge—some different and some the same or similar
to those noted at the AN level. Therefore, there is both a modification as well as a
preservation of the neural impulse patterns at the level of the CN.

Romand and Avan (1997) have generated an excellent tabular review of cell
types, connections, anatomical loci, and firing patterns for those interested in a comprehensive review of this information. This chapter will focus on only some of the key
PSTHs. The spherical and globular bushy cells in the AVCN yield "primary-like,"
"primary-like with notch" and "on" types of responses. The primary-like response is
similar to that observed in the AN. It is a pattern with a strong initial response followed by a plateau or gradual decrease in firing for the duration of the stimulus
(Figure 8.7). The primary-like with notch type offers the same response pattern as
the primary-like PSTH, but with a time period after the initial firing where there is a
sharp decrease in the neural activity. The on response is characterized by a single
burst of activity that stops after a few milleseconds even though the stimulus continues. The stellate or multipolar cells, found in the AVCN and the PVCN, usually display "chopper" and on responses. A chopper is a response that has periodic bursts of

● **Figure 8.7**

Five types of poststimulus time histograms from cells in the cochlear nucleus.

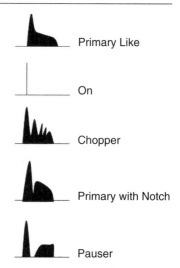

Primary Like

On

Chopper

Primary with Notch

Pauser

impulses throughout the duration of the stimulus—usually adapting somewhat over the time course of the stimulus. The octopus cells from the PVCN have only an on response. The pyramidal (fusiform) cells in the DCN can provide "pauser" and "build-up" responses. The pauser response is an initial response, followed by an arrestment of activity and then a resumption of firing that lasts for the duration of the stimulus. The build-up response increases in firing rate over the duration of the stimulus, usually in response to a short tone burst stimulus.

Frequency Representation

Frequency representation in the CN is quite distinct and follows the frequency representation that is seen in the AN. Specifically, the main AN branches that connect to the three main parts of the CN have a tonotopic representation, which is maintained in the CN. In humans the CN is more horizontal than it is in small animals. This means the tonotopic arrangement is likely to be slightly different in animal and human models. The low-frequency AN fibers project to the lateral regions of the CN, and the high frequencies to the medial regions of the DCN and the PVCN. The AVCN may have a slightly different arrangement, with the low frequencies being more lateral and ventral and the high frequencies being more medial and dorsal (Sando, 1965; Romand and Avan, 1997) (Figure 8.8). It is important to realize that much of the human interpretation in regard to tonotopicity is inferred and theorized based upon animal models, as

CLINICAL CORRELATE

It is important to realize clinically that if a lesion affects one or more of the cell types in the CN, then the derived impulse patterns (PSTHs) may not be generated, or if they are generated, they may be altered in some critical way. Since the impulse patterns convey important information about the stimulus to higher centers within the CANS, there may be either a total lack of information about the temporal details available or the presence of altered information for the higher centers of the brain to process. Either situation could create problems for the accurate perception of the stimulus. The difficulties encountered may not be great if the stimulus is simple (highly redundant), but if the stimulus is complex (having low redundancy), then insufficient processing of the signal at the CN may lead to poor identification or recogniton of the stimulus by higher (i.e., cognitive) areas of the brain. For example, subtle temporal characteristics needed for sound localization and hearing in background noise are functions that are dependent on fine temporal processing of acoustic information by the CN cells. If this temporal processing is not completed at the CN level, then difficulty localizing and hearing in noise could be a result. ●

● Figure 8.8

The tonotopic organization of the cochlear nucleus (transverse view). L = low characteristic frequency, H = high characteristic frequency.

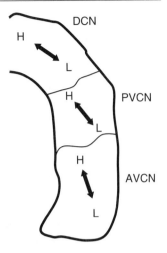

specific tonotopic mapping in the human model has not been done. Also, different animal species have slightly different tonotopic arrangements. Hence, the issue is not simple, and much misunderstanding surrounds frequency organization of the CN. However, it does appear that each segment of the CN has its own tonotopic arrangement. Therefore, connections from each segment of the CN carry frequency-specific information to higher levels of the CANS.

The tuning curves (TCs) of the fibers within the CN vary depending on the particular cell type. Generally, the tuning is similar to that noted in the AN, but in some cases the CN's TCs are broader and in other cases they are shaper (e.g., neural fibers in the DCN) than those seen in the AN. In the DCN, inhibitory sidebands may help sharpen the edges of the TCs, and there is generally sharper tuning at lower intensities than at higher intensities. (Rose, Galambos, and Hughes, 1959; Bourk, Mielcarz, and Norris, 1981; Spirou, May, Wright, and Ryugo, 1993).

Intensity Coding

As the auditory signal increases in intensity, there is a monotonic increase in the firing rate of most of the cells within the CN. This monotonic function is observed for the vast majority of the CN fibers, which tend to have a 30 to 40 dB dynamic range (Roullier, 1997). It has been shown, however, that some CN fibers have a much greater dynamic range for intensity, somewhere on the order of 80 to 90 dB (Rhode and Smith, 1986a,b). In the DCN specifically, neurons that have a non-monotonic output are relatively common (Roullier, 1997). It also has been demonstrated that CN fibers alter their firing rates in a stepwise manner by small amounts in response to a continuous tone that either increases or decreases in intensity (Moller, 1979). This finding relates to a possible physiological basis for intensity discrimination at this level of the CANS. The wide range of intensities that can be accommodated and the ability of the CN fibers to respond to subtle changes in intensity indicate the amazing capacity for intensity coding at this level of the CANS. As would be expected, based upon what was just mentioned, the CN is highly responsive to **amplitude-modulated** (AM) tones.

In a review of the function of the CN fibers in the processing of intensity cues, Moller (2000) discusses how the CN responds to AM tones. The CN has the ability to follow modulations closely over a 60 to 80 dB range. These fibers follow the envelope of the acoustic signal with fluctuating firing rates that depend upon the specific contour of that envelope. This is interesting in light of the fact that many CN fibers have only a 20 to 30 dB intensity dynamic range for steady-state acoustic stimuli.

The concept that neurons respond better to modulated than steady-state sounds will become a common theme as we proceed up the central auditory system. For the same AM sound stimulus, the CN yields a larger response than does the AN. The CN also has a wider range of modulations to which it responds than does the AN (Moller, 2000). The concept that stimulus change seems to result in more neural activity than stimuli that do not change is supported by the dynamics of the CN's responses to AM signals.

Some parts of the CN respond to a wide range of AM frequencies (modulation rates) from below 50 Hz to around nearly 1000 Hz, but overall the CN responds best to AM signals in the 300-Hz range (Moller, 1972). This is a relatively high modulation rate compared to neurons farther up in the auditory system. In general, as will be discussed later, optimal modulation rates decrease as one progesses up the auditory system. It is interesting to note that most commercial auditory steady-state response (ASSR) units employ modulation rates that are under 100 Hz. The ASSR, by way of brief introduction, is an auditory evoked potential that uses modulation of intensity (amplitude modulation [AM]) and/or frequency (frequncy modulation [FM]) to trigger a response. The responses obtained resemble the modulated signal and can often be tracked down to intensity levels close to the indiviudal's behavioral threshold for the stimulus. Currently, the ASSR is used on a limited basis in newborn screening.

CLINICAL CORRELATE

Most pediatric audiologists would agree that infants and toddlers tend to respond better (in sound field testing) to warble tones (tones that are either frequency or intensity modulated) than they do to pure tones. This common observation has been attributed to the idea that with pure tones there is the potential of a greater effect of standing waves within the testing area, which results in alterations in the strength of the test signal within the test environment (sound room). Therefore, infants do not respond as well as to pure tones as they do to warble tones since the strength of the pure-tone signals is likely to be more attenuated in some areas of the test environment than in others because of the effects of standing waves. This is probably true. However, we would submit that the reason infants respond better to warble tones than pure tones is more likely related to the fact that these stimuli result in more neurons responding within the CANS because of the signal modulation that exists in these types of test stimuli. This in turn would translate into better behavioral responses. ●

Temporal Functions

Temporal coding integrity is most often measured and judged by the ability of neurons to phase-lock onto a periodic stimulus. In small animals, many of the CN fibers can phase-lock onto tones of up to 3000 to 4000 Hz and often these fibers do so with greater precision than do the neural fibers of the AN (phase-locking as described here means that the neurons may not lock onto every cycle but maintain a locking sequence with integrity). Other fibers in the CN (i.e., those that have a chopper response) are more limited in their ability to phase-lock and can do so only for tones up to about 1000 Hz (Moller, 2000).

The best temporal coding in the CN seems to be linked to bushy and octopus cells because these cells have good synchronicity. The octopus cells with their abrupt "on" response and great stability of their first discharges allow for good coherence to the signal (Romand and Avan, 1997).

Rhode (1998) demonstrated that the AVCN has better temporal resolution than the AN for sequences of exponentially damped sinusoids in the chinchilla. However, for paired click stimuli, the timing of CN fibers was found to be similar to that seen in the AN (Parham, Zhao, Ye, and Kim, 1998). The DCN probably has poorer temporal resolution abilities than either the PVCN or the AVCN. This may be related to the fact the the DCN plays a major role in the processing of spectral information and as such is less involved in the processing of temporal information.

Speech Signals

Although recently there has been considerable interest in the investigation of the coding of speech signals at the CN, compared to what is currently known about the coding of other types of acoustic signals in the CN, there is not a great deal of information specific to the coding of speech stimuli. Recio and Rhode (2000) showed that most of the neurons in the VCN of chinchillas, with the exception of onset cells, respond to the presentation of vowels. The cells in the VCN provide good rate and place representation of vowel spectra. In addition, it has been observed that some cells in the CN, such as the bushy cells, lock on to the fundamental frequency of vowel sounds (Sachs and Blackburn, 1991). It is difficult to determine if these cells in the CN respond specifically to the speech characteristics of the signal or to the complex acoustic stimuli that compose the speech signal. Therefore, it is not known whether the CN processes speech signals in the same manner as it does other complex acoustic stimuli that are not speech, or whether the CN processes speech stimuli in some unique fashion that is distinctly different from the processing of nonspeech acoustic stimuli.

One early study showed similar temporal coding for speech sounds in the CN to that observed in the AN (Kiang, 1975). This early study relates what appears to be the commonly held assumption among auditory physiologists today: that the CN preserves much of the information that is passed on to it by the AN. The available evidence from experiments on animals conducted to date appears to support the hypothesis that there is not a major difference in the processing of speech sounds at the level of CN when compared to that which occurs in the AN (Kiang, 1975; Romand and Avan, 1997).

Binaural Processes

At first glance, the CN does not appear to be a structure that one would focus on if one were interested in studying binaural interactions within the CANS. However, as mentioned earlier, some communication may exist between the two CNs–at least in animals. There is evidence from animal studies that some neurons in both the ventral and dorsal CN respond to stimulation of either ear (Mast, 1973). In such cases it appears that ipsilateral stimulation is excitatory, while contralateral stimulation is inhibitory—certainly different from what is noted at higher levels of the auditory pathways.

In cats it appears that the DCN plays a role in sound localization in the vertical plane (May, 2000). Surgical lesions of the DCN, the dorsal acoustic stria, and the intermediate acoustic stria all have been shown to result in degradation of localization abilities in cats. Since the dorsal, ventral, and intermediate acoustic striae all contribute to the lateral lemniscus (LL) pathway and also have direct connections to the inferior colliculus (IC), these structures are believed to have important processing roles within the CANS that are critical to normal localization ability. Compromise of any of these structures or pathways is likely to result in decreased or altered localization ability. For optimal localization, each brainstem pathway must maintain its integrity, and the periphery must be intact to ensure good localization skills. The study by May (2000) discussed above raises some questions as to whether or not the CN is directly responsible for the processing of auditory information that would be critical for normal localization of a sound source. Damage to the VCN influences the timing and intensity cues processed at the CN these altered neural signals are then sent on to the superior olivary complex (SOC). Under these circumstances the SOC does not have the necessary inputs to correctly process the timing and intensity cues needed for accurate localization. Hence, one might conclude at least in one sense, that the CN's role in localization may not be any different from other structures within the (peripheral) auditory system (for example, the middle ear), where a conductive loss also compromises localization by creating timing and intensity problems at a lower level in the auditory system that are then passed on to the SOC.

Evoked Potentials

Evoked potentials (EPs) can be recorded both near- and far-field from the CN in animals and in humans. Near-field recordings from animals show a prepotential that occurs approximately 0.5 msec before the action potential (AP). The AP is sharp and highly repeatable. The EP waveform in animals is split into a prepotential and the AP, which is believed to be the influence of a postsynaptic potential that is observed in animals but not in humans (Bourk, 1976).

In humans, the CN is thought to contribute primarily to the generation of wave III of the ABR. In far-field recordings, wave III occurs about 2 msec after the AN's AP and is usually of a greater amplitude than the AP. Near-field recordings from the CN of humans during neurosurgery show a sharp negative peak at the same latency (about 3.5 msec) as wave III of the ABR. This negative peak is followed by a slow, large negative response probably propagated from the dendrites of the CN (Moller, Jannetta, and Jho, 1994; Moller, 2000).

Output of the Cochlear Nucleus

After the processing is completed in the CN, neural impulses travel to other nuclei along the auditory pathway on both sides of the brainstem. These ipsilateral and contralateral connections to nuclei higher in the CANS set up both sequential and parallel processing channels within the auditory system. The neural outputs from the CN take three primary routes: the ventral, dorsal, and intermediate acoustic striae (Helfert, Sneed, and Altschuler, 1991) (Figure 8.9). The DCN output fibers course along the **dorsal acoustic stria,** the AVCN fibers leave along the **ventral acoustic stria,** and the PVCN fibers exit via the **intermediate acoustic stria.** These striae are predominantly contralateral pathways, but some fibers travel ipsilaterally to synapse on various brainstem nuclei on the same side of the brainstem where the

● Figure 8.9

A drawing that focuses on the dorsal, intermediate, and ventral stria leaving the cochlear nucleus. DAS = dorsal acoustic stria, IAS = intermediate acoustic stria, VAS = ventral acoustic stria, IV = fourth ventricle, LL = lateral lemniscus, AVCN = anterior ventral cochlear nucleus, PVCN = posterior ventral cochlear nucleus, DCN = dorsal cochlear nucleus, LSO = lateral superior olive, MSO = medial superior olive, LNTB = lateral nucleus of the trapezoid body, VNTB = ventral nucleus of the trapezoid body, MNTB = medial nucleus of the trapezoid body, PO Nuc. = periolivary nucle.

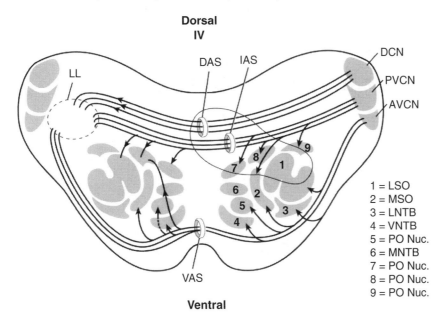

1 = LSO
2 = MSO
3 = LNTB
4 = VNTB
5 = PO Nuc.
6 = MNTB
7 = PO Nuc.
8 = PO Nuc.
9 = PO Nuc.

fibers originate (Pickles, 1988). These three striae also contribute to the fibers leaving the SOC laterally to help form the LL. Besides the acoustic striae, the CN has other fibers that go directly to the SOC and the IC via ipsilateral and contralateral routes (Moller, 2000). Davis (2002) has recently shown direct connections between the DCN and the central nucleus of the IC in cats. Hence, it is important to not only realize the existence of multiple connections to CANS nuclei above the level of the SOC, but to also realize that the acoustic striae compose the major auditory pathways exiting the CN.

The outputs of the CN can be linked to particular cell types. Most of the available information in this area of the brainstem is based on evidence derived from studies on small animals; however, it is likely that the output connections for humans are similar to those of animals (Cant, 1992). Romand and Avan (1997) have published a detailed account of output connections of the CN. The AVCN's spherical cells project ipsilaterally to the lateral superior olive (LSO). These cells also connect bilaterally to the medial superior olive (MSO) and the lateral nucleus of the trapezoid body (LNTB). Also in the AVCN, globular and bushy cells connect to the trapezoid body (TB) and periolivary nuclei (of the SOC) bilaterally. The AVCN's stellate cells addtionally project to the contralateral ventral nucleus of the lateral leminiscus (VNLL) and the IC. Also, the granular cells in the AVCN connect via an intrinsic route to the DCN in the CN complex.

The PVCN has stellate cells that input to the periolivary nuclei bilaterally. The PVCN's octopus cells project to the IC and VNLL contralaterally and the periolivary nuclei bilaterally. The DCN's vertical or corn cells project to other local areas of the CN, while its pyramidal cells course to the contralateral VNLL and IC (see Figure 8.10).

● **Figure 8.10**

The output connections of
the cochlear nucleus.

AVCN – Anterior Ventral Cochlear Nucleus
DCN – Dorsal Cochlear Nucleus
LNTB – Lateral Nucleus of the Trapezoid Body
LSO – Lateral Superior Olive
MSO – Middle Superior Olive
VNLL – Ventral Nucleus of the Lateral Lemniscus
PVCN – Posterior Ventral Cochlear Nucleus
IC – Inferior Colliculus
PON – Periovilary Nuclei

——————— Ipsilateral
– – – – – – – Contralateral

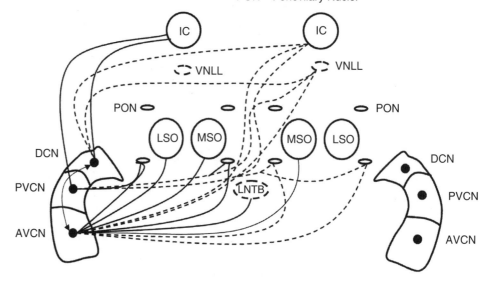

CLINICAL CORRELATE

Given the profuse ipsilateral and contralateral connections of the CN to the SOC, the LL fiber tracts, the nuclei of the lateral leminiscus (nLL), and the IC, both within and outside of the dorsal, ventral, and intermediate acoustic striae, it is understandable how lesions (especially intrinsic lesions) of the lower pons could devastate function of this region of the auditory system. It has been shown that the ABR is abnormal more frequently in cases of intrinsic brainstem lesions than in any other CANS disorder category (Musiek, 1991). Most acoustic tumors (extrinsic lesions) that either originate or extend medially into the CPA affect the CN (see Figure 8.11). These effects are difficult to separate from the effects of an acoustic neuroma that is limited to the IAM only. In the rare situation where the CN alone is affected by a disorder, the effects are noted ipsilaterally for both behavioral and electrophysiological central tests (Jerger and Jerger, 1974). Lesions that are located more to the midline of the low pons can affect the striae. These types of lesions, however, usually result in bilateral deficits on both ABR and behavioral tests of central auditory function (Musiek, Gollegly, Kibbe, and Verkest, 1988). ●

● **Figure 8.11**

A coronal view of the brain showing a large acoustic neuroma (arrow) on the left side. This would be considered an extrinsic brainstem tumor, as it has compressed and displaced the brainstem, undoubtedly compromising the cochlear nucleus (from Dublin, 1976, with permission).

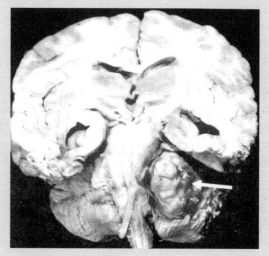

CLINICAL CORRELATE

It has been postulated that damage to the CN can affect peripherally driven auditory measures such as pure-tone thresholds. This concept was supported by early studies on **kernicterus**, which revealed effects in the CN but not the cochlea. Kernicterus is the pathological condition that can evolve if hyperbilirubinemia is not properly managed. Briefly, high bilirubin levels, especially if unconjugated, result in the staining of and damage to the nuclei in the brain. Although there can be damage to many of the nuclei within the brain, the CN (and other brainstem nuclei) seems to be a prime target for high bilirubin concentrations (see Dublin,

(continued)

● Figure 8.12

A central auditory test profile of a 10-year-old child who at birth had high bilirubin levels. This child was classified as having a learning disability with difficulties only in verbally based subjects. He also experienced several auditory problems, such as difficulty hearing in noise, following verbal directives, and so on. The behavioral central tests showed a deficit on frequency pattern perception (a) and the ABR tracings showed extended I–III and I–V intervals bilaterally (b). Nothing in this child's medical history other than the hyperbilirubin could be related to the abnormal test findings. C. Sent = competing sentences, D. Digits = dichotic digits, SSW = staggered spondaic words, LPFS = low-pass filtered speech, FP = frequency patterns. (Note: the frequency pattern score was obtained in a sound field.)

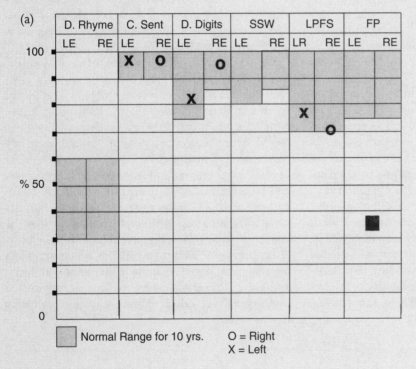

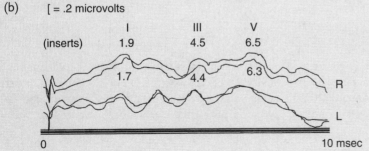

1974; Moller, 2000). There is some controversy over which bilirubin levels constitute risk; however, bilirubin levels greater than 15 mg/dl are of definite concern. One of the main concerns with hyperbilirubinemia is its potential to damage hearing, as it has been shown that high bilirubin levels compromise hearing secondary to damage to the auditory nuclei in the brainstem—especially the CN.

Kernicterus has typically been associated with high-frequency sensorineural hearing loss; however, other degrees and configurations of pure-tone hearing loss have also been reported (Matkin and Carhart, 1966). High-frequency hearing losses are most often associated with damage to the cochlea or sensory end organ. However, it is unlikely that the hearing deficit shown on the pure-tone audiogram in individuals with kernicterus is due to cochlear damage. There are three explanations for why hearing loss in kernicterus/hyperbilirubinemia is not likely to be cochlear in origin: (1) postmortem studies indicate that in cases of kernicterus, the cochlear structures are not damaged (Dublin, 1976), (2) normal OAEs have been commonly reported in cases of severe elevation of bilirubin levels (Rhee, Park, and Jang, 1999), and (3) cellular studies of the AVCN in patients with kernicterus have documented cell damage in the tonotopic area of 3000 to 8000 Hz of this structure (Dublin, 1986). Therefore, it is much more likely that in patients with kernicterus/hyperbilirubinemia, compromise of the CN influences the pure-tone hearing thresholds as opposed to any damage to the cochlea itself (Matkin and Carhart, 1966). Moreover, it is often the case that the ABR is abnormal in individuals with this condition in ways that are not necessarily consistent with a cochlear site of lesion. Moller (2000) reported that the I–III interwave interval is frequently extended in cases with hyperbilirubinemia, which would be more consistent with CN involvement as opposed to compromise of the cochlea. However, it should be noted that the evidence available in the literature indicates that the ABR findings for patients with kernicterus/hyperbilirubinemia are highly variable. Extensions of central conduction times, totally absent ABRs, and ABRs that are normal, all have been reported in subjects with this condition (Perlman, Fainmesser, Sohmer, Tamari, Wax, and Pevsmer, 1983; Nakamura, Takada, Shimabuku, Matsuo, Matsuo, and Negishi, 1985).

Hyperbilirubinemia and jaundiced conditions have also been associated with a condition known as auditory neuropathy (Starr, Picton, and Kim, 2001; Starr, Sininger, Nguyen, Michalewski, Oba, and Abdala, 2001) (see earlier discussion in this chapter). This association has been made primarily because many of the cases of hyperbilirubinemia with jaundice provide an audiologic profile that is similar to that noted in cases with **auditory neuropathy/dyssynchrony.** Perhaps there could be some secondary involvement of the AN in cases of high bilirubin levels, but it is important to realize that high bilirubin levels (based on pathological evidence) is primarily a disorder that affects brain tissue and not the AN (Dublin, 1986; Moller, 2000).

Figure 8.12 presents a case of a ten-year-old boy who had severe hyperbilirubinemia as a newborn. He had no other medical problems subsequent to this condition. However, in school he struggled with some subjects, such as reading, and was referred for evaluation of a possible central **auditory processing disorder** (CAPD/APD). As can be seen in the data presented in Figure 8.12, this young boy had an abnormal ABR, consistent with hyperbilirubinemia and CN involvement. He also had difficulty on a pattern perception test. It is believed that the abnormal findings noted at the time of his audiologic testing were related to residual effects from the high bilirubin levels that he experienced at birth, suggesting that the auditory deficits noted were a direct result of compromised auditory brainstem function. ●

CLINICAL CORRELATE

Another auditory disorder, tinnitus, might be associated with increased spontaneous activity measured at the DCN. Kaltenbach and Afman (2000) showed that after exposure to high levels of noise, there was an increase in the level of spontaneous activity (hyperactivity) of DCN neurons in hamsters that was equivalent to that observed in the DCN when a pure-tone signal was presented at a 20 dB

(continued)

sensation level. Further evidence that DCN hyperactivity is related to tinnitus has been recently reviewed (Kaltenbach, Zhang, and Finalayson, 2005).

The CN is also the site for implantation of electrodes for auditory brainstem implants, which are used in cases where cochlear implants are not viable, for example, when the AN is compromised, such as in cases with bilateral acoustic neuromas. The electrode complex of the brainstem implant is generally aligned with the ventral CN from a lateral surgical approach (to the ponto-medullary junction). This allows about a 3-mm by 10-mm area for placement of the electrode complex. Any placement that may be slightly in error may infringe upon the seventh (facial) and ninth (glossopharyngeal) cranial nerves as these nerves enter the brainstem in this area (Figure 8.13) (Klose and Sollmann, 2000). Because electrode placement on the lateral aspect of the ponto-medullary junction may result in facial or vestibular symptoms, there now has been a trend toward surgical placement of the electorode complex more dorsally. This more dorsal placement would cause direct stimulation of the DCN. ●

Figure 8.13

Lateral view of the human brainstem showing the area of the ventral cochlear nucleus with the elliptically drawn form indicating the approximate area and place where the electrode complex of a brainstem implant would be placed.

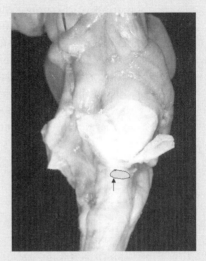

Neurotransmitters at the Cochlear Nucleus

There are several neurotransmitters in the CN. **Acetylcholine** (Ach) has been identified in the CN—especially in the granular cell area (Godfrey, Beranek, Carlson, Parli, Dunn, and Ross, 1990). This particular neurotransmitter may have differential excitatory and inhibitory effects depending on whether it is present in the VCN or the DCN (Caspary, Havey, and Faingold, 1983). **Gamma-amino-butyric acid (GABA)** and **glycine** are two inhibitory neurotransmitters found in the CN (see Romand and Avan, 1997 for review), whereas the main excitatory neurotransmitters in the CN are **glutamate** and **aspartate** (Wenthold, Hunter, and Petralia, 1993; Romand and Avan, 1997).

The Acoustic Startle Reflex and the Cochlear Nucleus

The **acoustic startle reflex (ASR)** is known in the field of audiology as a cursory, not precise, test for hearing sensitivity. In the past it has even served as a hearing screening test for infants. It is well known that a loud sound will result in an abrupt movement (jump) on the part of the individual who hears the sound. This type of response is often viewed as an indication that the structures of hearing are functional. The ASR, however, can indicate that other neural mechanisms in addition to those involved in hearing are functional. The information on hearing and nonhearing systems related to the ASR can be of value in neurologic assessments. The main reason that the ASR can be of value neurologically is related to the anatomy that underlies the response.

The understanding of the anatomy of the ASR has changed over the years as it has been studied more extensively. Currently the circuit involves obligatory hearing structures and connected neural pathways. The acoustic stimulus travels through the middle ear to the cochlea, where it is transduced into neural signals that are carried by the AN. The AN connects to the CN, the final auditory structure in the ASR circuit. From there the impulses pass from the CN to the ventral lateral pons and the pontine reticular formation (PRF). It appears that in small animals the DCN may bypass the ventral lateral pons and connect directly to the reticular formation of the pons (Meloni and Davis, 1998). The PRF then connects to spinal cord neurons via the medial longitudinal fasciculus, and these spinal neurons connect to muscles of the upper torso (Yeomens and Frankland, 1995). The latency of the ASR in humans has been shown to range from 10 to 150 msec, with much of this variance related to the type of stimulus, the recording techniques used, and the state of the organism at the time of stimulation (Koch, 1999). Of interest here is a study done by Parham and Willott (1990) that indicates that the IC plays a role in mediating an inhibition of the ASR. Although the IC is not an obligatory part of the ASR circuit, it does seem to influence its function.

SUMMARY

In summary, the CN complex is located at the postero-lateral aspect of the ponto-medullary junction within the brainstem. It is composed of three subdivisions, the AVCN, the PVCN, and the DCN, all of which are tonotopically arranged. There are a variety of cell types in the CN, with the principal types being pyramidal, octopus, stellate, globular, and bushy cells. These cell types are located in particular regions in the CN and make connections to other cell types in higher-order auditory structures. These cell types generate distinctive firing patterns, or PSTHs, to which they can be uniquely associated. These PSTH patterns provide an elaboration of the temporal processing of the acoustic stimulus that has been delivered to the CN by the AN. The TCs of the CN neurons differ from those of the AN fibers in an important aspect; that is, they show strong evidence of inhibitory influences. This inhibition contributes to the narrowing of tuning in the CN fibers—thus increasing their frequency selectivity. It is therefore likely that these temporal and spectral response properties affect the representation of complex signals such as speech. The CN and its connections are also important to normal binaural processes, including sound localization. Finally, the CN appears to play a major role in the generation of wave III of the ABR in humans.

Hyperbilirubinemia seems to have an affinity for damaging the CN and compromising the ABR. The CN is also often compromised by acoustic neuromas that grow into the CPA and by fourth ventricle hydrocephalus that expands the ventricles laterally and affects the function of the CN.

The output connections of the CN include both ipsilateral and contralateral connections to various nuclei within the SOC, the NLL, and the IC. The primary output connections, however, are contralateral connections traveling within the three main fiber bundles that exit the CN (the dorsal, intermediate, and ventral acoustic striae). Recent reports indicate that the CN may be the final auditory nuclei involved in the generation of the acoustic startle reflex. This is a motor response that is triggered by the presentation of an intense acoustic signal that triggers an afferent response within the auditory system that then triggers an efferent or motor response through the activation of afferent–efferent interneurons.

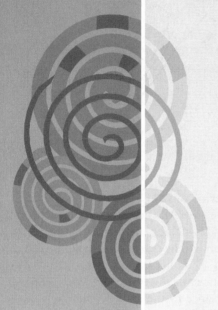

9

Superior Olivary Complex

Introduction

The **superior olivary complex** (SOC) is the next major group of nuclei after the cochlear nuclei in the ascending auditory pathways within the brainstem. These nuclei and their associated fibers are distributed in several areas of the caudal pons and are rather diverse in both their morphology and function. The SOC is the first place in the auditory system where binaural representation (left and right SOCs) from monaural input is noted. This binaural representation of sound at this level of the central auditory nervous system (CANS) sets up these nuclei for some interesting functions related to binaural fusion, perception of interaural timing differences, and sound localization and lateralization abilities. Clinically, the SOC is critical to many important functions that can be tested reasonably well audiologically by such procedures as **masking level differences** (MLDs), **interaural time differences** (ITDs), and **interaural intensity differences** (IIDs), as well as the **auditory brainstem response** (ABR). The SOC also plays a key role in the mediation of the **acoustic reflex** (AR).

ANATOMY OF THE SUPERIOR OLIVARY COMPLEX

General Aspects

The anatomy of the SOC includes a number of nuclei that are located in the medial to lateral ventral, caudal pons (in humans). Unlike most of the nuclei located within the auditory pathways of the brainstem, these structures are not situated close to the posterior or lateral surface of the brainstem. Rather, the SOC nuclei are located between the cochlear nuclei (CN) and the midline of the brainstem. The auditory nuclei comprising the SOC are relatively small, rather diffuse, and difficult to locate and approach surgically (Figure 9.1). Therefore, they have not been studied as extensively as some of the more surgically approachable nuclei in the brainstem.

The main nuclei in the SOC that are of relevance to the present discussion depend upon whether one is considering the anatomy of the nuclei represented in the human or the animal model (Schwartz, 1992; Moore, 2000). In the cat the SOC is located in the rostral medulla, and in the human it is located in the caudal pons. The main nuclei of the SOC (based

A transverse section through the rostral medulla* (one side) focusing on the superior olivary complex (SOC) (Note: the drawing is based upon the anatomy of the cat). LSO = lateral superior olive, MSO = medial superior olive, MNTB = medial nucleus of the trapezoid body, VNTB = ventral nucleus of the trapezoid body, VAS = ventral acoustic stria, LL = lateral lemniscus, PO = periolivary nuclei, DCN = dorsal cochlear nucleus, AVCN = anterior ventral cochlear nucleus, PVCN = posterior ventral cochlear nucleus, IV, fourth ventricle. *(The SOC in the human is in the caudal pons, but in the cat it is in the rostral medulla. Therefore, in using the cat model as the reference for this figure, showing the 'rostral medulla' area of the brainstem is appropriate.)

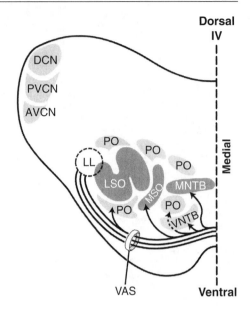

upon the cat model) include the **lateral superior olive** (LSO), which is the largest of the SOC nuclei, the **medial superior olive** (MSO), and the **medial nucleus of the trapezoid body** (MNTB). Additional nuclei include the periolivary nuclei and the lateral and dorsal nuclei of the trapezoid body. The periolivary nuclei, which are much smaller than the other SOC nuclei and are rather dispersed in their location within the SOC, and the lateral and dorsal nuclei of the **trapezoid body** (TB) are not considered with the same level of importance to the auditory function of the SOC as are the MSO, the LSO, and the MNTB.

Although the animal and human models of the SOC share many of the same nuclei, there are some notable differences. In humans, as is the case for the cat, the main anatomical nuclei in the SOC involve the LSO and the MSO. However, in the human model the MSO is larger than the LSO—the opposite of what is observed

● **F i g u r e   9 . 2**

Transverse view of the medial superior olive (MSO), the lateral superior olive (LSO), and the facial nerve (FN) tract in the chinchilla (Nissl stain) (courtesy of Tony Sahley).

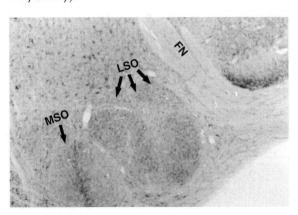

in the cat. Also, in the human model the LSO does not take on the appearance of an S-shaped segment as it does in small animals (Moore, 2000) (Figure 9.2). Other differences between the animal and human models include the MNTB, which in the human is a minor, ill-defined structure at best, as is also the case with the lateral and dorsal nuclei of the trapezoid body. The MNTB in cats, for example, is proportionally larger and better defined. Other differences include the observation that in humans the periolivary nuclei are much more prominent anatomical structures than they are in the cat and that the human MSO extends considerably further in a rostral direction than it does in animal models. The trapezoid body in humans can perhaps be best viewed as more of a fiber tract that connects the anterior ventral cochlear nucleus (AVCN) to parts of the SOC and the contralateral lateral lemniscus (LL). This tract is often termed the ventral acoustic stria. This stria, along with the intermediate and dorsal striae, crosses the midline of the caudal pons to connect the CN with the SOC and other parts of the brainstem pathway (see previous chapter) (for review, see Pickles, 1988; Helfert, Sneed, and Altschuler, 1991; Moore, 2000).

Neural Inputs to the Superior Olivary Complex

The ventral acoustic stria (VAS), which arises from the AVCN's spherical and globular cells, contains fibers that project to the MSO on both sides of the brainstem and to the LSO on the ipsilateral side (Helfert et al., 1991; Helfert and Aschoff, 1997). The VAS fibers coming from the AVCN's stellate (multipolar) cells also connect to some of the periolivary nuclei and trapezoid nuclei on both sides of the brainstem (Helfert et al., 1991). The intermediate acoustic stria (IAS) connects octopus cells of the PVCN to periolivary nuclei on both sides of the brainstem, but the dorsal stria from the DCN has only a few, or perhaps no, connections directly with the various nuclei of the SOC. Fibers originating from within the DCN have primary connections with auditory nuclei higher in the auditory nervous system. It is important to understand that the connections from the CN to the SOC through the ventral, intermediate, and possibly dorsal striae, along with the efferent neurons of the olivocochlear bundle, make up a heavy neural network of auditory fibers at the caudal part of the pons (see previous chapter for additional discussion of this topic).

Related Anatomy

In addition to the heavy auditory neural network found in the caudal pons, an important nonauditory anatomical structure needs to be introduced here. The fourth ventricle is located between the cerebellum and the brainstem and extends from slightly below the pontomedullary junction up to the midbrain. Laterally, it extends from the medial most aspect of one CN to the other. This means that the fourth ventricle lies in close proximity to the cochlear nuclei, the dorsal acoustic stria (and even the intermediate acoustic stria), and the olivocochlear bundle. As a result, pathologies that compromise the structure or function of the fourth ventricle may also result in secondary effects within the auditory structures of the SOC.

Cell Types

Helfert et al. (1991) has detailed the cell types of the SOC in the cat. The MSO has primarily multipolar and bipolar cells, whereas the LSO is made up mostly of one cell type: the principal, or fusiform, cell. There are also multiplanar and marginal cells found in the LSO, but three-fourths of the LSO cells are of the principal, or fusiform, type. Principal, or fusiform, cells are by far the most common in the MNTB, but stellate and elongate neurons are also found (see Schwartz, 1992).

Tonotopic Organization

The SOC, like other structures within the CANS, is tonotopically organized (Figure 9.3). In this section, only the LSO and MSO will be discussed, in terms of their frequency representations. In the cat, the lateral aspect of the LSO is the locus

● Figure 9.3

The lateral superior olive (LSO) and the medial superior olive (MSO) in the cat, showing the tonotopic organization of these two structures (H = high frequencies, L = low frequencies).

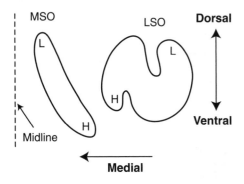

of the neurons that are specifically tuned to low-frequency sounds. As one moves in a medial direction on the LSO, the characteristic frequencies (CFs) become higher, with the highest frequencies being represented at the ventro-medial aspect of the LSO (see Helfert and Aschoff, 1997). The MSO's frequency arrangement is such that the high frequencies are represented toward the ventral end of the structure, with lower frequencies being represented at the dorsal end (see Helfert and Aschoff, 1997). In small animals, like the cat, the frequency range of the LSO and MSO are somewhat different, with the LSO accommodating more high frequencies than the MSO (for additional information, see Schwartz, 1992; Moore, 2000).

Projections from the Superior Olivary Complex

The SOC has both ipsilateral and contralateral connections to the inferior colliculus (IC) (Figure 9.4). The MSO neurons, for the most part, project ipsilaterally to the central nucleus of the IC (Adams, 1979). There are some MSO fibers, however, that connect to the contralateral IC and other collaterals that project to the (contralateral) dorsal nucleus of the lateral lemniscus (DNLL) (Schwartz, 1992). These latter connections are not major connections and may vary in regard to both numbers of fibers and specific anatomical connections in different species. The projections from the LSO are a little more complex than those of the MSO. Projections from the LSO are bilateral, with neurons from the lateral aspect of the LSO (i.e., lower frequency area) projecting mostly to the ipsilateral IC, whereas neurons from the medial aspect of the LSO (i.e., higher-frequency area) course primarily to the contralateral IC. There is also a difference in neurotransmitter content for ipsilateral and contralateral inputs to the IC. LSO projections to the ipsilateral IC are mostly glycinergic and inhibitory (Saint Marie, Ostapoff, Morest, and Wenthold, 1989), while the projections to the contralateral IC are excitatory and probably glutamatergic (Glendenning, Baker, Hutson, and Masterton, 1992). The projections from the

● Figure 9.4

The main output connections of the lateral superior olive (LSO) and medial superior olive (MSO) on the left side of the brainstem. (Note: the LSO is not S-shaped in this drawing, as the drawing is intended to reflect the general shape of the LSO in the human). Additional abbreviations: NLL = nucleus of the lateral lemniscus, I.C. = inferior collicullus.

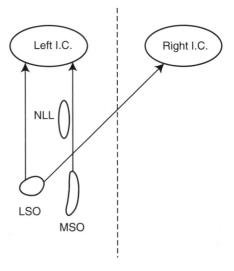

MNTB course to the LSO and other periolivary nuclei in the SOC (see Schwartz, 1992 for review). The MNTB to LSO projections are glycinergic and inhibitory. This is important since this inhibitory input underlies the "I" part of the "EI"-type responses of LSO neurons (see discussion on page 195) as well as their sensitivity to ILDs.

The output connections from the LSO have been viewed structurally as an acoustic chiasm (similar to the structural situation seen in the visual system, that is, the optic chiasm) (Glendenning, Hutson, Nudo, and Masterton, 1985). The acoustic chiasm involves the crossed connections that connect the LSO and the IC. Glendenning et al. (1985) used the term *acoustic chiasm* only with reference to the LSO projections and not the MSO projections, which are mostly unilateral.

CLINICAL CORRELATE

Because the SOC is located in a different region of the brainstem as compared to most brainstem auditory structures, it may be affected in different ways by various pathologies. **Extra-axial lesions** of the brainstem, such as those arising from the cranial nerves, especially acoustic (eighth) and fifth nerve tumors, will most likely not affect the SOC as much as the posterolateral auditory nuclei like the CN and the IC. On the other hand, lesions of structures such as the basilar artery on the ventral side of the pons may affect the SOC more directly than other auditory nuclei in the brainstem simply because the lesion would be closer.

Intra-axial lesions may compromise the function of the SOC and its connections to a considerable degree. Since intra-axial lesions arise from within the brainstem, there often could be direct effects on the SOC if the lesion was in the lower pons. This is best supported by the high sensitivity (>95%) of the ABR to intra-axial lesions of the brainstem (Chiappa, 1983; Musiek, 1991). Intra-axial lesions of the low pons could easily affect the MSO, LSO, trapezoid body, and periolivary nuclei directly. These lesions could also compromise the dorsal, ventral, and intermediate striae that carry impulses from the CN complex to the SOC. Since the SOC plays a key role in generating the ABR waves and in mediating the acoustic reflex, it is common to see abnormalities in both of these audiological measures for intra-axial lesions.

Binaural interaction measures associated with auditory tests such as masking-level differences (MLDs) or interaural timing tests are often abnormal when the SOC is damaged. The SOC is designed to integrate, compare, and analyze timing information from the two ears. Hence, binaural interaction tests are well suited to challenge the functions of this structure. These kinds of tests will be discussed further in the next section. ●

PHYSIOLOGY OF THE SUPERIOR OLIVARY COMPLEX

Interaural Interaction, Localization, and Lateralization

The SOC plays a key role in the **localization** and **lateralization** of acoustic information. In addition, one of its key functions is to receive auditory information that is presented to both ears and combine this information into a "fused" auditory perception. All of these processes require complex binaural interactions that are accomplished in a variety of ways. The foundation for such 'binaural' processes lies in the fact that the SOC is the first place in the auditory system where the inputs from the two ears converge. This convergence allows the SOC to analyze differences in the neural impulses that represent important information such as the time of arrival and intensity levels of the original auditory signals that have arrived at the two ears. Moore (2000) relates that the SOC is responsible for recreating the auditory spatial field. Although the entire auditory system contributes in some way to localization

The development of a clinical test known as the binaural fusion test, although not high in clinical utility, was based on some key SOC functions (Matzker, 1959). This procedure involved filtering speech so that one ear received low band-pass segments of the original test stimuli and the other received high band-pass segments of the original signals. Listening to the segments presented to only one ear does not permit accurate perception of the signals. However, when listening to both ears, the speech signals are understood if the SOC appropriately fuses the stimuli. If the SOC does not appropriately fuse the signals, the speech segments are not understood, indicating dysfunction of the SOC fusion process. This test procedure can only be used reliably when the auditory periphery is intact. This concept of fusion at the SOC may be related to the binaural interaction component (BIC) of the ABR, which is discussed later in this chapter. ●

and lateralization, the SOC certainly plays a key role early on in the temporal course of these functions. Also, the SOC codes intensity, frequency, and temporal parameters of the acoustic stimulus, just as is done in the CN. Unfortunately some of these basic parameters of hearing have not been studied as extensively within the SOC as they have for other structures of the central nervous system. This is probably related to the fact that it is difficult to access this structure for close investigation because of its location and size. Nonetheless, some intriguing functions are associated with this structure.

The **fusion** of information from each ear is a key function that has been approached perhaps more from a clinical than from a basic science perspective. It is reasonable to expect that before the analysis of interaural time or intensity differences can take place, there needs to be an integration of the information from the two ears for comparison of the timing and acoustic similarities and differences. Fusion of information at the SOC offers the auditory system information that is likely to be meaningful and more readily processed at higher levels within the central nervous system. It has been shown that if this fusion does not occur at this level of the central nervous system, then the information arriving from the two ears may be perceived inaccurately (Matzker, 1959).

If the SOC is the first and key player in localization and lateralization, then its neurons should be extremely sensitive to interaural time and intensity differences (Joris and Yin, 1995). Discerning small time and intensity differences is the basis for localization in auditory space and for lateralization of a sound image in one's head. Animals and humans have amazing ability to localize sound sources along the horizontal plane. It has been shown that under ideal conditions humans can discern a 5 to 10 μsec time difference between ears (Tobias and Zerlin, 1959). This ability to discriminate such small time differences helps explain the excellent localization ability noted in humans with normal auditory function.

Although timing differences play an important role in localization and lateralization processes, intensity cues also may play a role and these intensity cues can interact with timing information in regard to localization and lateralization. It is well known that there is a time–intensity trade-off in lateralization processes. That is, a sound leading in time from one side of the head can be offset by a more intense sound from the other side to provide a midline image (Deatherage and Hirsh, 1959). Another manner of relating this concept is that if signals are presented to each ear at the same time, but one of the signals is presented at a higher intensity level than the other, the localization and lateralization would be to the side with the higher-intensity signal.

At the level of the SOC, inhibition may also play an important role in sound localization. As summarized by Fitzgerald (2002), the MSO of mammals receives inputs from the CN on both sides as well as from other structures in the SOC. While many of these inputs are excitatory, some are inhibitory with this inhibition mediated by the neurotransmitter glycine. By treating MSO neurons that had strong interaural timing difference (ITD) responses with strychnine, which blocks glycine, the ITD sensitivity was shown to be severely reduced. This suggests a key role for inhibition in the MSO and therefore an effect on sound localization. That is, inhibitory fiber actions in the MSO enhance the interaural timing differential (one of the key processes underlying sound localization), and as a result, the ability to localize a sound source is improved.

There is also inhibitory input from the MNTB to the LSO that converges with the excitatory input from the CN to produce ILD sensitivity in LSO neurons.

Good localization and lateralization skills can be of benefit in hearing in noisy rooms or environments (this is often referred to as the **cocktail party effect**).

Quick and accurate localization of the sound source in noisy environments helps the listener focus on the important auditory signal and allows better application of auditory filtering and suppression processes to minimize the distracting auditory signals. In a noisy environment, it is possible for an individual with normal auditory function to hear conversations because the noise and the speech signals often have different spatial origins that can be processed with binaural hearing processes. On the other hand, monaural hearing conditions render spatial discriminations of the noise and speech difficult; therefore, hearing becomes a challenge under these listening conditions (Boehnke and Phillips, 1999).

The SOC has a wide array of neurons that are sensitive to interaural time and intensity differences, as well as other neurons that help define left and right inputs and associated auditory fields. These differential functions are related to the fact that the neurons within the SOC have different response patterns. Some demonstrate an excitatory response (i.e., a neuronal firing rate that increases above the spontaneous rate), while others demonstrate an inhibitory response (i.e., a neuronal firing rate that decreases below the spontaneous rate) or a response pattern that is unaffected by certain inputs (i.e., no change in the spontaneous rate) (see Helfert and Aschoff, 1997 and Rouiller, 1997 for discussion).

Rouiller (1997) provides an excellent explanation of these neurons in the auditory system and has used the following conventions to identify the function of the neurons.

E: excitatory neuron

I: inhibitory neuron

O: a neuron that is not influenced by input

This letter labeling scheme is used for both contralateral and ipsilateral inputs to a neuron in such a way that when two letters appear in tandem within a description, the following classification system is used: the first letter indicates the influence of the contralateral ear and the second letter indicates the effect of the ipsilateral ear. Therefore, the following combinations are possible.

EE: a neuron that increases its firing rate for signals presented to either ear

EI: a neuron that is excitatory to input from the contralateral ear and inhibited by stimuli to the ipsilateral ear

IE: a neuron that is inhibitory to input from the contralateral ear and excited by stimuli to the ipsilateral ear

EO: a neuron that is excitatory to input from the contralateral ear but is not influenced by input from the ipsilateral ear

OE: a neuron that is not influenced by input to the contralateral ear but is excited by stimuli to the ipsilateral ear

Rouiller (1997) relates that within the MSO approximately 65% of the neurons are of the EE type, another 25% (or so) are EI- or IE-type neurons, and the remaining 10% (or so) are EO neurons. In the LSO the majority of neurons are of the IE type, with only a small proportion of the fibers being the EO type. The interaction of excitatory and inhibitory inputs has been demonstrated by Boudreau and Tsuchitani (1970). They showed that an IE neuron located in the LSO of a cat would decrease its firing rate with the introduction of a contralateral stimulus. When the contralateral stimulus was turned off and the ipsilateral stimulus remained present, the neuron fired strongly (see Figure 9.5). More important, this could show that the IE neuron is sensitive to interaural time differences in one manner and EI neurons are sensitive to ITDs in the opposite manner.

● Figure 9.5

Depiction of the manner in which the firing rate of a cell in the LSO is influenced by acoustic stimulation to the contralateral ear (based on data from Boudreau and Tsuchitani, 1970).

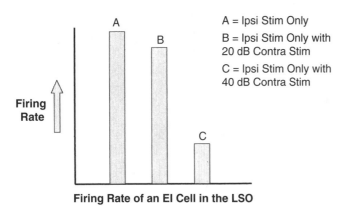

A = Ipsi Stim Only

B = Ipsi Stim Only with 20 dB Contra Stim

C = Ipsi Stim Only with 40 dB Contra Stim

Firing Rate

Firing Rate of an EI Cell in the LSO

A classic study showed that MSO neurons are highly sensitive to interaural time differences, but that MSO neurons respond better to interaural time differences for low-frequency sounds than for high-frequency stimuli (Galambos, Schwartzkopff, and Rupert, 1959). The LSO neurons respond to a wide range of frequencies but appear to be better equipped to respond to interaural level differences than time differences. The LSO seems to have neurons that are for the most part excitatory to ipsilateral and inhibitory to contralateral stimulation (Joris and Yin, 1995; see also Moore, 2000). It has been suggested that for high-frequency stimuli, differences in intensity levels rather than time of arrival might be the more useable acoustic cue to signal the source of a sound. However, it is important to realize that LSO neurons can also be ITD sensitive, either to ITDs in the carrier signal or to ITDs in the envelopes of different types of acoustic signals (see Joris and Yin, 1995).

CLINICAL CORRELATE

The MSO is the largest of the SOC nuclei in humans. Hence, one might assume that it is a major player in regard to function at this level of the CANS. A clinical test known as masking-level differences (MLDs) has much to do with ITDs and the SOC's ability to process such ITDs (Hirsh, 1948) (lesion studies will be discussed later). MLDs require that a target signal (tones or speech) be presented along with noise to both ears simultaneously. Testing is conducted under two conditions: (1) when the phase of the target and the noise are similar at each ear (i.e., in-phase) and (2) when the phase of one of the signals (either the target or the noise) is presented at a different phase angle while the other stimulus remains in-phase between the two ears. When targets (tones or speech) and noise are presented in-phase (S_oN_o) to each ear, a certain level of intensity is required for the subject to hear the target. However, if the targets or noise are presented out-of-phase with each other ($S_\pi N_o$ or S_oN_π), there will be a release from masking and the subject will be able to hear better than in the former test condition. The difference in dB between these two measures is the MLD. It is now well known that MLDs are considerably larger for low-frequency than for high-frequency stimuli (Hirsh, 1948). It is not unusual to obtain MLDs for a 500-Hz tone at 12 to 15 dB, while for a 2000-Hz tone they could be as small as 3 dB. MLDs are related to the fact that the auditory system (in particular, the SOC) is sensitive to phase differences between the ears. These phase differences are translated into interaural time differences. At high frequencies, the phase differences are small (in reference to time) and much of the differential timing information is too brief for the neurons to respond to in an accurate manner. This is why MLDs are conducted primarily with low-frequency tones (usually 500 Hz) or low-frequency speech signals (spondees or consonant-vowels) (Noffsinger, Martinez, and Schaefer, 1985). Hence, what Galambos et al. (1959) were seeing physiologically in the cat (see earlier discussion) has also been witnessed clinically in humans for many years.

Clinically, the MLDs, sometimes termed BMLDs (bilateral masking level differences), can be utilized in the detection and delineation of lower brainstem dysfunction (see Noffsinger et al., 1985 for review). The use of MLDs for this purpose is consistent with the SOC's differential timing functions. These functions and the site at which they are mediated are well demonstrated by the classic study of Lynn, Gilroy, Taylor, and Leiser (1981), who studied four populations with MLDs using CVs (consonant–vowels) as the stimuli. The groups included normals; a group of patients with lesions of the auditory areas of the cerebrum; a group with lesions of the upper pons, midbrain, or thalamus; and a group with lesions confined to the pontomedullary region. As can be seen in Figure 9.6, the MLD was reduced only in the

(continued)

Figure 9.6

The mean masking level difference (MLD) for consonant-vowel stimuli for three populations of patients with brain lesions at various levels of the auditory system and one control group (y-axis label = masking level difference in dB) (based on data from Lynn et al., 1981).

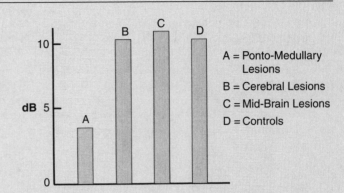

A = Ponto-Medullary Lesions
B = Cerebral Lesions
C = Mid-Brain Lesions
D = Controls

pontomedullary group, while the other groups performed similarly in regard to their release from masking. This study demonstrates the clinical value of using MLDs to determine the functional integrity of the low brainstem auditory structures. It also provides insight as to the mediation site of MLDs.

In a second study, Noffsinger and his associates (1985) shared data showing the clinical value of MLDs in defining lesions of the low brainstem. The sensitivity of MLDs to brainstem dysfunction associated with specific lesion sites was reported to range from 50 to 100%. Granted, these clinical research findings indicate a wide range of performance for the diagnostic use of MLDs; however, it is clear that MLDs can be affected by lesions that compromise the integrity of the SOC. ●

The ABR and the Superior Olivary Complex

The SOC makes a major contribution to the ABR. Waves I and II of the ABR are generated by the auditory nerve (AN), with the CN contributing to the generation of wave III. Therefore, the only ABR waves remaining that are used clinically are waves IV and V. The morphology of waves IV and V is such that these two waves are often fused into what is known as a IV–V complex. Moller and colleagues studied the ABR generator sites in humans and have provided some key information about the ABR and the SOC (Moller, Jho, Yokota, and Jannetta, 1995). These researchers observed strong neural responses correlating to wave IV of the ABR in the region of the SOC. As a result of these findings, these investigators argued that wave IV of the ABR was most likely generated, for the most part, from SOC structures at or close to midline in the brainstem.

CLINICAL CORRELATE

Clinical evidence has supported the SOC as a probable generator of wave IV of the ABR (see Musiek, Gollegly, Kibbe, and Verkest, 1988 and Musiek, Baran, and Pinheiro, 1994 for reviews). A relevant case is that of a middle-aged patient who suffered a mini-stroke of the caudal pons in the midline that extended laterally on each side but that did not involve the CN or the lateral lemniscus tract on either side of the brainstem. As can be seen in Figure 9.7, waves I, II, and III of the ABR are all normal, but the IV–V complex has been delayed significantly. The findings from this case correspond well with the concept of the ABR wave IV being generated by midline SOC

(continued)

structures. This case also argues for wave III originating from the CN, which was unaffected by this lesion.

Noffsinger and colleagues (1985) have suggested that the ABR and MLD have similar neural generators and support this idea with a study that revealed good correlations between abnormal ABRs and abnormal MLDs for patients with low brainstem lesions. ●

● Figure 9.7

(a) The ABR from a patient with a caudal, midline, pontine lesion as described in the text (modified from Musiek, 1988).
(b) A sketch of the levels of the brainstem's ascending auditory pathways with the lesion depicted as a black oval.

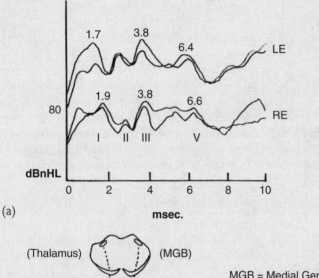

(a)

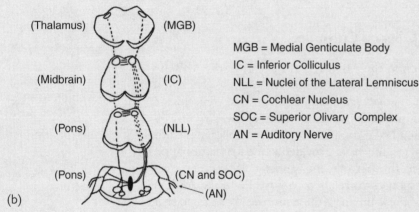

(b)

MGB = Medial Genticulate Body
IC = Inferior Colliculus
NLL = Nuclei of the Lateral Lemniscus
CN = Cochlear Nucleus
SOC = Superior Olivary Complex
AN = Auditory Nerve

Binaural Interaction Components of the ABR: Relationships to the SOC

Another ABR measure that can be used to assess SOC function is the binaural interaction component (BIC). If ABRs are recorded from the right and left ears independently and the responses are summed, a combined waveform is derived that is approximately twice the amplitude of either of the individual waveforms derived from the ears. However, if the ABR is derived with a stimulus that is presented to both ears simultaneously (i.e., a binaurally presented stimulus), the waveform is greater in amplitude than the ABRs obtained monaurally but smaller in amplitude than the ABR obtained from the summed right and left ear responses. The difference between the

● **F i g u r e 9 . 8**

Derivation of the binaural interaction component (BIC) of the ABR. Left and right ear ABRs are added together, which effectively doubles the amplitude of the waves. An ABR derived with a binaural stimulus (BIN) is obtained, and the amplitudes for waves I, II, and III are similar to those for the added waveform; however, the amplitudes for the later waves are slightly attenuated in the binaural condition. Hence, when the binaural waveform is subtracted from the added waveform there is a difference wave for the later waves, which is the binaural interaction component (BIC).

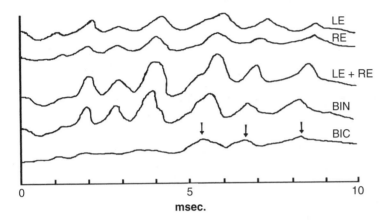

binaural ABR and the ABR summed from the two ears is referred to as the BIC (see Figure 9.8). It is important to note that the BIC does not occur for waves I, II, or III of the ABR, but only for the later waves (IV, V, VI, and VII) and only when they can be recorded reliably (see McPherson and Starr, 1995). If the SOC is the first loci of binaural convergence, then the BIC findings would support the SOC as contributing to the generation of the ABR waves occurring after wave III.

Pratt and colleagues (1998) recorded the BIC in patients with pontine lesions. This study showed the BIC to be more sensitive to pontine involvement than the regular ABR procedure. Based upon a careful analysis of the lesion sites for their subjects, Pratt and colleagues suggested that the BIC components were generated from the ventral caudal TB (ABR wave IV), the ventral TB (ABR wave V), and the rostral LL (ABR wave VI).

Tuning Curves and Cell Response Types in the Superior Olivary Complex

In the MSO, poststimulus time histograms (PSTHs) take the form of primary and primary-like with a notch. The LSO has chopper-type and primary-like PSTHs. The tuning curves (TCs) in the SOC nuclei (which include the TB and periolivary nucleus in addition to the MSO and LSO) demonstrate great variability, ranging from broad to narrow TC functions. However, the MSO and LSO have mostly narrow TCs with good sensitivity (Guinan, Guinan, and Norris, 1972; Rouiller, 1997). As one would expect, neurons in the SOC have good phase-locking properties, with some neurons locking on signals of up to 2 to 3 kHz (Rouiller, 1997). This good phase-locking is consistent with expectations for neurons that have good interaural timing properties. It is also a requisite characteristic for nuclei that

CLINICAL CORRELATE

Although the BIC of the ABR appears to hold great promise as a clinical tool for assessing auditory brainstem involvement, it has not yet been used to any great degree clinically. Perhaps the reason for this lack of clinical use is that the BIC is easily influenced by asymmetrical hearing loss, which is translated into ABR waveforms that are different for left and right ears (see Hall, 1992 for discussion). The procedure, however, appears to have a potential application as test of brainstem integrity, but its efficacy for this purpose awaits more clinical trials. ●

contribute to the components of the ABR, as the neural responses of the cells (i.e., firing rates) within these structures need to be both fast and highly synchronous for the evoked-potential (EP) response to be generated.

Intensity Coding at the Superior Olivary Complex

The intensity functions (rate-level or rate-intensity functions) of the neurons in the SOC are highly complex and are frequently dependent on the interaction of binaural inputs; that is, the neural functioning of many SOC neurons varies depending upon the nature of their responses to binaural stimuli (e.g., EI, IE, EE) and the precise locus of the stimulus source. Some neurons in the SOC have rate-level functions reaching maximum discharge rates at about 80 dB sound pressure level for monaural stimuli. Hence, even for monaural stimulation some SOC neurons have large dynamic intensity ranges (see Boudreau and Tsuchitani, 1968). In addition, the rate-level functions for many neurons in the SOC are not linear, as only small increases in firing rate are noted at both low and high intensities as the intensity level is increased. In a classic study by Goldberg and Brown (1969), binaural stimulation of neurons in the SOC of the dog resulted in a markedly higher firing rate than did monaural stimulation, especially at high intensities. This supports the classic concept that it is at this level of the CANS where binaural processing of the auditory signal first occurs. It is also at this level and beyond where it is common to see binaural representations of stimulus characteristics and complex interactions among the SOC neurons. Because the SOC has many excitatory and inhibitory interacting neurons, it would be likely to see both increases and decreases in firing rate in the SOC for binaural stimuli that vary in intensity and spatial orientation.

Interaural Timing and the Superior Olivary Complex

The auditory neurons in the SOC are highly sensitive to interaural time differences (ITDs). These ITDs form the basis, at least in part, for localization and lateralization processes (see Irvine, 1992 for review). Interaural timing is also a key factor in discriminating phase differences, such as in BMLDs. Classic physiologic studies have shown that the nerve cells in the SOC are sensitive to ITDs as brief as 10 μsec (Galambos et al., 1959). These ITD values are similar to the 5 to 10 μsec values reported for behavioral measures in humans by Tobias and Zerlin (1959). These measurements of extreme sensitivity to ITDs are most interesting when compared to the latency of response of nerve fibers (EI and IE cells) in the SOC. Galalmbos et al. (1959) have reported latency measures of approximately 5 to 7 msec for SOC fibers. Interestingly, this range of latency measures is similar to the latency range for wave IV of the ABR. Wave IV is believed to be generated in the SOC region and tends to occur in the 4.5 to 5.5 msec range when derived at moderately high intensities.

It is important to realize that although intensity and phase differences at the two ears can translate into ITDs, some cells in the SOC respond only to ITDs, others only to interaural intensity differences (IIDs), and others to either time or intensity differences at the two ears (Pickles, 1988). It is also critical to understand that neurons that are so finely tuned to time and intensity disparities at the two ears (such as the SOC) can easily be deceived by problems in the auditory periphery or CN. Therefore, compromise at lower levels in the auditory system, especially if the compromise is limited to one ear or if it is bilaterally asymmetric, can result in processing difficulties at higher levels in the auditory system since these more rostral structures will be receiving disrupted input. For example, a conductive, cochlear, or AN-based unilateral hearing loss typically results in poor localization and/or lateralization abilities.

Neurotransmitters in the Superior Olivary Complex

Glutamate decarboxylase (GAD) is an excitatory neurotransmitter that is found in the LSO, MSO, and TB in many small animals. There appear to be some species differences for small animals for γ-aminobutyric acid (GABA), an inhibitory neurotransmitter, which is also found in a number of structures (LSO, MSO) of the SOC. A large number of LSO cells contain glycine, which like GABA is inhibitory. The MSO has relatively high levels of aspartate and glutamate, making it a structure with more excitatory neurotransmitters than the LSO (Wenthold, 1991; Helfert and Aschoff, 1997). The LSO has both glycinergic and glutamatergic outputs to the IC, with the glycinergic in the uncrossed and glutamatergic in the crossed projections. The crossed, glutamatergic projection is probably as strong as the uncrossed, glycinergic projection. Hence, there is an excitatory crossed system balanced by an inhibitory noncrossed system. It is the difference in neurotransmitters between the crossed and uncrossed projections that amplifies the chiasm-like properties of the LSO projections (Glendenning et al., 1992). The MSO projection is not considered to be part of the acoustic chiasm. The MSO projection is almost completely uncrossed.

CLINICAL CORRELATE
LESION STUDIES OF THE SOC

Animal Studies   Some key lesion studies in animals support what has been said thus far about the function of the SOC. These studies are primarily related to EPs and sound localization tests. The SOC is certainly a contributor to the ABR; however, it is important to realize that animal ABRs are slightly different than those recorded from humans. Wada and Starr (1983) provided evidence that damage to the TBs of the guinea pig and cat altered wave III of the ABR, and Achor and Starr (1980) also showed marked effects on the ABR waveform by lesioning the TB in cats. These studies indicate that the TB and SOC are critical for the appropriate conduction of impulses through the auditory brainstem pathways as well as for the generation of specific EPs.

Gaining access to the various nuclei of the SOC is difficult. This is the likely reason why the TB, which is the most accessible of the SOC structures, is the SOC structure most often used for experimentation in animal studies (Irvine, 1986). It has been shown that sectioning of the TB in cats results in reduced sound localization abilities. The extent to which localization was compromised in these animals depended to some degree upon the size of the lesion. Small lesions of the TB created only mild deficits and the animals could be retrained to near normal performance. Large lesions of the TB resulted in localization deficits that were similar to those seen when one cochlea was ablated (Moore, Casseday, and Neff, 1974). Interestingly, sectioning of the commissure of the inferior colliculus did not result in anywhere near the extent of the localization deficits that were seen with TB sectioning (Moore et al., 1974).

Jenkins and Masterton (1982) in a series of ablation experiments on the TB showed the TB to be critical for binaural integration. They demonstrated that damage to the TB eccentric to one side would yield bilateral or ipsilateral acoustic space deficits. Lesions to higher auditory brainstem structures resulted in deficits only in the contralateral acoustic space. These findings are consistent with what is commonly observed for behavioral central auditory tests administered to humans with lesions in this same area of the CANS (Musiek et al., 1988).

(continued)

Human Studies There have been a number of studies on the effects of lesions in the region of the SOC on the ABR in humans (see Chiappa, 1983 and Musiek et al., 1994 for reviews). It seems clear that in humans, waves I, II, and III of the ABR are generated by structures before the SOC. In humans, lesions are not as specific as those induced in animals and therefore some liberty must be taken in the discussion of lesion effects. Levine and colleagues (1993) showed abnormal ABRs in patients with multiple sclerosis (MS) plaques affecting the SOC. Pratt et al. (1998) extended these earlier findings showing abnormal BICs for the ABR in SOC lesions.

Griffiths and colleagues reported a case of a midline lesion of the pons at the level of the SOC with excellent magnetic resonance imaging (MRI) documentation (Griffiths, Bates, Rees, Witton, Gholkar, and Green, 1997). The authors claimed that the crossed inputs to the SOC were prohibited with this lesion, leaving only the ipsilateral inputs to the SOC. It was also stated that the TB was involved. The patient complained of having great difficulty detecting the direction of moving sounds, such as a train approaching and continuing to pass by him. In addition, this patient could not determine which of three telephones in a room was ringing in spite of the fact that the three phones were separated by considerable distance. Specialized, experimental auditory testing revealed a mild impairment of making judgments on fixed timing differences and locating a sound that moved around the head.

Levine et al. (1993) and Furst et al. (2000) showed ITD difficulties and poor lateralization of binaurally presented sounds (with small IIDs and ITDs) for subjects with lesions of the SOC (including the TB). The results of these human studies are consistent with the animal studies mentioned earlier (i.e., Moore et al., 1974).

The MLD, or BMLD, test procedure is one that focuses on phase changes to propagate a release from masking effect. It has been well shown that the MLD is dependent on the functional integrity of the SOC. However, the appropriate release from masking is also dependent on normal function of the auditory system up to and including the SOC (Levine, Gardner, Fullerton, Stufflebeam, Furst, and Rosen, 1994).

Given the findings reviewed above, it is recommended that if dysfunction of the SOC is suspected, tests such as the ABR, ABR with BIC measures, MLDs, and interaural timing measures should be considered. Although currently there are no feasible clinical tests of sound localization ability, this function would be clearly affected in cases where the SOC was compromised. ●

THE ACOUSTIC REFLEX

The anatomy and physiology of the acoustic reflex (AR) are important parts of the SOC. The AR could have been presented as part of the discussion of anatomy and physiology of the middle ear, the cochlea, the AN, and the CN, as the AR encompasses much more than just the SOC. The entire auditory periphery, as well as branches of the auditory and facial nerves and a number of structures within the low brainstem must be intact for the AR to take place. The AR has become an important clinical tool for evaluation of the functioning of the middle ear, cochlea, CN, and low auditory brainstem. AR anatomy and physiology, therefore, are highly relevant for the clinician.

Anatomy of the Acoustic Reflex Arc

At the outset, it should be stated that two muscle tendons within the middle ear contribute to the overall AR in many animals. These muscle tendons are the stapedius and tensor tympani. However, in humans it appears as though only the contraction of the stapedius tendon contributes in a significant manner to the AR. The stapedius muscle is innervated by a branch of the facial nerve (seventh cranial nerve) and connects to the posterior aspect of the neck of the stapes bone (see Borg, 1973; Moller, 2000).

The AR pathway begins in the external ear where sound enters the auditory system. The middle ear directs the sound into the cochlea and from the cochlea the electrical impulses are imparted to the AN. The AR pathway involves primarily the ventral cochlear nucleus, and from there one set of fibers courses directly to the facial nerve motor nucleus ipsilaterally and another set of fibers travels through the TB and on to the LSO and MSO on the other side. From the SOC there are (bilateral) connections to the motor nucleus of the facial nerve. Hence, there are both ipsilateral and contralateral inputs to the facial nerve motor nuclei. The efferent pathway leading from the facial nerve nuclei to the facial nerve courses through the inner auditory meatus (IAM) (medial to lateral) and out into the middle ear, where a branch (stapedius nerve) is sent to the stapedius muscle (Borg, 1973; Brask, 1978; Moller, 2000) (Figure 9.9). Most of this anatomy is based on experiments done on the rabbit (Borg, 1973). The more central connections, especially in humans, are not as well understood (Hall, 1985). The AR in humans involves only a small portion of the caudal brainstem. Hence, the AR does not reflect the physiology of the mid or upper pons and therefore is limited in its diagnostic application to the area of the caudal pons.

Physiology of the Acoustic Reflex

There have been a number of explanations offered as to what is the functional significance of the AR. The main one that has been advanced is that it protects the cochlea from high-intensity sounds by attenuating the sounds before they can cause damage to the cochlea (Borg, 1973). When the stapedius contracts, the middle ear impedance increases and sound transmission through the middle ear is reduced, thus attenuating the sound. Moller (2000) discusses the AR as a control system for input to the cochlea. At high intensities the stapedius contraction is greater, while at lower intensities the contraction

● **F i g u r e   9 . 9**

Anatomy of the acoustic reflex with the acoustic stimulus presented to the left ear.

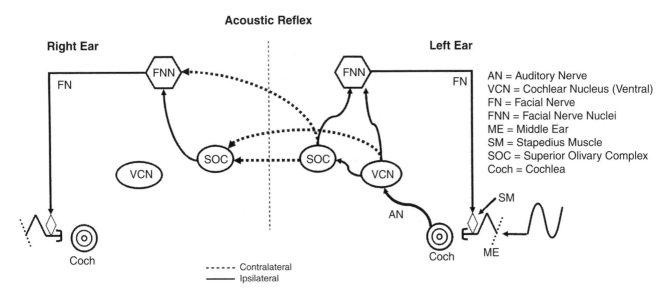

is less or absent. Hence, this may be viewed as somewhat of a compression system.

Laterality of the Acoustic Reflex

The AR is a consensual reflex. That is, stimulating one ear (at a sufficient intensity level) results in the stapedius contraction bilaterally. This, as described above, is based on the fact that afferent tracts coming from the CN travel ipsilaterally to connect to the motor nucleus of the facial nerve and contralaterally to connect to the motor nucleus of the facial nerve on the other side of the brainstem via the SOC. Connections from the afferent fibers on both the ipsilateral and the contralateral sides of the brainstem connect to the motor nuclei of the facial nerve that are also located on both sides of the brainstem. If the entire system is intact, the stapedius muscles on both sides of the head contract.

CLINICAL CORRELATE

The contralateral AR requires that the neural connections across the midline of the brainstem be intact. Therefore, as pointed out by Jerger, Jerger, and Mauldin (1972), a midline brainstem lesion of the caudal pons will disrupt the contralateral AR. However, a midline brainstem lesion (if it does not extend laterally) will

Figure 9.10

(a) Pure-tone thresholds and (b) acoustic reflexes from a patient with a brainstem lesion as discussed in the text. Acoustic reflex levels are presented in dB of hearing level.

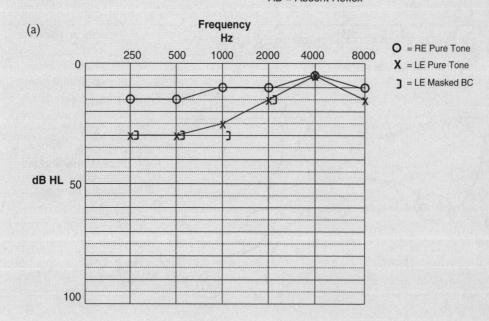

(b)

	Right Ear				Left Ear			
	500 Hz	1000 Hz	2000 Hz	4000 Hz	500 Hz	1000 Hz	2000 Hz	4000 Hz
Ipsilateral	105	100	105	AB	AB	AB	AB	AB
Contralateral	AB	AB	AB	AB	110	110	AB	AB

AB = Absent Reflex

(a)

O = RE Pure Tone
X = LE Pure Tone
] = LE Masked BC

(continued)

allow an ipsilateral reflex to be present as long as the AN, CN, and the facial nerve and its nuclei are intact. It is possible to have an ipsilateral response negated by a brainstem lesion, but the lesion would have to be located at the lateral brainstem encompassing the ipsilateral cochlear nuclei and/or the ipsilateral facial nerve nuclei.

Figure 9.10 displays the audiogram and AR test results for a young adult with a midline pontine le-sion with an inferior-lateral extension to the left. Note that the ipsilateral left reflexes are absent even at high frequencies, while the ipsilateral right ear reflexes are present at three frequencies. Contralateral reflexes are absent or elevated for both ears. This pattern is consistent with midline brainstem involvement with extension to the left lateral brainstem. ●

Intensity and the Acoustic Reflex

One of the key measures of the AR is its threshold. As would be expected, there is some variability in threshold measures. Most studies indicate that normal AR thresholds for humans are in the 80 to 90 dB hearing level (HL) range with little effect of frequency over a 250 to 4000 Hz range. The ipsilateral reflex threshold may be reached at slightly lower levels than contralateral thresholds (see Wilson and Margolis, 1999). The measured amplitude of the AR (the degree of movement of the ossicular chain and eardrum caused by the contraction of the stapedius muscle) increases as a function of intensity level. However, there is less change in amplitude at intensities just above threshold and at high intensities (Moller, 1962; Wilson and McBride, 1978). Bilateral stimulations result in the largest amplitudes, followed by ipsilateral and then contralateral stimulations (Moller, 1962).

CLINICAL CORRELATE

Individuals with acoustic nerve or low brainstem lesions often show elevated AR thresholds or no responses. The sensitivity and specificity of the AR for discriminating cochlear from eighth nerve lesions is around 80% (Olsen, Bauch, and Harner, 1983). These measurements are somewhat dependent on the frequency of the acoustic stimulation, with higher frequencies yielding better hit rates.

It is critical to remember that the AR has an efferent component as well as an afferent component and its presence is dependent on a normally functioning facial nerve. If the facial nerve is compromised, it may be the reason for an abnormal AR response (see Silman and Silverman, 1991 for review).

Cochlear hearing loss can result in an absent AR, but usually this requires considerable hearing loss. Most individuals with less than a 45 dB HL sensorineural hearing loss of cochlear origin have an AR at less than 105 dB HL. If one measures AR thresholds in sensation level (SL) rather than HL, then most individuals with cochlear involvement have AR thresholds at reduced SLs (Popelka, 1981; Jerger et al., 1972).

Using the AR to measure the integrity of the cochlea, AN, or brainstem connections is dependent upon the presence of a normal tympanic membrane and middle ear system. The presence of a conductive hearing loss significantly limits the chances of observing an individual's AR. For example, Jerger, Anthony, Jerger, and Mauldin (1974) have shown that 40% of patients with conductive losses of 20 dB HL do not have an AR, and this percentage rises to 80% for patients with conductive hearing losses of 40 dB HL. ●

Latency of the Acoustic Reflex

The latency of the AR can be measured as a change in the ear's acoustic impedance. It is usually measured from the onset of the stimulus to the onset of the response. What constitutes the onset of the AR influences the latency measure. For example, some investigators accept any change in acoustic immittance, whereas others may require an amplitude change of 90% of the maximum (see Wilson and Margolis, 1999). Generally, stimuli that are higher in frequency and/or intensity result in shorter latencies. Moller (2000) reported that AR latencies can range from 25 to over 100 msec, and Clemis and Sarno (1980) reported AR latencies around 100 msec for normal control subjects. Recording AR latencies using electromyography (EMG) procedures yields much shorter time periods (on the order of 10 msec) than those recorded using traditional electroacoustic measures (Perlman and Case, 1939).

CLINICAL CORRELATE

AR latency is a clinical measure that deserves a close look from a diagnostic perspective. When it was first introduced as a potential clinical measure, the ABR procedure was gaining in popularity. As a result of the increased focus on the ABR, little investigative effort was directed at establishing the utility of the AR latency measure. A few reports from the early 1980s did, however, show AR latencies to be of value in separating cochlear from eighth nerve lesions (Clemis and Sarno, 1980; Jerger and Hayes,

1983). For example, AR latencies for patients with confirmed acoustic tumors were found to be more than twice the latencies measured in normals or in patients with cochlear hearing loss (Jerger and Hayes, 1983). Hence, there is some limited evidence that AR latency may be a good differential measure, but further work needs to be done—especially methodologically (see discussion above)—before the latency of the AR can be used as a diagnostic measure with proven efficiency. ●

CLINICAL CORRELATE

If dysfunction at the level of the SOC were suspected in a given patient, a battery of tests that would challenge this portion of the auditory system could be (and should be) constructed. The battery of tests might include the ABR (and if possible, the BIC of the ABR), MLDs, ipsilateral and contralateral reflexes, and some form of ITD test. This type of focused audiological test battery would require high integrity of the structures of the SOC and should uncover any abnormalities existing within this structure. ●

SUMMARY

The SOC is located in the caudal pons and is composed of two main nuclei, the LSO and MSO, as well as the nuclei of the trapezoid body and several periolivary nuclei groups. The SOC receives most of its input from the CN via the dorsal, intermediate, and ventral acoustic striae, with the preponderance of neural inputs to the SOC arising from the contralateral CN. The main cell types in the SOC are stellate (multipolar), bipolar, and fusiform cells, although other cell types are also found in the SOC. The LSO and MSO are tonotopically organized and have relatively sharp TCs. The SOC represents the first location in the auditory system where there is binaural representation of auditory signals, and this sets the stage for localization and lateralization of sound sources. These binaural processes are possible since the cells located in the SOC are highly sensitive to small time differences and level differences between the ears, and this provides potent cues for the localization and lateralization of a sound. The SOC also plays a key role in fusing or integrating information from the two ears and it is the likely the generator for wave IV of the ABR. The ABR is usually abnormal when the SOC is affected, as is often the case in intra-axial brainstem lesions. The output of the LSO of the SOC forms what has been referred to as an acoustic chiasm as the neural fibers course from the SOC to connections in the nuclei of the LL and IC. Finally, the SOC is the site of the most rostral aspect of the acoustic reflex arc. The presence of an AR within the auditory system requires major participation of the SOC along with its associated connections in the brainstem.

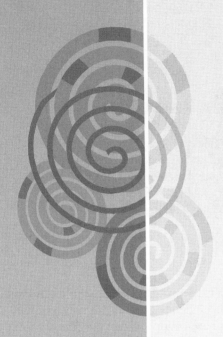

10

The Lateral Lemniscus and Inferior Colliculus

Introduction

This chapter will combine reviews of the lateral lemniscus (LL) and the inferior colliculus (IC) (Figures 10.1, 10.2, 10.3). It is reasonable to discuss these two anatomical areas in the same chapter since the LL has not received as much research or interest as other anatomical areas in the auditory system. Therefore, in the interest of efficiency it seemed practical to combine the discussion of the LL and IC. Also, in many ways the LL and IC are closely associated not only anatomically, but also physiologically. The neural fibers running through the LL represent the major auditory pathway that associates the two major subdivisions of the brainstem: the pons and the midbrain.

The IC, which is located in the midbrain region, is perhaps the most recognized and best studied structure in the ascending auditory pathway. Because of its relatively easy accessibility, a large quantity of information has been generated about its structure and function in animals. In humans, the investigation of the structure and especially the function of the IC is gaining momentum; however, it remains a challenge.

ANATOMY OF THE LATERAL LEMNISCUS

The LL encompasses three major auditory structures that will be discussed here. The LL tract is a major brainstem pathway for the auditory system (Figures 10.1 and 10.2). Two nuclei groups in the LL will also be discussed; these have been termed the ventral nucleus (VNLL) and the dorsal nucleus (DNLL). The LL pathway is formed by fibers arising from the (contralateral) cochlear nucleus (CN) that combine with fibers running from the ipsilateral superior olivary complex (SOC), immediately lateral to the lateral superior olive (LSO). This large fiber tract courses rostrally and dorsally along the lateral-most aspect of the pons before it terminates in the IC. The LL contains both afferent and efferent fibers and is about 3 cm in length in the adult human brain. About three-fourths of the way up the pons is a commissure, termed the **commissure of Probst**, that connects the nuclei of the LL (Musiek and Baran, 1986; Parent, 1996). The LL's lateral position in the pons makes it vulnerable to extrinsic lesions originating from cranial nerves VIII, VII, and V (auditory, facial, and trigeminal).

● **Figure 10.1**

The human upper pons and midbrain (dorsal view). I = inferior colliculi, 2 = lateral lemniscus, 3 = brachium of the inferior collicullus, 4 = medial geniculate body, 5 = superior colliculi, 6 = thalamus (pulvinar).

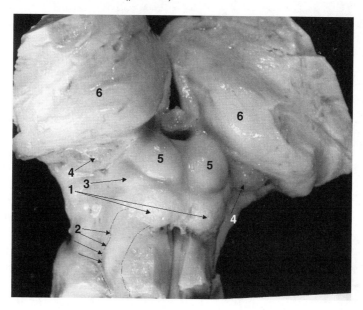

The VNLL and DNLL are the two main nuclei within the LL, but a postero-medial and an intermediate nucleus have also been defined (see Helfert and Aschoff, 1997). The latter two nuclei do not appear to have major auditory functions associated with them. Therefore, these two nuclei will not be discussed here. The VNLL is positioned more caudally and is more of an elongated structure than is the DNLL. The DNLL is in turn located immediately caudal to the caudal-most aspect of the IC. Both of the LL nuclei are surrounded by fibers of the LL (Figure 10.2) (Roberts, Hanaway, and Morest, 1987).

The VNLL receives afferent inputs from mostly contralateral tracts, with one of the key contributors being the ventral cochlear nucleus (VCN), with inputs from both the anterior-ventral and posterior-ventral portions of this nucleus (AVCN and PVCN). There are also some afferent connections from the ipsilateral medial nucleus of the trapezoid body (Glendenning, Brunso-Bechtold, Thompson, and Masterton, 1981; Parent, 1996). The VNLL may also receive some fibers from various segments of contralateral SOC, but interestingly it does not have any known inputs from the contralateral nuclei of the LL (Buser and Imbert, 1992).

The DNLL receives more inputs from lower structures and the contralateral LL nuclei than does the VNLL (Glendenning et al., 1981; see Schwartz, 1992 for review). The DNLL has bilateral inputs from the LSO. It also receives input from the ipsilateral medial superior olive (MSO), ipsilateral VNLL, contralateral VCN, and contralateral input from the other DNLL via the commissure of Probst. The commissural connection between the two DNLL is a relatively substantial neural connection. Although many of the ascending afferent fibers within the auditory system terminate and/or course through the LL, it is important to realize that there are a substantial number of ascending fibers from the CN and SOC that bypass both the DNLL and VNLL (Figure 10.2).

● Figure 10.2

(a) The main ascending neural connections of the lateral lemniscus and inferior colliculus. (b) Contralateral projections to the lateral lemniscus and inferior collicullus from more caudal auditory nuclei. (c) Ascending neural projections to the lateral nucleus (LN) of the inferior collicullus. VNLL = ventral nucleus of the lateral lemniscus, DNLL = dorsal nucleus of the lateral lemniscus, LL = lateral lemniscus, CP = commissure of Probst, IC = inferior colliculus, CIC = commissure of the inferior colliculus, BIC = brachium of the inferior colliculus, MGB = medial geniculate body, SOC = superior olivary complex, CN = cochlear nucleus, RF = reticular formation, DCN = dorsal cochlear nucleus, NDC = nucleus of the dorsal column.

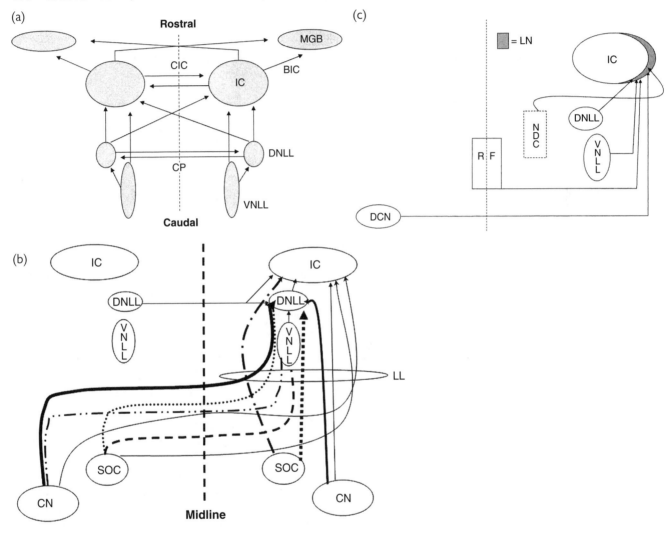

● Figure 10.3

(a) The anatomical areas of the inferior collicullus (horizontal section). (b) The perisaggittal section of the superior and inferior collicullus. ICC = central nucleus of the inferior colliculus, CIC = fibers of the commisure of the inferior collicullus, LN = lateral nucleus, CC = caudal cortex, DC = dorsal cortex, DMN = dorsal medial nucleus, SC = superior colliculus, L = lateral, D = dorsal, M = medial, V = ventral.

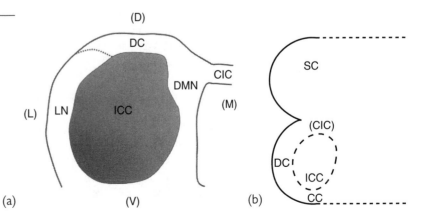

Cell Types

The cell types found in the nuclei of the LL vary depending on the species of animal investigated. In bats the VNLL is composed primarily of multipolar, globular, and elongated cells, whereas the cell types found in the DNLL include globular, elongated, and ovoid cells (Covey and Casseday, 1986). These cell types can be further categorized by their soma size, ranging from small to large (Kane and Barone, 1980; Adams, 1981).

PHYSIOLOGY OF THE LATERAL LEMNISCUS

Cell Discharge Patterns

Not as many types of discharge patterns are associated with the nuclei of the LL as there are for other brainstem nuclei. The firing patterns of the cell types in the VNLL are often "onset" and "sustained discharge" patterns (Batra and Fitzpatrick, 2002), whereas many of the DNLL cells demonstrate "chopper-type" poststimulus time histograms (PSTHs) (Aitkin, Anderson, and Brugge, 1970).

Tonotopic Organization

It was originally believed that the VNLL had low frequencies represented at its dorsal aspect and high frequencies at its ventral aspect (Brugge and Geisler, 1978). However, more recent findings suggest that the tonotopicity of the VNLL is not as well organized as in lower auditory nuclei or even as well as in the DNLL (Helfert, Sneed, and Altschuler, 1991). In addition, some novel findings are emerging that suggest that the tonotopic arrangement in the VNLL may resemble a corkscrew. Merchan and Berbel (1996) refer to this as a "helicoid" organization. The DNLL has high and low frequencies represented in the ventral and dorsal regions, respectively (Aitkin et al., 1970; Brugge and Geisler, 1978; see Helfert et al., 1991 for review). The complexity of the tonotopic organization in the VNLL and DNLL across animal species makes it difficult to predict what it might be like in the human.

The tuning curves (TCs) in the VNLL are believed to be quite broad, at least based upon investigations of TCs in the bat (see Helfert et al., 1991; Buser and Imbert, 1992). A recent study by Batra and Fitzpatrick (2002) suggests the VNLL may have varied frequency tuning. This seems to be consistent with the rather ill-defined tonotopicity of the VNLL noted above. It therefore may be reasonable to conclude that the tuning of the DNLL and VNLL is less sharp and more variable than is commonly observed at lower levels in the auditory system (e.g., low brainstem and auditory nerve).

Temporal and Binaural Aspects

The VNLL has been shown to have precise phase-locking ability, usually to the onset of a stimulus (at least in the bat). These types of rapid onset responses seem to play a key role in temporal processing either at this level or for transference to higher levels of the system for processing (Covey and Casseday, 1986). The VNLL appears to have a relatively large portion of cells that are sensitive to interaural time differences (ITDs). Also in the VNLL are some cells that are responsive only to ipsilateral ear stimuli, others that respond only to contralateral ear stimuli, and some that are responsive to binaural stimulation (Helfert and Aschoff, 1997; Batra and Fitzpatrick 2002). The DNLL has a large number of neurons that are responsive to binaural input and interaural intensity differences (IIDs). As in the SOC, there are EI and IE cells (see Chapter 9 for a description of these cell types) in the LL that may contribute to localization cues (Brugge, Anderson, and Aitkin, 1970; see Helfert and Aschoff, 1997 for review).

Neurotransmitters

The main neurotransmitters of VNLL are glycine and γ-aminobutyric acid (GABA). The DNLL has a high proportion of GABA and much smaller amounts of glutamate. The DNLL does receive glutamatergic inputs, but its outputs are nearly all GABA (see Helfert and Aschoff, 1997).

Role of the Lateral Lemniscus in the ABR

In humans, the nuclei of the LL play an important role in the generation of the auditory brainstem response (ABR) (Moller, 2000). Moller's work on generator sites of the ABR waveform in humans indicates that the predominant wave used in ABR applications (i.e., wave V) arises largely from neural activity in the LL. More precisely, it is suggested that the sharp positive peak known as wave V is primarily generated by the LL, although lesser contributions from other brainstem auditory structures are also likely (Figure 10.4).

● **F i g u r e   1 0 . 4**

A normal ABR obtained for high-intensity clicks. Wave V is likely generated by the lateral lemniscus but it may also receive a contribution from the inferior collicullus (IC). The IC may also contribute to the generation of the negative wave, Vn.

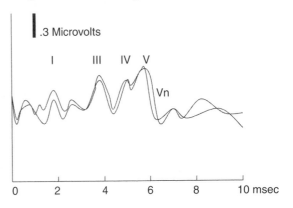

CLINICAL CORRELATE

Figure 10.5 presents audiological data for a clinical case study that is relevant to the present discussion because it highlights several key points. The patient was a young adult with a large trigeminal tumor on the right side, who presented with complaints of difficulty hearing in noise and intolerance to loud sounds. Test results revealed normal pure-tone thresholds and excellent speech recognition bilaterally at the time of testing. However, electrophysiological test results uncovered some abnormalities. The ABR for the right ear was abnormal because the interaural latency difference (ILD) was 0.6 msec, with wave V for the right ear lagging behind the latency noted for the left ear (see Figure 10.5). Also, the IV–V complex was much smaller in amplitude than wave I, and the I–III interval was extended on the right side. Since

the trigeminal nerve arises from the lateral aspect of the brainstem about midway up the pons, it was likely that the LL was involved (as well as other brainstem structures located more caudally and rostrally) in this patient. It is significant that wave V on the right side was both delayed in latency and compromised in amplitude given what we know about the generator sites (see discussion in accompanying text). Involvement of other auditory structures was supported by other electrophysiological and electroacoustic measures. The contralateral acoustic reflexes were absent, with right ear stimulation indicating auditory involvement at lower levels within the brainstem. In addition, involvement of auditory structures caudal to the LL was also supported by the I–III extension noted during ABR testing. ●

(continued)

● Figure 10.5

(a) The ABR and contralateral acoustic reflexes of a young adult patient who had a trigeminal nerve tumor on the right side. The patient's audiogram was normal bilaterally. Symptoms included tinnitus on the right side, intolerance to loud sounds, and difficulty hearing in noise. The ABR was normal for the left ear but showed an abnormal interaural latency difference (ILD) with the delay on the right. The IV–V complex was less than half the amplitude of wave I for the right ear. The contralateral acoustic reflex was elevated or absent for the right, indicating involvement of the caudal pons. (b) The anatomical effect of the lesion based on radiologic data is shown in the drawing of the brainstem pathway. The trigeminal nerve exits the lateral brainstem about halfway up the pons; hence, the lateral lemniscus was likely involved as well as neighboring auditory structures.

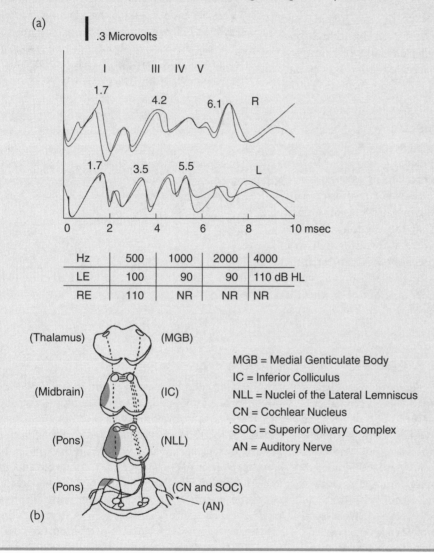

Hz	500	1000	2000	4000
LE	100	90	90	110 dB HL
RE	110	NR	NR	NR

MGB = Medial Geniculate Body
IC = Inferior Colliculus
NLL = Nuclei of the Lateral Lemniscus
CN = Cochlear Nucleus
SOC = Superior Olivary Complex
AN = Auditory Nerve

ANATOMY OF THE INFERIOR COLLICULUS

The IC along with the superior colliculus (SC) are recognized as four spherical mounds (two on each side) resembling pearls in the dorsal midbrain. The IC and SC occupy practically all of the dorsal aspect of the midbrain, with the SC located immediately rostral to the IC. The IC is bordered caudally by the DNLL. In the adult human brain, the IC is approximately 0.5 cm in diameter (Figures 10.1, 10.2 and 10.3).

It is generally recognized that there are three main divisions of the IC (Rockel and Jones, 1973). These include the central nucleus (ICC), which is bordered dorsally by the highly laminated dorsal cortex and laterally by the external (or lateral) nucleus (in humans this is referred to as the lateral zone). The lateral area of the IC has fibers that form the brachium of the IC (Geniec and Morest, 1971). In their work on the human IC, Geniec and Morest (1971) also defined a caudal cortex and a dorso-medial nucleus (the latter has also been noted in many animal models). Oliver and Morest (1984), while defining the cellular components of the IC, saw the need to further parcel the IC into additional divisions. These includ-

CLINICAL CORRELATE

Masterton, Granger, and Glendenning (1992) demonstrated the relative importance of the ipsilateral versus the contralateral LL in several hearing processes by sectioning the LL that was either ipsilateral or contralateral to the intact ear in a group of monaurally hearing cats. Sectioning of the contralateral pathway yielded more deficits for tasks involving tone and noise detection than did sectioning of the ipsilateral pathway. For frequency discrimination tasks, the contralateral LL seemed to provide better performance than did the ipsilateral LL, especially at lower test frequencies (performance was similar if the ipsilateral was or was not intact). For intensity discrimination tasks, the ipsilateral and contralateral conditions yielded similar results, but in spite of the similarity of results between the two test conditions, the results were usually not within the normal range of performance as demonstrated by matched controls. These findings suggest that the LL must be intact on both sides of the brainstem to provide optimum hearing—even for such basic auditory processes as tone detection. Moreover, the results demonstrated that compromise of the LL situated either ipsilaterally or contralaterally to the stimulated ear resulted in deficits for intensity discrimination proportionally greater than those for tonal detection. However, frequency modulation (FM) discrimination seemed to be handled well if just the contralateral lemniscus was intact. Although not documented experimentally in humans, it is anticipated that similar deficits are likely to exist in patients with compromise to the LL. ●

ed the pars centralis, the pars medialis, and the pars lateralis (for a detailed review regarding these anatomical segments of the IC, see Oliver and Shneiderman, 1991).

The IC (and its divisions) is the key auditory region in the midbrain and is essentially an obligatory connection for afferent fibers arising from lower brainstem structures. The dorsal and the external (also termed lateral) regions are less well organized auditorily and have some somatosensory representations. At this level, it is noteworthy that there is a division between the main (or perhaps classical) auditory pathway, which encompasses the ICC, its inputs, and its thalamic projections, and the nonclassical pathway, which involves the dorsal and lateral segments and their connections (Caird, 1991). The nonclassical auditory pathway, like the classical auditory pathway, continues to the medial geniculate body (MGB).

Afferent Inputs

Inputs to the IC come from the contralateral CN, SOC, and DNLL and the ipsilateral LSO, MSO, DNLL, and VNLL. Some neural inputs to the IC also arise from the ipsilateral CN (see Ehret, 1997 for review). The VNLL provides the largest single source of input to the ICC, based on numbers of cells retrogradely labeled from IC injections of horseradish peroxidose (HRP0) (Brunso-Bechtold, Thompson, and Masterton, 1981).

In animals, the connections from the LSO to the IC form an acoustic chiasm (similar to the crossing pattern in the visual system) (Glendenning and Masterton,

1983). The acoustic chiasm is composed of the low-frequency fibers projecting ipsilaterally to the IC and the high-frequency fibers crossing contralaterally to the IC (for further information, see Chapter 9). It is believed that the ipsilateral connections are inhibitory (glycinergic) and the contralateral inputs are excitatory (glutamatergic) (Glendenning and Masterton, 1983).

Output of the Inferior Colliculus

The main output tracts of the IC run ipsilaterally via the brachium of the IC to the MGB (Winer, 1992; de Ribaupierre, 1997; Moller, 2000). This is a large afferent fiber tract that courses rostrally and laterally to the MGB. There are also contralateral connections from the IC to the MGB, but these are fewer in number than those found in the ipsilateral tracts. The other major output of the IC is through the commissure of the IC. Specifically, the ICC projects to the ventral MGB (pars ovoidea) and to the posterior nucleus of the thalamus. The fibers from the dorsal and medial IC project to the ventral MGB. Most of the crossed fibers of the IC course to the medial division of the MGB (see next chapter). It is the authors' interpretation that the crossed fibers leave the IC via its commissure in some, but not all, cases.

Cell Types

Interestingly, there is considerable consistency in terms of cell types in the IC across species (see Oliver and Shneiderman, 1991 for review). There are essentially two cell types in the IC: disc-shaped cells and stellate cells (Geniec and Morest, 1971; Oliver and Morest, 1984). The disc-shaped cells are the most common type of cells in the IC, with the stellate cell types being more common in the dorsal cortex. The stellate cells can be subdivided into two categories: simple and complex. The simple cells are characterized by large oval dendritic fields, whereas the complex cells have medium-sized dendritic fields with a higher frequency of branching than the disc-shaped cells.

PHYSIOLOGY OF THE INFERIOR COLLICULUS

The IC is essentially an obligatory synapse for most of the fibers arising from lower auditory nuclei in the brainstem. Therefore, considerable information has to be processed by the IC in regard to time, intensity, frequency, and spatial domains. As Ehret (1997) explains, the IC cannot be viewed as a simple relay station to higher auditory centers, but rather, it is a complex group of nuclei that encode important information in new and different ways than is done in the lower auditory structures.

Tonotopicity and Frequency Characteristics

The IC is highly tonotopic, with well-defined iso-frequency sheets. The laminae in the IC form the basis for the tonotopic organization and correlate to the iso-frequency sheets in the IC (Parent, 1996). Moore, Semple, and Addison (1983) provide some nice examples of the iso-frequency strips in the ferret. In the IC of the house mouse, the low frequencies are located dorso-laterally and the high frequencies are located ventro-medially (Stiebler and Ehret, 1985; see also Ehret, 1997 for review) (Figure 10.6).

A variety of tuning curves (TCs) have been noted in the IC (Aitkin, Webster, Veale, and Crosby, 1975; Caird, 1991). The majority of TCs are sharp, but there also TCs that are multi-peaked and have relatively broad response characteristics. The broad and multipeaked TCs may arise from stellate cells that cross one or more of the laminae within the IC (hence, they cross one or more iso-frequency contours). These TCs have inhibitory sidebands, which are more often noted in animals that are anesthetized.

Ozesmi and colleagues implanted electrodes in the ICs of rats and stimulated these animals with tonal frequencies of 1, 2, 4, 6, and 8 kHz at 70 dB SPL (Ozesmi, Ascioglu, Suer, Golgeli, Dolu, and Sahin, 2002). No differences were noted in the latencies or amplitudes of the responses for these frequencies. This indicates that the latency differences across frequencies commonly noted at more caudal recording sites may not necessarily be maintained at the IC level. It should be noted that the frequencies in this study were quite low for the rat. Perhaps if higher frequencies were employed, the latencies may have been influenced. On the other hand, ABR recordings from humans show greater latencies for a negative wave V and wave VI (when these waves can be obtained) for 500-Hz tone pips than for higher-frequency tone pips. It is likely that the IC plays some role in the generation of negative wave V and wave VI of the ABR (see Moller, 2000 for review), and therefore, in humans it does have a latency–frequency relationship.

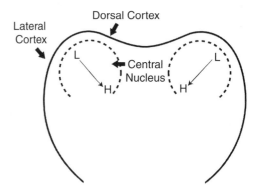

● **Figure 10.6**

The tonotopic organization of the central nucleus of the inferior colliculus. H = high frequencies, L = low frequencies.

Intensity Coding

As is now well known, both monotonic and nonmonotonic rate-intensity functions are represented in IC neurons. Some neurons increase their firing rates with intensity increases over a wide range of intensities (60 to 80 dB) and others "roll over" in regard to their rate–intensity functions, with intensity increases as small as 10 dB above threshold (Popelar and Syka, 1982; Rees and Palmer, 1988). Ehret and Merzenich (1988) showed that average spike rates for neurons in the IC are greater for tonal stimuli than for noise stimuli over a wide intensity range (−5 to 115 dB SPL). The intensity range that elicited the highest discharge rate was between 45 and 55 dB SPL, on average. It has been suggested that these response patterns may be related to a critical band code and the reestablishment of the frequency-place code at this level of the CANS (Ehret and Merzenich, 1988).

Temporal Processes and Amplitude Modulation

Most of the temporal processing studies on the IC center on amplitude modulation (AM), binaural interactions (discussed later), phase-locking, and physiological correlates to gap detection. It is of interest that the IC is the first level in the auditory nervous system that has neurons that are sound-duration sensitive (Faure, Fremouw, Casseday, and Covey, 2003). This specific neural characteristic probably contributes to the IC's ability to respond to temporal changes in a sound stimulus, such as that which is needed for accurate gap detection perception. Electrophysiological recordings from

● **Figure 10.7**

Depiction of the neuronal correlate to a gap detection task. Gap detection acuity is dependent on how quickly "responding" neurons shut down at the beginning of the gap and how quickly they respond to the beginning of the subsequent sound stimulus.

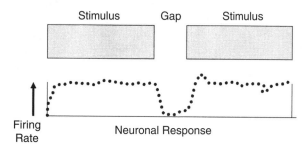

mouse IC neurons have shown gap detection functions similar to those that are obtained behaviorally (Walton, Frisina, Ison, and O'Neill, 1997). Single unit recordings from the IC in the mouse also show a physiological correlate to changing stimulus characteristics in a gap detection paradigm (Barsz, Benson, and Walton, 1998). Increasing stimulus rise and fall time increases gap thresholds, spike latency, and response strength for a given gap width. The ability of single and multiple units to shut down and turn on to follow the gap temporally is a critical physiologic characteristic (Walton, Frisina, and O'Neill, 1998) (see example in Figure 10.7).

Phase-locking of the neural fibers within the IC is not as prominent as it is for auditory neurons within the lower brainstem nuclei. Nonetheless, it is present and IC neurons can respond to the phase of low-frequency stimuli

CLINICAL CORRELATE

Walton and associates (1998) found that as mice aged, fewer IC units responded appropriately to small gap intervals in auditory stimuli. Hence, the average gap detection threshold increased as the animals aged. This finding is insightful in that it may help explain many of the subtle, but significant, auditory problems often noted in the elderly human population. ●

quite well (600 Hz and lower), but fewer IC fibers can phase-lock on signals above 600 Hz compared to more caudal auditory neurons (Kuwada, Yin, Syka, Buunen, and Wickesburg, 1984).

It has been known for some time that some IC neurons respond better (in terms of firing synchronization and response amplitude) to AM tones than to steady-state tones (see Moller, 2000). These modulation-sensitive neurons are relatively common in the IC. There are neurons in the IC of the rat that can respond to AM rates up to 500 Hz; however, the firing rates of these neurons tend to drop off quickly after an AM rate of 200 Hz is reached. In addition, some evidence suggests that the overall intensity of the stimulus has some effect on the response of IC neurons for AM rates up to 50 Hz, but that intensity has little effect on the performance of these fibers at higher modulation rates (Rees and Moller, 1987). As expected, greater modulation depths for AM stimuli tend to result in greater neural synchronization among the firing patterns of the IC fibers (Rees and Sarbaz, 1997). It has been demonstrated that some neurons in the IC have a preferred modulation depth of 100% (i.e., yielding the greatest response magnitude) (Poon and Chiu, 1997; see Joris, Schreiner, and Rees, 2004 for review).

CLINICAL CORRELATE

For optimal clinical use, auditory steady-state responses (ASSRs) are generally assessed using a 100% amplitude-modulated signal (this is referred to as maximum modulation depth). This procedure is typically followed to ensure the best possible response in a clinical setting since fully modulated stimuli evoke the greatest neural synchronization (see discussion in accompanying text). ●

CLINICAL CORRELATE

In the current clinical use of ASSR there are recommended AM rates. These recommended rates are based upon empirical data from humans that were obtained using specific recording techniques. These data provide useful information, but it may not be very specific. As we can see from information just mentioned, the IC has neurons that are sensitive to a certain stimulus modulation rate—meaning that populations of neurons may respond maximally at these AM rates. It must be realized, however, that not all neurons respond optimally to these AM rates. This could mean that by utilizing various AM rates, subpopulations of groups of neurons might be evaluated using ASSR techniques that otherwise would not be assessed if only a single AM rate is used (John, Dimitrijevic, van Roon, and Picton, 2001). ●

Spike discharges from IC neurons for AM signals are greater for the rising, as opposed to the falling, phase of the AM signal. However, it is important to take into account the shape of the AM, as this will influence the nature of the cells' responses (Poon and Chiu, 1997). In the IC there is good synchronization to AM signals, but modulation transfer functions are not as high in frequency modulation as noted in lower brainstem sites such as the CN (Rees and Moller, 1983).

CLINICAL CORRELATE

The 40-Hz steady-state response was measured in cats that had lesions induced in both ICs. Although the waveforms and the phase of the responses were essentially maintained in these experimental animals, the amplitude was markedly reduced (approximately 40%) (Tsuzuku, 1993). This could be interpreted to mean that the timing of the 40-Hz response was maintained but that fewer fibers responded synchronously. ●

A characteristic that has been discussed regarding a neuron's ability to respond to AM signals is that of response regularity (Rees and Sarbaz, 1997). There are both regular and irregular response neurons. The "regular" neurons are those that have intrinsic oscillations that help provide a "regular response," such as is noted in a "chopper" PSTH or other cells with similar types of responses. The "irregular" neural units do not have the same tendency to respond in the same manner to tone burst stimuli as do the regular units, but interestingly these units seem to respond to AM signals better than do the regular units. The "irregular" neurons are more synchronous in their firing patterns and they maintain responses at higher intensity levels than do the regular units. Therefore, it would follow that the irregular units within the IC are the ones that probably contribute to the AM responses in regard to far-field recordings such as those recorded in the clinical ASSR.

Response latencies of the IC are of great interest to clinical researchers as well as to basic scientists. Langner and Schreiner (1988) measured response latencies of the IC in the cat. In this study, which used a 60 dB SPL tone as the stimulus, response latencies ranged from 4 to 50 msec, with the majority of the fibers responding in the 10 to 14 msec range. This wide range of responses is likely representative of both excitatory and inhibitory influences within the neurons of the IC. Moller (2000) and Moller and Jannetta (1982) reviewed their work on near-field recordings from the IC in humans during neurosurgery. Moller and Jannetta (1982) used a 5-msec, 2000-Hz, 95 dB SPL tone that produced a slight positive response that was then followed by a large negative response. The positive peak occurred at about 7 msec, and the large negative peak varied in latency and morphology but usually occurred somewhere in the vicinity of 10 msec. In far-field recordings, the IC may contribute to the positive wave V noted in the ABR—but only minimally. A greater contribution from the IC is to the negative wave V of the ABR. The negative wave V usually occurs at between 6 and 7 msec for a click stimulus at intensities in the 80-dB nHL range.

CLINICAL CORRELATE

There has been much debate and misunderstanding about the relationship between the IC and the generation of wave V for the ABR. Wave V, for the most part, is generated by the nuclei of the LL. However, neurons at different levels of the brainstem and the auditory nerve may also contribute to the wave V response (see Moller, 2000 for review). Some of the still-lingering misconceptions about the IC as the pri-

mary generator site for wave V come from early reports on the ABR that suggested wave V was generated by the IC (in humans). The presumed link between neural activity within the IC and the generation of wave V was somewhat logical when one considered the latency of wave V and the fact that wave V was the largest peak within the ABR waveform, which matched with the fact that the IC was the largest auditory nuclei

Figure 10.8

An ABR (a) from a young adult with bilateral lesions of the inferior colliculus as shown in the MRI (b). There appears to be some compromise of the IV–V complex bilaterally. Since there was no damage that could be seen caudal to the inferior colliculi radiologically, it appears that the IC may contribute to some degree to the generation of wave V of the ABR when it is conventionally recorded.

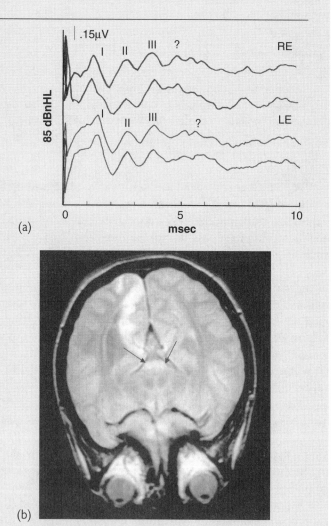

(continued)

group in the brainstem pathway. However, subsequent work in humans by Moller and his associates during neurosurgery indicated that the IC was probably not the primary generator of the ABR wave V (Moller and Jannetta, 1982; Moller, Jho, Yokota, and Jannetta, 1995; Moller, 2000).

A number of clinical reports of patients with lesions in the area of the IC have shown essentially normal ABRs, including a normal wave V and/or IV–V complex (Jerger, Neely, and Jerger, 1980; Musiek, Gollegly, Kibbe, and Verkest, 1988). On the other hand, other studies have shown some abnormalities in wave V or the IV–V complex in patients with involvement of the IC (Hirsch, Durrant, Yetiser, Kamerer, and Martin, 1996; Musiek, Charette, Morse, and Baran, 2004). In many, if not all, of these latter studies, however, there was not isolated involvement of the IC.

We recently reported ABR results for a case in which there was a highly specific lesion involving both ICs (Musiek et al., 2004). In this case it appeared that wave V may have been present but that it was severely compromised in terms of its morphology for both ears. Figure 10.8 presents the ABR waveforms for this patient. Inspection of the waveforms reveals that the latency of wave V may have been extended slightly, but the morphology of the IV–V complex is such that it is difficult to isolate a definitive peak. In analyzing these waveforms, it seems that much of the compromise of wave V may have been related to a lack of negative slope for wave V. This patient was totally "centrally" deaf for about a week but then started hearing environmental sounds. Eventually the patient achieved normal pure-tone thresholds; however, even when this was the case, his auditory discrimination was poor, as was his understanding of speech in noise. Hirsch et al. (1996) provided a report of a specific lesion to one IC, which resulted in a definite compromise of wave V of the ABR. Clearly, these cases document the major role the IC plays in many aspects of hearing. ●

Binaural Activity and Sound Localization

Many studies have been conducted on localization and binaural processing related to localization in reference to the IC. Many of these are rather extensive and complex studies that are beyond the scope of this chapter. Ehret (1997) provides an excellent review of these studies for the reader who is interested in more than the cursory overview that will be provided here. As was the case with the neural excitation patterns noted for SOC neurons, there are IC neurons that respond to various binaural situations. The EO neurons are the units that respond to monaural stimulation to the contralateral ear. Binaural responses (EI and IE) are neurons that are sensitive to acoustic stimulation of both ears, and EE units are those that are responsive to monaural stimulation for either ear. The EI neurons in the IC are especially sensitive to cues for localization, of which there are two components; ITD and IID neurons. As discussed in the previous chapter, the ITD units are those that are sensitive to interaural time differences and the IID units are those that are sensitive to interaural intensity differences, which of course is the basis for localization and lateralization. It should be stated, however, that EE units can also be sensitive to ITDs. Irvine (1986), in reviewing studies of the cat IC, found that 25% of IC neurons are monaural EO units and 75% are binaural units, of which 30 to 40% are EI units.

Aitkin (1988) showed that ITD and IID neurons generate variable firing rates as the azimuth of the sound source (i.e., its position along the horizontal plane) is varied. Some IC neurons are selective to certain azimuths and clearly respond best to those source angles (Aitkin, Pettigrew, Calford, Phillips, and Wise,

CLINICAL CORRELATE

It has been shown that humans with lesions in the region of the IC demonstrate below normal performance on both interaural intensity and time judgments (Furst et al., 2000). These findings suggest that these procedures would be useful for administration to patients with expected involvement in the upper brainstem region. Unfortunately, such procedures have not been used extensively in the clinical arena to date, largely because of the lack of commercially available clinical tests that assess these processes. ●

1985). Despite the sensitivity and organization of time and intensity difference by neurons in the IC, there are no spatial maps of the IC in mammals (Ehret, 1997). Perhaps one of the reasons for the lack of spatial maps is the lack of neurons that are sharply tuned to spatial information independent of sound intensity within this structure (see Ehret, 1997).

One of the best-known clinical tests and research tools tapping binaural interaction processes is the binaural masking-level difference (BMLD) procedure. Briefly, the procedure involves diotic listening to tones (or speech) in the presence of broadband noise. By changing the relative interaural phase of either the noise or the tones (speech) from an in-phase to out-of-phase condition, a release from masking occurs. This allows better hearing in noise. Palmer, Jiang, and McAlpine (2000), who recorded responses from low-frequency IC neurons in guinea pigs using a BMLD paradigm, showed a 4 to 7-dB increase in neural response for 500-Hz tones when the phase was changed from the in-phase to the out-of-phase condition. This indicates a correlation between what is observed in humans and the functioning of the low-frequency neurons in the IC of guinea pigs (see previous chapter for additional discussion of this topic).

CLINICAL CORRELATE

A number of clinical studies have documented the role the IC plays in sound location. A patient with a hemorrhage of the dorsal midbrain was tested for sound localization ability by Litovsky, Fligor, and Tramo (2002). This patient, who had a normal and symmetrical pure-tone audiogram, showed a deficit in sound localization identification in the hemi-field contralateral to his IC lesion. In our own patient with lesions of both ICs (discussed earlier), there was a marked sound field localization problem to the degree that this patient could not correctly localize acoustic stimuli emanating from speakers positioned at 45° to the left and 45° to the right. Over time, however, this patient's localization abilities improved. This finding was similar to that reported in a study on rats where bilateral IC lesions were induced and localization ability in the sound field was tested (Zrull and Coleman, 1996). The animals in this study showed significant deficits on the localization paradigm following lesioning of the ICs, but these deficits lessened with time. ●

Neurotransmitters of the Inferior Colliculus

Glutamate decarboxylase (GAD), GABA, and glycine are neurotransmitters all found in the IC. As noted in other auditory brainstem structures, glutamate is excitatory, while GABA and glycine play a more inhibitory role in auditory functions (Adams and Wenthold, 1987).

CLINICAL CORRELATE

It is interesting to note that Palmer and associates (2000) drew a correlation between an increase in neural responses in the IC with the phase changes and associated responses (i.e., the release from masking) commonly noted in humans when taking the BMLD test. However, a classic study (as discussed in Chapter 9) by Lynn and his colleagues that compared the effects of caudal pontine lesions, rostral pontine lesions, and lesions of the midbrain in humans revealed little effect of the more rostral lesions on the BMLD, whereas in the patients with lesions of the low pons, there was a marked effect on the release from masking measure (Lynn, Gilroy, Taylor, and Leiser, 1981). These findings are somewhat at odds with each other, and as such, raise some interesting questions. Lynn and his associates used speech stimuli (consonant-vowels), while Palmer and associates (2000) used tonal stimuli. Could the differences noted in these two investigations be related to the nature of the stimuli employed to assess the BMLD, or could the differences be related to some underlying physiological differences in the ICs of the animals (guinea pigs) versus humans? Answers to these questions will need to await further clinical investigation. ●

(continued)

SUMMARY

The LL pathway, its associated nuclei, and the IC represent the main auditory pathway and auditory structures within the brainstem above the level of the SOC. The LL is a fiber pathway positioned laterally in the pons that courses to the IC in the midbrain. The nuclei of the LL are termed the ventral and dorsal lateral lemnisci and are located in the upper pons. The VNLL receives mostly contralateral inputs, whereas the DNLL has mostly bilateral inputs. Tonotopically, both LL nuclei show high-frequency responses ventrally and low frequencies dorsally. The frequency selectivity of the neurons in the LL is not as sharp as those noted in more caudal auditory brainstem structures. Perhaps the LL and its nuclei are best known for their major contribution to wave V of the ABR. Finally, it should be noted that the LL has a commissure (Probst), which functionally connects the LL on both sides of the brainstem.

The IC is known as the largest structure in the auditory brainstem pathway. It receives input either directly or indirectly from essentially all of the more caudally situated auditory structures in the brainstem. The IC has a central nucleus that is made up of disc-type cells. This central nucleus has a tonotopic organization, with the low frequencies represented dorsal-laterally and the high frequencies represented ventro-medially. A wide variety of TCs are measured from the IC, with some of these being multipeaked. The IC is especially known for its variety of rate-intensity functions. Some neurons reach maximum firing rates at 5 to 10 dB above threshold and "roll over" at higher intensities, whereas other neurons have a large dynamic range for intensity. Neurons within the IC have been shown to have a strong response to both AM and FM signals, responding maximally to modulation frequencies under 200 Hz. The IC is also active in binaural processing and contains both binaurally and monaurally sensitive cells. Interaural timing and intensity-sensitive cells in the IC help provide the foundation for the ability of humans, as well as other species, to track sound sources that move. The IC also demonstrates a predictable neural response to gaps in auditory signals. Finally, clinical studies with patients with lesions affecting the IC have clearly established the importance of this structure in overall hearing processes, as damage to it has been shown to result in major deficits in auditory function.

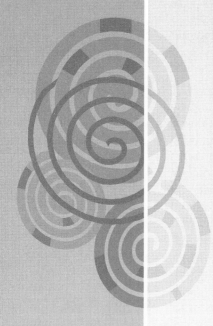

11 The Medial Geniculate Body and Auditory Thalamus

Introduction

The next major auditory structure in the ascending auditory pathway after the inferior colliculus (IC) and its brachium is the medial geniculate body (MGB). This chapter focuses primarily on the MGB, but it will also include a brief discussion of three other thalamic nuclei that are known to be responsive to acoustic stimuli, the **posterior nucleus** (PN) group, the **pulvinar**, and the **reticular nucleus** (RN). These nuclei increase the recognized auditory responsive area of the thalamus, which means that auditory dysfunction caused by damage to the thalamus becomes more probable although still relatively rare. Therefore, clinicians should be aware that damage to any of these four thalamic structures (MGB, PN, pulvinar, and RN) could result in some form of auditory compromise. Also, it is important to recognize that at this level of the auditory system there exists some anatomical and physiological diversity within the neuronal populations comprising these auditory nuclei that is not typically observed in the auditory nuclei located lower in the auditory system. Although many of the neurons at this level of the ascending auditory system respond to auditory stimuli, multimodality neurons additionally respond to other (nonauditory) stimuli, sending outputs to or receiving inputs from nonauditory structures within the central nervous system.

ANATOMY OF THE MEDIAL GENICULATE AND THE AUDITORY THALAMUS

The thalamus is a relatively large oval structure that is rostral and lateral to the brainstem axis. In the adult human the thalamus measures about 3 cm along its anterior to posterior axis and about 1.5 cm along its lateral to medial and caudal to rostral axes (Barr, 1972). The observation of the various segments of the thalamus depends on which view of the thalamus one takes. If one takes a latero-posterior, superior view, one can observe most of the nuclei of this structure. The internal medullary lamina divides the thalamus into lateral, medial, and anterior segments, with the lateral segment being the largest. The lateral-most aspect of the thalamus borders the internal capsule and contains the thinly layered reticular nucleus that is separated from the more medial nuclei of the lateral side by the external medullary lamina. Also, the anterior nucleus lies on the lateral side (between the "Y" branches of the internal lamina), along with the ventral anterior,

Figure 11.1

Posterior view of the human midbrain and thalamus.
1 = inferior colliculus, 2 = superior colliculus, 3 = medial geniculate body (MGB) (dashed outline), 4 = branchium of the inferior colliculus, 5 = the pulvinar of the thalamus. The arrows indicate the pathway of the brachium of the inferior colliculus, which can be seen in this picture as a slight bulge between the inferior colliculus and the medial geniculate body.

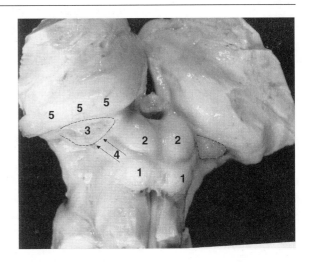

lateral dorsal, ventral lateral, lateral posterior, and ventral posterior nucleus groups. In the posterior segment is the pulvinar, with the lateral and medial geniculate located on its caudal aspect. On the medial side of the internal medullary lamina lies the medial nucleus (Netter, 1958; Barr, 1972). The MGB is the main auditory structure situated within the thalamus (Figures 11.1, 11.2, and 11.3).

The MGB can be viewed in the human brain by removing the cerebellum and observing the posterior aspect of the midbrain, specifically the IC. Lateral and rostral to the IC is the brachium of the IC that can be followed to an oval structure on the underside of the posterior thalamus, namely the MGB. Immediately lateral to the MGB is the lateral geniculate. The PN group of the thalamus is essentially anterior and rostral to the MGB and is divided into several segments (ventral, lateral, medial). The RN is rostro-lateral to the MGB. The RN's anterior portion is dedicated to somesthetic neurons, the posterior-dorsal portion to visual fibers, and the postero-ventral to auditory fibers (Winer, 1992; Parent, 1996).

Figure 11.2

A right thalamus. 1 = reticular nucleus, 2 = external medullary lamina, 3 = postero-lateral nucleus, 4 = ventral lateral nucleus, 5 = ventral anterior nucleus, 6 = pulvinar, 7 = lateral posterior nucleus, 8 = lateral dorsal nucleus, 9 = internal medullary lamina, 10 = medial nucleus, 11 = anterior nucleus, 12 = midline nucleus, 13 = medial geniculate body, 14 = lateral geniculate body (based on Netter, 1958).

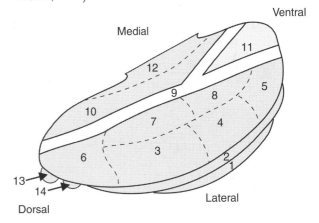

Figure 11.3

Transverse section of the medial geniculate body (MGB) in man showing the three main segments of this structure and the tonotopic arrangement of the ventral segment. H = high frequencies, M = mid frequencies, L = low frequencies.

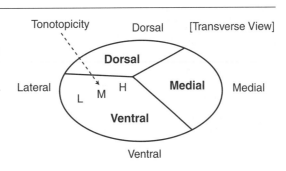

Morest (1964, 1965a) identified three major divisions of the MGB: the ventral, medial, and dorsal divisions. This anatomical categorization was initially based on morphological differences observed among the cells found in the three subdivisions of this structure, but later it was altered to reflect differences in the specific types and arrangements of the neural connections associated with the three subdivisions (Morest, 1965b). The ventral portion is highly auditory and the neurons are quite homogeneous (Figure 11.3). In the central segment of the ventral portion of the MGB is an area termed the pars ovidea. This is the area of the MGB that is most responsive to auditory stimuli.

Neural Inputs

De Ribaupierre (1997) discusses three ascending systems that input into the auditory thalamus: the tonotopic system, the diffuse system, and the polysensory system. The tonotopic system's input to the MGB comes from the central nucleus of the IC (ICC). These ascending fibers connect to the PN of the thalamus and the ventral division of the MGB. The diffuse system courses from the pericentral nucleus of the IC and inputs primarily to the dorsal MGB. The polysensory system courses from the external (or lateral) nucleus of the IC and connects to the medial division of the MGB (Figure 11.4).

Winer (1992) also reviews the neuronal inputs to the MGB. The brachium of the IC is the main pathway for the IC to MGB connection. The brachium of the IC essentially becomes the medial aspect of the MGB and sends fibers to the other sections of the structure (Morest, personal communication). The main input from the ICC is

● Figure 11.4

The main afferent inputs from the inferior colliculus to the medial geniculate body (MGB). IC = inferior colliculus, central = central nucleus of the inferior colliculus, MGB = medial geniculate body. The connections between the IC and MGB are primarily via the brachium of the IC and the inputs from outside of the central nucleus (lateral and dorsal regions of the inferior colliculus) are likely part of the nonclassical auditory pathway.

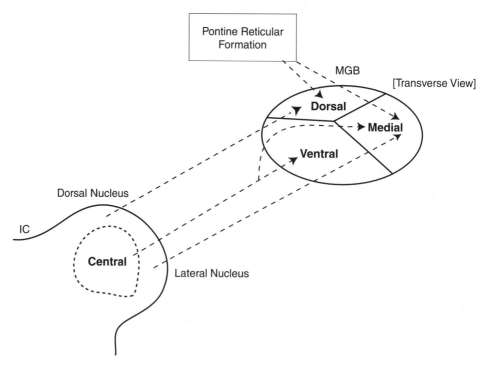

to the ventral portion (including the pars ovidea) of the MGB. This connection is from one highly auditory area in the IC to another highly concentrated auditory area in the MGB. The ventral division also receives input from the dorsal-medial IC. The dorsal and medial divisions of the MGB receive inputs that originate for the most part from areas outside the ICC, as shown in Figure 11.4. These latter connections contribute to what has come to be known as the nonclassical auditory pathway. These neural connections to the medial and dorsal divisions of the MGB have some auditory fibers, but in addition, they have many nonauditory neurons.

It is probably fair to say that most of the crossed inputs from the IC and lower brainstem nuclei end up in the medial division of the MGB, although there is some uncertainty about this (Pickles, 1982; Winer, 1992). However, it should be noted that most of the afferent inputs from the IC to the MGB are not crossed.

The PN group of the auditory thalamus receives some of its auditory input from the IC (Winer, 1992; de Ribaupierre, 1997). The RN of the thalamus is in the loop of the thalamo-cortical connections and feedback to the IC (Winer, 1992). This feedback loop is likely to contain efferent neurons and may be a part of the efferent system (see Chapter 15). The MGB also contributes to the nonclassical auditory pathway. The dorsal and medial segments of the MGB are polysensory and are generally considered part of the nonclassical pathway. This nonclassical auditory pathway also contributes (inputs) to the pulvinar (see Ehert and Romand, 1997 for discussion).

Neural Outputs

The neural outputs from the MGB, in general, course through the basal ganglia, specifically the internal capsule where some fibers connect to two structures (i.e., caudate and putamen), which border the internal capsule on both sides (Figures 11.5, 11.6, and 11.7). The ventral portion of the MGB takes a pathway

● **Figure 11.5**
_____

The main cortical connections of the medial geniculate body.

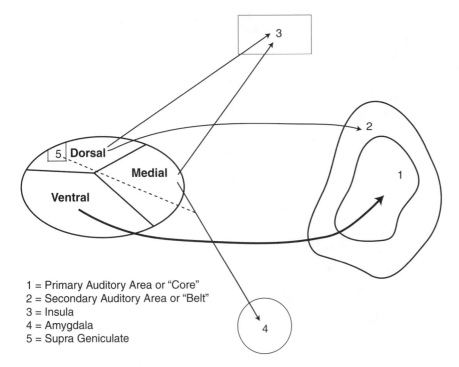

1 = Primary Auditory Area or "Core"
2 = Secondary Auditory Area or "Belt"
3 = Insula
4 = Amygdala
5 = Supra Geniculate

● **Figure 11.6**

The authors' proposed pathways of neurons projecting from the medial geniculate to cortical areas. One is a sublenticular pathway, which is a well-known pathway. The other pathway courses more rostrally, ascending through the internal capsule and potentially leading to the inferior parietal lobe and possibly the insula. AC = auditory cortex, LP = lenticular process, MGB = medial geniculate body.

AC = Auditory Cortex
MGB = Medial Geniculate Body
LP = Lenticular Process
TH = Thalamus

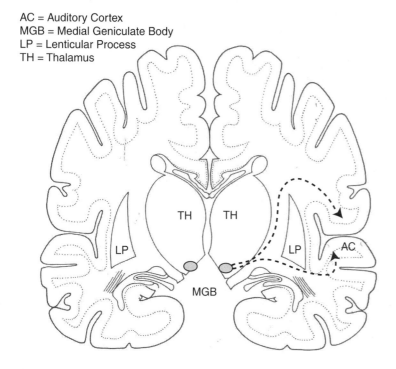

● **Figure 11.7**

The superior temporal plane. Arrows show the pathways of medial geniculate neurons through the internal capsule leading to the cortex. 1 = internal capsule, 2 = external capsule, 3 = insula, 4 = Heschl's gyrus, 5 = planum temporale, 6 = caudate, 7 = thalamus, 8 = lenticular process.

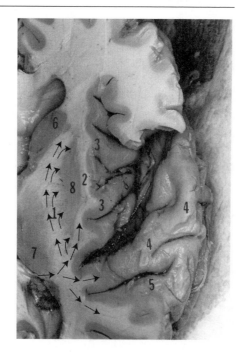

through the internal capsule and then courses in a lateral direction to the primary auditory area (Heschl's gyrus). This fiber tract is essentially all auditory fibers (Waddington, 1984). The pulvinar and PN project their polysensory neurons to the parabelt areas of the auditory cortex (see Chapter 12) (Hackett, Stepniewska, and Kaas, 1998).

Another pathway from the MGB (probably from the suprageniculate or medial nucleus) courses along the inferior internal capsule and proceeds in an anterior direction alongside but medial to the optic tract before running laterally under the putamen to the external capsule, from which it connects to the insula. These fibers are auditory, somatosensory, and possibly visual (Streitfeld, 1980; Musiek and Baran, 1986). The dorsal division of the MGB takes the common internal capsule route to the secondary auditory areas of the cortex, as well as the insula. There may also be some connections to the primary auditory areas (Streitfeld, 1980; Winer, 1992; de Ribaupierre, 1997).

Another output connection from the MGB (probably fibers from the medial division) courses to the amygdala (Russchen, 1982). This connection has become a much studied one in recent years because of the relationship between emotion and auditory anatomy. Specifically, the fibers from the medial division of the MGB connect to a striatal field involving the dorsal archistriatum, which is also termed the amygdala (LeDoux, 1986). In addition to its connections to the cortex and amygdala, the MGB projects to the posterior area of the caudate. Auditory fear-conditioning experiments contributed to our understanding of this anatomy. In these experiments, the animals (usually rats) were conditioned to a sound that created a fear response, and then they underwent ablations of the auditory cortex. Follow-up testing subsequent to cortical ablation revealed essentially no effect on the conditioned fear response. However, when the MGB was ablated, the fear response was totally lost, indicating the importance of the MGB and its relay to the subcortical areas, specifically the amydala, in this response pattern (LeDoux, 1986; Yaniv, Schafe, LeDoux, and Richter-Levin, 2001).

Cell Types

There are two main cell types in the ventral portion of the MGB. These include large bushy cells and small stellate cells (Morest, 1964; see Winer, 1992 for review). In contrast, Winer and Morest (1983) found cell types in the medial and dorsal divisions of the MGB that were highly diverse and included different types of stellate, bushy, tufted, and elongated nerve cells. These two divisions within the MGB (i.e., medial and rostral) have auditory sensitive neurons, but they also have many neurons that are nonauditory (mostly somatosensory) in nature. This composition of auditory and nonauditory fibers is somewhat different than what is observed in the ventral division, which appears to contain only auditory responsive fibers. In a recent study, however, two types of cells were defined in the ventral division of the MGB of the rabbit (Cetas, Price, Velenovsky, Crowe, Sinex, and McMullen, 2002). Type I cells were defined as those with thick dendrites and diverse appendages, and type II cells had thin dendrites and small spines. For the most part, type 1 cells were auditory responsive cells, whereas the type II cells were largely nonauditory cells. However, both types were acoustically responsive and yielded onset, offset, and sustained response patterns to auditory stimuli.

PHYSIOLOGY OF THE MEDIAL GENICULATE BODY AND AUDITORY THALAMUS

Frequency Information

The discussion of the tonotopic organization of the MGB will focus on the ventral division, since this division contains the majority of the auditory fibers within the thalamus and is considered part of the classic ascending auditory pathway. Reference will be made to other structures in the auditory thalamus only when the physiology of these structures is important to the discussion at hand.

The tonotopic organization of the ventral segment of the MGB was first elucidated by the discovery of a layered arrangement of dendrites (Morest, 1965a) and then by the sequencing of the best frequencies that were recorded by Woolsey (1964). In the cat, it was observed that the low frequencies were located in the lateral aspect of the ventral component of the MGB and that the high frequencies were situated in the medial aspect of this structure (see also Aitkin and Webster, 1971, 1972) (Figure 11.3). The PN also has a tonotopic arrangement with representation of low to high frequencies running in a rostral to caudal direction within this region (Imig and Morel, 1985).

Tuning curves (TCs) recorded from the ventral segment of the MGB show a wide variety of types, with up to five categories of TCs being identified (Morel, Rouiller, de Ribaupierre, and de Ribaupierre, 1987). The TCs from the MGB have been classified as broad, narrow, multipeaked, and atypical. There are two atypical types of TCs within the PN and RN. One is a TC that is relatively sharp for both high- and low-frequency stimuli and the other is rather board, at least in comparison to the TCs noted in other auditory structures. Imig and Morel (1985) demonstrated relatively narrow TCs for the PN, whereas the RN has been shown to have rather broad TCs (Villa, 1990). It seems safe to state that the MGB, PN group, and RN of the auditory thalamus in some manner retain the frequency information that has been processed and passed on from the auditory nuclei located more caudally in the auditory system (i.e., the midbrain and pons). The wide range of types of TCs found within the auditory structures within the thalamus possibly reflects the capacity of these structures to process various types of inputs along the frequency domain.

Intensity Aspects

Intensity coding at the MGB generally falls into two categories: **monotonic** and **nonmontonic** (Dunlop, Itzkowic, and Aitkin, 1969; Rouiller, de Ribaupierre, Morel, and de Ribaupierre, 1983). These two response patterns are similar to the types of intensity responses observed in auditory nuclei located within the pons and the midbrain. However, there are some notable differences in the proportions of monotonic and nonmonotonic cells found in the MGB and in auditory nuclei located more caudally. In the MGB, about one-fourth of the cells are monotonic and three-fourths are nonmonotonic (Roullier et al., 1983). Some of the monotic fibers in the ventral part of the MGB have an intensity range of 60 to 80 dB, but other monotic fibers within the structure begin responding only at high intensity levels. The combination of these two types of monotonic fiber types extends the dynamic range of this structure. The nonmonotonic fibers are characterized by varied dynamic ranges for intensity coding; however, they generally shut down at higher intensities (see de Ribaupierre, 1997).

Another measurement of intensity effects has to do with the latency of the spike discharges. It is well known that for the auditory nerve and lower brainstem nuclei, as the intensity of the stimulus increases, the latency of the response decreases. However, at the MGB, only 38% of the cells follow this course; the others do not necessarily respond to intensity increases in the typical fashion (see de Ribaupierre, 1997).

Temporal Responses

Rouiller, de Ribaupierre, and de Ribaupierre (1979) and de Ribaupierre (1997) have published experimental results and reviews that address the temporal coding of auditory information within the MGB. Temporal coding within the MGB, specifically within the ventral segment of the MGB, is slightly different than that noted at the lower nuclei within the central auditory nervous system. Only about 10% of the neurons in the MGB (ventral division) can phase-lock onto tones up to 1000 Hz, with the vast majority of the neurons in the MGB limited in their phase-locking ability to tones at or under 250 Hz. In contrast to these capacities, neurons in the low brainstem and auditory midbrain have the ability to phase-lock at much higher frequencies (see earlier chapters for discussion).

Another type of temporal processing can be determined by how well neurons can respond to repetitive transients (clicks). The majority of cells within the MGB can respond to several hundred clicks per second. However, some cells of the MGB do not respond at all and others respond or fire only between clicks. Perhaps the most interesting firing patterns are found among some selective neurons that fire to groups of clicks rather than to individual stimuli (de Ribaupierre, 1997). Finally, it should be noted that the available evidence suggests that temporal coding is better preserved in the ventral portion of the MGB than it is in the medial or dorsal portions of this structure (Lennartz and Weinberger, 1992).

Rouiller and colleagues (1979) categorized five types of responses from cells in the ventral portion of the MGB. The most common response type is the "on" response, which demonstrates activity only at the onset of an abrupt, short stimulus. There is also a sustained response (termed a "through" response), which continues for the entire duration of the stimulus, and an "off" response, in which firing occurs only at the termination of the stimulus. A fourth category is the "late" response category, which is essentially a delayed response in which firing occurs following the onset of the stimulus and terminates before the offset of the stimulus. The last category is the "sustained suppression" response, which is most likely an inhibitory response that is initiated after the onset of the stimulus and continues throughout the duration of the stimulus. He (2001) showed that the on type of response is the most common of the MGB responses. This investigator was able to attach some specific anatomy to the on and off responses, showing that on responses were found at the core of the ventral segment and that off responses were more likely to be situated toward the fringe of this area, close to the boundaries of the other divisions.

An exploration of the manner in which the temporal coding of strings of transient stimuli is handled in the MGB helps reveal more information about the temporal coding processes in this structure (see de Ribaupierre, 1997 for review). Rouiller and colleagues have developed a classification system for the coding of cell responses based upon their response patterns to repeated transients (Rouiller, de Ribaupierre, Toros-Morel, and de Ribaupierre, 1981). The classification developed includes four categories of cell response patterns. The most common are the synchronous responses in which the cells lock onto each individual transient. These responses are limited by the rate of presentation. There are also global responsive cells that fire at the onset and/or offset of a train of transient stimuli and other cells that fire in between the clicks in a train. These latter cells are thought to be inhibitory in nature, with the clicks triggering the inhibitory responses. Finally, some cells in the MGB simply do not respond to series of transient stimuli. The last three types of cells mentioned are in the minority within the MGB, with the cells that provide synchronous responses clearly in the majority. A consideration of these categories reveals certain physiological characteristics associated with MGB neurons. The lockers (i.e., fibers that fire synchronously) show good temporal integrity that is critical for processing speech and acoustic patterns. Other cells (e.g., those that fire between stimuli in a train) are likely inhibitory responses, which showcase this important auditory process in the temporal domain. The cells that are nonresponders may reveal cells that are waiting in "reserve" for situations when either there is damage to the other types of cells or when other unique types of stimuli are presented. Finally, the global responsive cells may provide more neural activity at the beginning or end of the stimulus—perhaps an important process in facilitating the response to onset of sound and then back to silence. Interestingly, it appears that the PN group has similar temporal processing properties as the ventral nucleus of the MGB (de Ribaupierre, 1997). These varied firing patterns clearly point to a diversity in the response patterns of the neurons within the MGB and auditory thalamus.

Binaural Coding

The MGB and other auditory areas of the thalamus are active in sound localization and lateralization. It has been shown that the majority of the cells in the auditory areas of the MGB show various types of binaural interactions that are critical for localization and lateralization (Calford, 1983; de Ribaupierre, 1997). In a recent report, Cetas et al. (2002) showed that in the ventral segment of the MGB 53% of the cells were the EE type, 27% were the EO type, and 20% were the EI type (see Chapter 9 for specification of these various cell types). Similar findings have also been reported by de Ribaupierre (1997). Ivarsson, de Ribaupierre, and de Ribaupierre (1988) showed that in the ventral MGB, there were cells sensitive to both interaural time and intensity differences (ITDs, IIDs). In this study, there were cells that responded to small and large IIDs and cells that responded to ITDs that varied considerably in their response characteristics. These researchers additionally found that a large portion of the cells in the PN were sensitive to localization cues, similar to those in the ventral MGB. Finally, de Ribaupierre (1997) reported an inability to locate cells in the ventral MGB that responded to specific points in auditory space. This would indicate that auditory space maps may not exist in the ventral MGB.

Comparison of Selected Physiologic Properties of the Main Divisions of the MGB

Calford and Aitkin (1983) overviewed the key physiologic properties of the various segments of the MGB for comparative purposes. The ventral portion has good frequency selectivity, while the dorsal and medial segments have relatively poor frequency selectivity. The dorsal segment has short latencies in response to acoustic stimuli, while the dorsal and medial segments have long latencies and/or variable latencies to sound onsets. The ventral portion of the MGB is tonotopically organized, but it is difficult to determine organized tonotopicity in the dorsal and medial segments. This relegation of distinct physiologic properties to different nuclei within the MGB is consistent with the observation that the MGB and thalamus have two pathways, with the classic auditory pathway involving the ventral segment and the nonclassical pathway involving the dorsal and medial portions of the MGB as originally suggested by the pioneering neuroanatomical studies of Rassmussen (1964), Winer and Morest (1983), and Morest (1965b).

Pathological Aspects

A review of the literature reveals a paucity of information as to what happens to auditory function when the MGB is damaged. Given what is known about the function of the MGB, there is no reason to expect that auditory function remains unaffected by compromise of the auditory substrate within this structure (see Table 11.1); however, only a few cases with MGB involvement have been studied. It must be remembered that not all lesions of the thalamus necessarily affect auditory processes. The thalamus is relatively large and some areas are not auditory; hence, damage to nonauditory areas of the thalamus may not yield auditory deficits.

● **Table 11.1**

Summary of the expected test findings for a number of audiologic test procedures in patients with damage to the medial geniculate body.

Test Procedure	Expected Results
Pure-tone thresholds	No effect
Speech recognition	No effect
Dichotic listening	Reduced scores for the ear contralateral to the side of the MGB lesion
Frequency patterns	Questionable, possible bilateral deficits
Auditory brainstem response	No effect
Middle latency response	Reduced amplitude of the Na-Pa response with ear and electrode effects variable
Late potentials	Reduced amplitude of the N1, P2, and P3 responses with ear and electrode effects variable

Behavioral studies in animals where the MGB was systematically damaged have demonstrated effects on frequency discrimination and sound localization abilities (Jenkins and Masterton, 1982; Heffner and Heffner, 1984). An earlier study by Glassman, Forgus, Goodman, and Glassman (1975) showed a compromise for both click and tone discrimination in animals with large lesions of the MGB, while more recently, Peiffer, Rosen, and Fitch (2002) demonstrated that animals with small lesions of the MGB had difficulty with temporal processing tasks such as rapid ordering of two acoustic elements.

Some of the evoked potentials (EPs) routinely used in the clinical assessments of auditory function are likely to be affected by damage to the MGB (and the auditory thalamus). Specifically, compromise of the middle latency response (MLR) may be expected since the thalamo-cortical pathway and the RN play a role in the generation of this response. In addition, compromise of the later auditory EPs could be

CLINICAL CORRELATE

It has been demonstrated that humans (children) with language problems and/or dyslexia often have difficulty performing temporal processing tasks such as those discussed above (Tallal et al., 1996). Postmortem studies of the brains of individuals with dyslexia have revealed anatomical differences in the MGB compared to the brains of controls. Specifically, dyslexic brains had more smaller and fewer larger neurons on the left side of the brain than on the right side when compared to the cell distribution seen for individuals without reading disability (Galaburda and Eidelberg, 1982). These results suggest that the MGB in dyslexics may have an anatomical correlate to the abnormal auditory processing often noted in children with this common reading abnormality. ●

CLINICAL CORRELATE

A few studies have examined the effects of lesions of the MGB on auditory processing (Berlin, Cullen, Berlin, Tobey, and Mouney, 1975; Hugdahl, Wester, and Asbjornsen, 1991; Fischer, Bogner, Turjman, and Lapras, 1995; Wester, Irvine, and Hugdahl, 2001). There were some common features among the subjects studied in these investigations as well as in the experimental procedures used to assess auditory function that may provide some important insights into the functioning of the MGB. In all but one of the cases studied in these four investigations, the involvement was unilateral and all four of the studies included some type of dichotic test measure. The collective results of these investigations revealed a marked deficit for dichotic listening in the ear contralateral to the lesioned side for all of the cases studied. This finding was consistent with the clinical research results for a number of other patients who had lesions in the upper pons, midbrain, subcortex, and/or cortex (Musiek, Baran, and Pinheiro, 1994). The classic finding for the patients studied by Musiek et al. (1994) was a deficit in the ear contralateral to the lesion. It appears that lesions of the MGB show similar laterality effects;

that is, deficits are noted in the ear contralateral to the lesioned MGB.

Based upon the results of the studies discussed above, it is fair to predict that when the MGB is involved to a significant degree, dichotic listening will be severely compromised in at least one ear. This compromise in function may be related to the fact that little auditory information reaches the auditory cortex on the same side of the brain as the lesioned MGB (i.e., if the lesion affects a significant portion of the MGB). The consequence of this type of compromise may not be limited to the lack of input (or severely reduced input) from the auditory pathway on the lesioned side (which would result in the "classic" contralateral ear deficit since the major crossover of fibers occurs at lower levels within the central nervous system). It may also result in freeing up neural substrate for the processing of auditory information arising from the other pathway (i.e., the contralateral pathway originating at the ipsilateral ear and crossing over in the region of the SOC). Under these circumstances, it is possible that the "good" ear could perform even better than expected, as was the case with the subjects from the Wester et al. (2001) study. ●

predicted since reduced or dysynchronous input from the thalamus is likely to affect the generation of these responses. However, it should be noted that a review of the literature has failed to uncover any studies documenting abnormalities in the later EPs associated with compromise limited to the MGB and auditory thalamus.

Two investigations in the early 1990s showed that lidocaine injections into the ventral and caudo-medial MGB, as well as in the RN of guinea pigs, created a midline change in the MLR (McGee, Kraus, Littman, and Nicol, 1992; Kraus, McGee, Littman, and Nicol, 1992). A number of other studies have also documented the contribution of the MGB to the MLR (see Kraus, Kileny, and McGee, 1994 for review). It is important, however, to understand that the MGB is not the sole generator of the MLR. The RN, the auditory cortex, and the neurons along the thalamo-cortical pathway also contribute to the MLR (Kraus et al., 1994); hence, abnormalities may also be found with compromise to one or more of these structures.

Near-field EPs with recordings directly from the MGB in humans have been performed and have provided insightful information. Yvert and associates, in an investigation of patients with epilepsy who had electrodes implanted for measuring ongoing EEG activity, recorded neuroelectric activity from an electrode placed in the MGB at its lateral aspect (Yvert, Fischer, Guenot, Krolak-Salmon, Isnard, and Pernier, 2002). These investigators observed a negative potential at 13 msec and two positive potentials at 21 and 29 msec when a moderate intensity stimulus was used to elicit a response. In addition to these potentials, the waveforms also had cortical potentials interspersed between them. In an earlier investigation, Velasco and colleagues recorded responses from humans with implanted electrodes and reported response latencies ranging from about 6 to 16 msec that were interpreted as

CLINICAL CORRELATE

Harada and colleagues showed abnormal MLRs and 40-Hz potentials in a group of patients with thalamic lesions (Harada, Aoyagi, Suzuki, Kiren, and Koike, 1994). Most often the deficit was noted when the ear contralateral to the lesioned thalamus was stimulated. This trend, however, was not consistent for all of the subjects studied. Musiek et al. (1994) also documented an abnormal MLR in a patient with a left-sided thalamic lesion, but these researchers found no notable laterality effects for their patient. Fischer and colleagues (1995) employed both psychophysical methods and EPs to evaluate a patient in which the MGB and IC were excised on the left side. The middle and late auditory EPs showed no response from either ear for the electrode placed over the left hemisphere, while the responses over the right hemisphere were normal for both right ear and left ear recordings. In this patient, the ABR was abnormal, with an extended wave V for the right ear only, which is most likely related to the involvement of the IC on the left side. The dichotic listening results were similar to those reported by Berlin et al. (1975), Hugdahl et al. (1991), and Wester et al. (2001); however, in this patient there was a complete extinction of contralateral ear (i.e., right ear) responses rather than simply a contralateral ear deficit as was noted for the patients in the other studies. Obviously, with this case it is difficult to comment specifically on the role that the MGB may have played in the auditory deficits that were noted since the IC as well as the MGB had been excised. However, this case does help demonstrate the extent of the auditory compromise that might be expected if there is extensive unilateral damage to thalamic and midbrain structures. The EP and dichotic measures in this patient were consistent with the "absence" of information outflow from the MGB to the cortex and subcortex on the left side. ●

coming from the MGB (Velasco, Velasco, Almanza, and Coats, 1982). Yirmiya and Hocherman (1987) recorded near-field EPs from neurons of a rhesus monkey that was required to perform an auditory discrimination task. The auditory EPs that were recorded were increased in amplitude and were associated with motor movement, suggesting a sensori-motor interaction.

CLINICAL CORRELATE

The contribution that the MGB makes in regard to clinical auditory EPs remains unclear. However, the studies by Velasco et al. (1982) and Yvert et al. (2002) may provide some basic information that could be useful in guiding the clinician. Both the ABR and the MLR are electrophysiological measures that could reflect some activity within the MGB. Waves VI and VII of the ABR, although not used clinically because of their inconsistencies, might reflect some early MGB activity as suggested by Velasco and associates (1982). Also, the negative potential recorded by Yvert et al. (2002) in patients with epilepsy using near-field electrodes could be what is commonly termed the Na wave for the MLR. Granted, the 13-msec latency noted by these researchers is a little early for the Na response, but given the difference in the recording techniques (i.e., near-field versus far-field), slight differences might be expected. It is also conceivable that the two positive potentials recorded by Yvert and colleagues from the MGB may contribute to the Pa response noted during conventional MLR recordings, as this response can occur with latency in the range from the low 20s to low 30s msec. However, in spite of these observations, it is likely that the Pa response is generated more by neural activity within the auditory cortex and thalamo-cortical pathways (see Kraus et al., 1994) than by activity within the MGB.

Since the MGB is an obligatory connection in the auditory pathway from the IC to the auditory cortex, it undoubtedly influences the physiological activity noted at the thalamic level and higher. However, which EP or psychophysical test (or tests) may best capture its function is difficult to determine. It is important to consider that the MGB not only represents an obligatory relay station within the central auditory nervous system, but that it also is a point of convergence of the auditory neurons arising from the more caudal auditory nuclei within the auditory system. Therefore, it is likely that lesions of the MGB have marked effects on many behavioral and electrophysiological tests of higher auditory function. ●

Neurotransmitters

The predominant inhibitory neurotransmitter associated with the MGB is γ-aminobutyric acid (GABA), which is also found in the RN and in the PO group. Also found in the MGB are excitatory neurotransmitters. The main excitatory neurotransmitter in the MGB is glutamate. Inputs from the IC to the ventral MGB use glutamate and GABA for excitatory and inhibitory transmission, respectively. Cortical inputs from the MGB are thought to be glutamatergic and excitatory, while local interneurons are inhibitory and use GABA (Schwartz, Tennigkeit, and Puil, 2000; Li, Phillips, and LeDoux, 1995).

SUMMARY

The MGB is located on the underside of the posterior thalamus. Its main afferent input is from the brachium of the IC on the ipsilateral side and it is anatomically divided into three parts (the ventral, dorsal, and medial segments). The greater concentration of auditory fibers is within the ventral segment, but both the dorsal and medial parts contain some auditory fibers. In addition to the MGB, three other major structures located within the thalamus have considerable auditory responsive substrate. These include the PN, the pulvinar, and the RN. Frequency representation in the MGB is revealed by a tonotopic organization with a progression from low to high frequencies in a lateral to medial manner in the ventral segment (i.e., the major auditory segment of the MGB). The MGB has a wide variety of TCs, including narrow, broad, and multipeaked forms, and intensity is coded in the MGB by both monotonic and nonmonotonic fibers. Some fibers within the MGB only respond to high intensities, whereas others fire over low- to mid-intensity ranges. The combination of these two fiber types increases the overall dynamic range of the structure. Most MGB fibers phase-lock onto tones at or below 250 Hz, and some MGB fibers also can lock onto transients presented in rapid succession (up to several hundred per second). Other fibers have what appear to be complex interactions for trains of transient stimuli, possibly indicating inhibitory interactions or more global responses.

The MGB and other auditory areas of the thalamus are active in sound localization and lateralization. Cells in the MGB are sensitive to IIDs and ITDs, and this sensitivity to interaural time and intensity differences is the basis for this structure's contribution to localization and lateralization. Substantial evidence in the literature shows that damage to the MGB clearly affects sound localization ability in animals.

Clinical research on patients with documented lesions of the MGB have shown contralateral ear deficits on dichotic listening measures, with most of the cases reported showing considerable deficits. The use of the middle latency response (MLR) may be the best clinical EP to define deficits related to damage of the MGB at this point in time. This opinion is offered based upon clinical experience since little empirical data is currently available to support this statement.

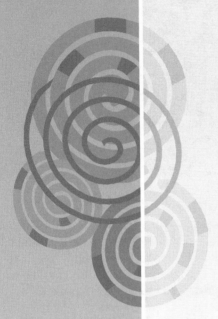

12

The Auditory Cortex and Subcortex

Introduction

As was described in the previous chapter, the medial geniculate body (MGB) and other thalamic auditory areas provide input to the auditory subcortex (subcortical white matter and basal ganglia regions) and cortex. The auditory cortex has been studied rather extensively because it is large, accessible, and of obvious import to overall auditory function in both animals and humans. Less attention has been directed toward the investigation of the structure and function of the subcortical structures; however, some interesting information is emerging that helps detail the role of the auditory subcortex in normal and disordered auditory function.

This chapter will focus on the cortical and subcortical structures involved in hearing, and to the extent that it is possible, the discussion will focus on the human model. A number of investigative approaches can provide insights as to areas of the cerebrum that are responsive to acoustic stimuli. For the most part, the auditory cortex and subcortex have been defined through (1) the mapping of electrical responses (including electromagnetic responses), (2) the microscopic analysis of cell types, (3) the documentation of pathological effects and observations, and (4) the application of imaging techniques and morphological studies. Although much of the early work on the auditory cortex and subcortex used animal models, there has been an increased interest recently in the study of the human auditory cortex. Along with this growth in interest in the human brain has come an increased understanding of how the human and animal cerebrums may be similar and how they may be different.

Probably the largest difference in structure and function of the brains of animals and humans can be found at the level of the cortex. Therefore, new techniques that allow the investigation of the structure and function of the human brain are desirable; however, it is also important to understand both the strengths and shortcomings of studying only the human brain. In animals, relatively precise lesions can be induced experimentally. With humans, however, lesion sites are limited to those that are the result of disease or trauma, and these are usually far less precise, limiting one's ability to link auditory dysfunction with a specific site of lesion. On the other hand, the human brain clearly serves as the best model for clinical correlation since interspecies differences often exist, thereby restricting the application of at least some of the findings from animal studies to the human model.

● **Figure 12.1**

Coronal view of the human cerebrum.
1 = internal capsule, 2 = thalamus, 3 = caudate,
4 = globus pallidus, 5 = putamen, 6 = external
capsule with claustrum, 7 = insula, 8 = superior
temporal gyrus, 9 = Sylvian fissure, 10 = middle
temporal gyrus, 11 = inferior temporal gyrus,
12 = corpus callosum, 13 = lateral ventricle,
14 = inferior parietal lobe. This picture of the
brain also shows the gray and white matter.

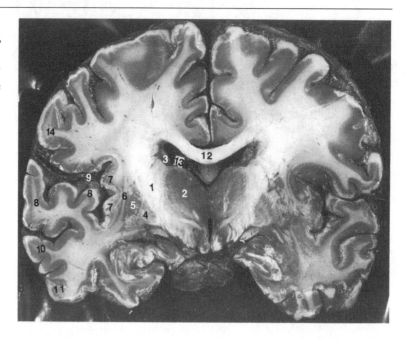

ANATOMY OF THE AUDITORY CORTEX AND SUBCORTEX

Inputs to the Auditory Cortex and Subcortex

The auditory cortex and subcortex receive neural input from the MGB. The pathway from the MGB to the cortex is complex. This pathway is often referred to as the **thalamo-cortical pathway.** For the most part, the MGB fibers that reach the auditory cortex do so by running through the **internal capsule,** but some fibers take a sublenticular route. The internal capsule is a large white-matter pathway that runs from the subcortical areas to the cortex. A coronal view shows the internal capsule running rostrally and then laterally to the thalamus and caudate and medially to the globus pallidus and putamen (Figure 12.1). A lateral view of the internal capsule shows it to be a fan-like structure reaching out to all areas of the cerebrum (Figure 12.2). The internal capsule at its rostral-most position connects to and crosses with other fibers in the subcortical white matter of the parietal lobe. This area, or matrix, of nerve fibers is termed the **corona-radiata** (Waddington, 1984).

From a transverse view, the internal capsule can be segmented into an anterior segment and a posterior segment. The posterior segment is the area where most of the auditory fibers are located; however, auditory fibers can also be found in the anterior segment (Waddington, 1984).

The connections from the MGB to auditory areas of the cerebrum were discussed in the previous chapter but

● **Figure 12.2**

Saggital view of the human brain showing the fan-like appearance of the radiation fibers running rostrally via the internal capsule (from Waddington, 1984, with permission).

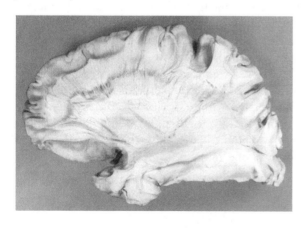

will be briefly reviewed here. The ventral portion of the MGB takes a pathway through the internal capsule and then courses laterally to the **primary auditory area (Heschl's gyrus)**. Fibers from the MGB (probably from the suprageniculate or medial nucleus) run along the inferior internal capsule and proceed anteriorally alongside (but medial to) the optic tract before coursing laterally under the putamen to the external capsule where they connect to the insula. The dorsal division of the MGB takes the common internal capsule route to the secondary auditory areas of the cortex, as well as to the insula. There may also be some connections from the dorsal portion of the MGB to the primary auditory areas (see previous chapter) (Jones and Powell, 1970; Waddington, 1984).

It is customary when describing the auditory cortex that there is a designation of the primary and secondary auditory areas. However, as neuroanatomists and neurophysiologists have learned more about the auditory cortex and as they have tried to adapt the primate anatomical model to the human model, the primary versus secondary distinction has become somewhat blurred. Therefore, it is difficult to state with any degree of certainty whether some or all of the secondary areas are "less auditory" than the primary areas—especially in humans. Brodmann's area 41 has been considered the primary auditory region in the human for many years, with other areas being considered secondary areas.

Auditory anatomists and physiologists such as Rose and Woolsey made the primary–secondary distinction over 50 years ago based on cytoarchitectonic studies. This information was supported by thalamo-cortical connectivity and physiology, and therefore the primary–secondary concept was well-grounded. More recently, Merzenich, Knight, and Roth (1975) showed that the primary auditory area (determined physiologically in animals) varied according to the fissural pattern and that the fissural pattern varied greatly across the animals they studied. To compound the complexity of this issue, new functional imaging studies on humans showed structures and areas responding to acoustic stimuli that are different from and additional to those that have been presumed to be the auditory areas of the brain based upon earlier data (Hall, Hart, and Johnsrude, 2003). Although there was and continues to be high variability of detailed information on primary and secondary auditory regions, it appears that such an anatomical configuration does exist in the cerebral cortex. That is, there is a central, or core, auditory region that represents the primary auditory area and it is surrounded by belts that are secondary or associated regions, at least in some animal species. Adapting this information to the anatomy of the human brain is at this stage difficult (at least for these authors), but it is important to embrace the concept of primary (core) and secondary (belt) regions even though one cannot provide direct anatomical boundaries of these areas in the human brain. In animals cytoarchitectonic and physiological data can be used to distinguish the primary and secondary areas. Unfortunately, similar data for the human brain does not exist. In the discussion that follows, the term *auditory cortex* will be used to refer to the cortical

CLINICAL CORRELATE

The auditory fibers that course through the internal capsule on their way from the MGB to the auditory cortex represent an important anatomical region from a clinical perspective. This anatomical region represents a bottleneck in the auditory pathway, which is similar in many respects to that seen in the auditory nerve (AN) (see Chapter 7). In the internal capsule, especially in the posterior segment of this structure, a convergence of the vast majority of the auditory fibers eventually leads to the auditory areas of the cerebrum. This concentration of auditory fibers in this area of the central auditory nervous system (CANS) means that a lesion in this region could have a dramatic effect on central auditory function. A lesion in the posterior internal capsule could deprive both the primary and secondary auditory areas of the brain of input from the MGB. For this reason, it is important that audiologists understand the key role of the internal capsule in regard to auditory function. ●

areas that have auditory functions (i.e., both the primary and secondary areas). When the discussion focuses on the primary, or core, auditory cortex, this terminology will be used.

The auditory cortex is the **gray matter** on the peripheral surface of the brain. The width of the cortex ranges from about 1.5 to 4.5 mm, with the thickest areas being found over the crests of the convolutions and the thinnest areas in the depth of the sulci (Carpenter and Sutin, 1983) (Figure 12.1). Following the concept of **neural arborization** in the brain, there are far more auditory responsive neurons in the cortex than any other area of the brain. This rather simple and well-known fact argues strongly for an increased load of auditory processing at the cortical level.

The **cortex** is composed of six layers that are defined by different cell types and cell arrangements. The current specification of these layers is based upon the early work of Campbell (1905). However, much of the information presented here is based upon Winer's (1984a,b,c, 1985) subsequent descriptions using the cat model that describe well the six layers of the auditory cortex. Layer I is defined as a cell-poor zone with axons located superficially and terminal dendrites found deeper in the layer. Layer II is described as having a high number of small pyramidal cells. Large pyramidal cells and tufted multipolar (fusiform) cells are found in layer III, whereas layer IV is characterized by mostly stellate cells and a few pyramidal cells, with the larger cells located more deeply in this layer. Layer V can be divided into two sublayers: a cell-sparse layer located superficially and a cell-dense layer located deeper in the layer. Some large pyramidal cells also characterize this layer. Finally, layer VI contains many pyramidal cells that are organized in a rather complex arrangement.

In layers V to II, the neurons are arranged in columns, and the columns in the left hemisphere are generally wider than those in the right hemisphere. This organization fits well with some gross anatomical findings that have documented an asymmetry in the brain in the area of the **planum temporale** (Geschwind and Levitsky, 1968; Aitkin, 1990).

The inputs and connections to the neurons in the various layers are highly varied. Neurons from the thalamus (auditory) connect primarily to cortical neurons in layers III and IV (see Aitkin, 1990). Neurons in layer II seem to be involved in various interconnections within the primary auditory cortex and they typically have little neuronal communication outside this area (Mitani, Shimokouchi, Itoh, Nomura, Kudo, and Mizuno, 1985). Layer III contains neurons from the primary auditory area that take a callosal route to the other hemisphere (Code and Winer, 1985). Layer V neurons connect to lower auditory (cortical-thalamic, cortical-collicular) and nonauditory areas, as do the neurons in layer IV. Layer VI has some callosal neurons (Kelly and Wong, 1981).

Auditory Cortex Location

The auditory areas of the cortex and subcortex in the human brain have not been fully delineated at this time. Defining the extent and boundaries of the auditory cortex is an evolving situation. There is, however, some general (but often not specific) agreement as to what constitutes the cortical and subcortical areas of the auditory system. In reviewing a number of studies, including recent research investigations using functional magnetic resonance imaging (fMRI), it is striking that Celesia's early work (1976) defining the auditory cortex has been so insightful and that it is in at least general agreement with the findings of more recent studies. As more emphasis is placed on understanding the anatomy of the human auditory cortex, new questions continue to arise, which indicates that our knowledge of the structure and function of the auditory cortex and subcortex may not be as advanced as was once believed.

The location of the boundaries of the primary and secondary areas of the auditory cortex is an evolving and controversial issue. In humans, Brodmann's area 41 has been considered the primary auditory area. This area overlaps much of Heschl's gyrus. The Brodmann maps are nearly 100 years old and new information—especially from functional imaging studies—may have altered what is considered the primary auditory cortex in humans. Hall, Hart, and Johnsrude (2003) have provided information that defines the primary auditory cortex, or core, region as the more medial two-thirds of Heschl's gyrus (see later section on "core-belt" concept). The anterior border of the primary area is defined by the transverse temporal sulcus, and the posterior border by Heschl's sulcus. Based on cytoarchitectonic and functional imaging findings, the primary area may extend into and slightly past the neighboring sulci. It is the view of the authors of this book that many other areas (as will be defined later) often considered to be secondary areas may in fact be more active than the primary area for certain kinds of auditory processes. Therefore, in the discussions that follow, these other auditorily responsive areas of the brain will also be referred to as auditory cortex. However, when the need to identify an area of the cortex as specifically the primary or core area arises, the use of this alternative terminology will be employed (see Figure 12.3).

The auditory cortex from a lateral view exposes many of the structures that are involved in auditory functions. The **Sylvian or lateral fissure** is a focal point. This fissure lies between the rostral-most aspect of the superior temporal gyrus (STG) and the inferior aspect of the frontal and parietal lobes (Figure 12.3a).

Figure 12.3

(a) Lateral view of the left hemisphere showing (arrows) the Sylvian fissure. (b) Horizontal section of the human brain with a focus on the temporal plane. 1 = internal capsule, 2 = external capsule (with claustrum), 3 = insula, 4 = Heschl's gyrus, 5 = planum temporale, 6 = caudate, 7 = thalamus, 8 = putamen (c) Horizontal section of a human brain that defines the primary auditory, or core, area (within the dotted boundaries). Ins = insula, HG = Heschl's gyrus, PT = planum temporale (Note: The arrows are pointing to the temporal sulcus [anterior] and Heschl's sulcus [posterior].) (Based on Hall et al., 2003.)

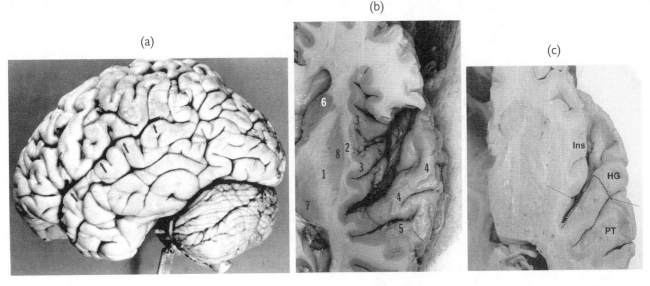

● Figure 12.4

(a) Lateral view of the left hemisphere of the human brain. A = superior temporal gyrus, B = supramarginal gyrus, C = angular gyrus, D = postcentral gyrus, E = precentral gyrus, F = insula, G = Heschl's gyrus, H = planum temporale. (b) Drawing of the lateral aspect of the brain depicting the auditory responsive areas on the surface of this structure. 1 = superior temporal gyrus, 2 = supramarginal gyrus, 3 = inferior parietal lobe, 4 = inferior–posterior frontal lobule, 5 = anterior segment of the angular gyrus.

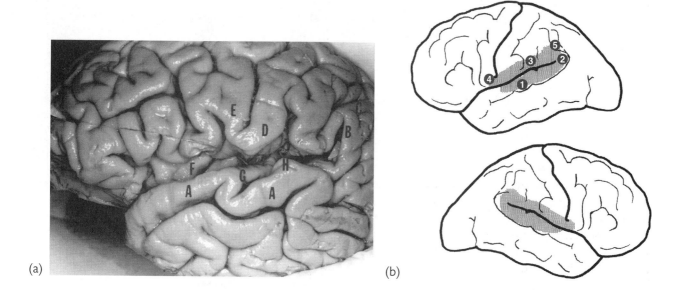

(a)   (b)

The Sylvian fissure begins at a location in the brain where the anterior frontal and temporal lobes clearly separate and it continues posteriorly to the **supramarginal gyrus**. The Sylvian fissure can run a relatively straight course in an anterior to posterior direction or it may change course in its posterior-most aspect, usually posterior to Heschl's gyrus, and turn either upward or downward (Rubens, 1977). In some cases the Sylvian fissure will take a sharp turn upward (rostrally) (this is often termed the ascending ramus, or **planum parietale**), whereas in other cases, it may take a turn downward (caudally) (often termed descending ramus) (Figures 12.4 and 12.5). The exact course of an ascending ramus may affect the morphology of the auditory structures along the posterior aspect of the Sylvian fissure (Rubens, 1977). Key components that can be seen from a lateral view of the auditory cortex include the posterior two-thirds of the STG (a good marker here is the **vein of Labbe,** which is in the region where the auditory area begins anteriorly), the supramarginal gyrus, the anterior part of the **angular gyrus**, the inferior aspect of the postcentral gyrus, the precentral gyrus, and the posterior-inferior frontal gyrus (Musiek, 1986; DeArmond, Fusco, and Dewey, 1989). In addition to these auditory structures, some portions of the middle temporal gyrus may also be acoustically responsive.

A major portion of the auditory cortex in humans is located on the superior temporal plane (STP), which is defined by the temporal bank of the Sylvian fissure. If the frontal and parietal lobes were removed and one looked down on the brain, the STP would be observed in its entirety (Figure 12.3b). Located on the STP are Heschl's gyrus and the planum temporale (Figure 12.3b,c). Heschl's gyrus is positioned in the posterior one-fourth to one-third of the STP. Located immediately posterior to Heschl's gyrus is the planum temporale. Because of the close proximity of these two structures, Heschl's gyrus is sometimes difficult to discern from the planum temporale.

● Figure 12.5

Lateral view of human brain, with the arrows pointing to a sharply ascending ramus.

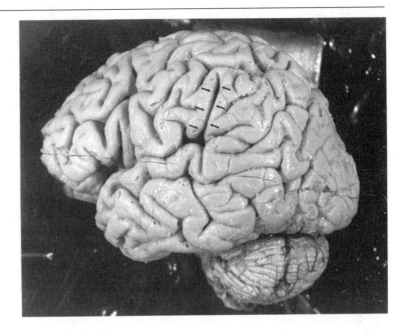

A number of recent papers have raised questions as to the exact anatomical location of Heschl's gyrus (Penhune, Zatorre, MacDonald, and Evans, 1996; Leonard, Puranik, Kuldau, and Lombardino, 1998; Schneider, Scherg, Dosch, Specht, Gutschalk, and Rupp, 2002). Anatomical questions surrounding the location of Heschl's gyrus concern variances in the number of gyri and the anatomical markers that define the anterior aspect of this structure (i.e., the anterior sulcus of Heschl's gyrus, also termed the anterior temporal sulcus) and the posterior aspect (i.e., Heschl's posterior sulcus, which separates Heschl's gyrus from the planum temporale).

Heschl's gyrus can be described as a relatively small gyrus that courses posterio-medially along the STP, while the planum temporale is shaped like a piece of pie (the crust is the lateral cortex and the pointed area is the medial cortex) that courses latero-medially. As just mentioned, the sulcus between Heschl's gyrus and the planum temporale is sometimes referred to as **Heschl's posterior sulcus**—a designation that appears to be appropriate. The identification of Heschl's gyrus and the planum temporale is difficult at times because there can be more than one Heschl's gyrus. When there is more than one gyrus, the division is noted by a small sulcus known as Beck's intermedius sulcus or the sulcus intermedius. Two and even three Heschl's gyri have been reported in some individuals (Campain and Minckler, 1976; Musiek and Reeves, 1990). In addition, asymmetries for the number of gyri on the left and right sides of the brain have also been reported (Campain and Minckler, 1976). Some studies have additionally shown an asymmetry in the size of Heschl's gyrus between the two sides of the brain, with the left side being larger than the right, but other measurement techniques have yielded somewhat varying results (Campain and Minckler, 1976; Rubens, 1977; Musiek and Reeves, 1990; Penhune et al., 1996). Recent MRI-based information has indicated greater gray matter volume for Heschl's gyrus on the left side than on the right side of the brain for most individuals (Rademacher, Morosan, Schormann, Schleicher, Werner, Freund, Zilles, 2001). Interestingly, this has not been found to be the case for professional musicians, who tend to show more symmetry in the gray matter volumes for their right and left transverse gyri and who additionally exhibit an overall greater volume of gray matter than do controls (Schneider et al., 2002). Finally, MRI studies have shown greater overall volume for the left primary auditory cortex compared to the right for most normal subjects (Penhune et al., 1996).

The "Belt-Core" Concept

Recently there has been increased interest in defining the main areas of the auditory cortex into **"belt" or "core" regions** (Hackett, Stepniewska, and Kaas, 1998; Kaas and Hackett, 1998; Kaas, Hackett, and Tramo, 1999; Hackett, Preuss, and Kaas, 2001). This approach has been attractive because it is based on both primate and human studies. The core and belt regions are essentially located on the STP and STG (see Hackett et al., 2001) and encompass the planum temporale, Heschl's gyrus, and a region immediately anterior to Heschl's gyrus (Figure 12.6). The core can be viewed as the "primary" auditory area as mentioned earlier (Figure 12.3c) and the belt and core areas from an anterior–posterior perspective occupy the posterior two-thirds of the temporal plane and gyrus (see Figure 12.6). Core and belt areas have been defined based on studies of macaque monkey and human brains. The core is, with some minor variations, located between the **posterior (Heschl's) sulcus** and **anterior temporal sulcus of Heschl's gyrus** and does not extend to the peripheral fringe of the temporal plane laterally or to the insula medially. The core is further divided into three sections: the rostral temporal (RT), which is anterior; the rostral (R), which lies between the other two segments; and the (AI), which is the posterior sigment of the iore posterior-most section. The belt that is medial to the core is composed of three segments: the rostral temporal medial (anterior), the rostral medial (middle), and the caudal medial (posterior) segment. The lateral belt has four divisions: the rostral temporal lateral, the anterior lateral, the medial lateral, and the caudal lateral. A **parabelt region** is also located on the surface of the STG; this has two divisions: the rostral and caudal parabelts (Hackett et al., 2001).

The core is composed of **koniocortex**, and the belt areas are composed of para–koniocortex or pro-koniocortex (Hackett et al., 2001).

Intrahemispheric Connections of the Primary Auditory Cortex

The primary auditory area has profuse connections directly and indirectly within its own hemisphere. There appears to be a hierarchy among the auditory fibers of the primary auditory cortex, with neural connections first occurring within the immediate area of Heschl's gyrus before the fibers connect to

● **Figure 12.6**

Schematic of the auditory cortex revealing the core and belt concepts of this anatomy. The arrows indicate the flow of impulses starting at the core area and proceeding to the belt and parabelt areas. M = medial, L = lateral, R = rostral, C = caudal.

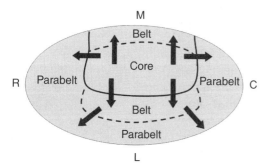

regions of the auditory cortex outside this area. This concept was discussed by de Ribaupierre (1997), who referred to these connections as "within" module and "outside" module connections. In addition to within module connections with auditory areas of the brain, Heschl's gyrus has a variety of connections to other areas of the brain. Which connections are used in the processing of an auditory event depends on the nature of the stimuli and the nature of the auditory task at hand (de Ribaupierre, 1997).

The classic view of neural impulses first accessing the primary auditory area of the brain, followed by being conducted posterior to **Wernicke's area,** and then being directed anteriorally to the frontal lobe via the arcuate fasciculus may be valuable in defining the neural connections of Heschl's gyrus. There is evidence from primate research that lesioning the primary auditory area results in degenerative effects in the posterior STG (Seltzer and Pandya, 1978). The STG has multisynaptic pathways that course caudally to medially to rostrally and then in reverse (Jones and Powell, 1970; Seltzer and Pandya, 1978). These auditory connections from the primary area do not reach as far as the temporal pole, as few auditory responsive fibers have been noted there (Jones and Powell, 1970). There are also connections to the superior temporal sulcus (Streitfeld, 1980) and to the insula and frontal lobe, many of which are reciprocal (Forbes and Moskowitz, 1977; Streitfeld, 1980).

The anatomical constructs of the core and belt designations for the auditory cortex may further define the connections of this structure. As expected, the main input from the ventral MGB is to the core, while the dorsal and ventral MGB connect primarily to the belt regions (Kaas and Hackett, 1998; Hackett et al., 2001). It appears that the belt and parabelt areas also receive input from the core. The latencies to acoustic stimuli at the belt area are later than those noted for the core; hence, it appears that the belt receives impulses secondary to the core and as such may indicate a second stage of processing (Kaas and Hackett, 1998, Hackett et al., 2001). The belt areas connect to prefrontal, parietal, and other temporal areas of the brain (Pandya, 1995; Hackett et al., 1998; Hackett et al., 2001).

The planum temporale is located on the STP directly posterior (dorsal) to Heschl's gyrus. The planum temporale shares the acoustic (Heschl's) sulcus anteriorly (ventral) with Heschl's gyrus and it extends to the end point of the Sylvian fissure immediately anterior to the supramarginal gyrus (Figures 12.3a and 12.4a). In some cases, there is a segment of the Sylvian fissure, the posterior ascending ramus, that turns rostrally into the parietal lobe. This is often termed the planum parietale and is often not considered to be part of the planum temporale (Rubens, 1977). The planum temporale is sometimes considered to be part of Wernicke's area and it has been shown to be sensitive to a variety of types of acoustic stimulation (Binder, Frost, Hammeke, Rao, and Cox, 1996; Johnsrude, Giraud, and Frackowiak, 2002).

Perhaps one of the most famous neuroanatomical discoveries involving the planum temporale was Geschwind and Levitsky's (1968) finding that this structure is larger in the left hemisphere than in the right hemisphere in most humans. These investigators reasoned that if the left hemisphere is the dominant hemisphere for speech and the planum temporale is in the region of Wernicke's area, the planum temporale may be the anatomical correlate to receptive language functions in humans. Other anatomical studies subsequent to Geschwind and Levitsky's have yielded essentially the same results (Wada, Clarke, and Hamm, 1975; Steinmetz, Rademacher, Huang, Hefter, Zilles, Thron, and Freund, 1989; Musiek and Reeves, 1990).

Geschwind and Levitsky (1968) reported the mean length of the left planum temporale to be 3.6 cm compared to 2.7 cm on the right, and subsequent studies have reported grossly similar measurements (Wada et al., 1975; Musiek and Reeves, 1990). This finding on the gross anatomy of the planum temporale has triggered considerable research on brain asymmetry and laterality (see Figure 12.3b). The asymmetry in the planum temporale has also been documented via MRI techniques for children 3 to 14 years of age (Preis, Jancke, Schmitz-Hillebrecht, and Steinmetz, 1999). These findings, when considered in the context of the other studies mentioned, indicate that the relative asymmetry noted in humans does not change with increases in age or brain size. In addition, the results for the Preis et al. (1999) study revealed that girls tend to exhibit a more prominent left–right planum temporale asymmetry than boys.

Insula

The **insula (island of Reil)** is a cortex under a cortex. This structure lies deep in the Sylvian fissure under the operculum and is covered by segments of the temporal, frontal, and parietal lobes. The insula can be observed directly by removing segments of these brain lobes (Figure 12.7). There are several gyri and sulci in the insula. These include the anterior, medial, and posterior short gyri and the anterior and posterior long gyri, all of which are divided by distinct sulci (Ture, Yasargil, Al-Mefty, and Yasargil, 1999). Like Heschl's gyrus and the planum temporale, the insula is larger on the left side than on the right side of the brain in humans (Mesulam and Mufson, 1985). The insula is emerging as a structure that plays a role in central auditory function, although the specifics of this function are not yet well understood (Bamiou, Musiek, and Luxon, 2003). The insula also plays a role in visceral, motor, vestibular, and somatosensory functions (Augustine, 1985, 1996).

Based on its **cytoarchitectonics**, the insula can be parceled into three belts running from anterior to posterior (Rivier and Clarke, 1997). The anterior third of the insula is composed of agranular cells, the middle third of dysgranular cells, and the posterior third has well-defined granular cells. The cytoarchitecture for the posterior insula aligns with what would be expected in a primary sensory area (Bamiou et al., 2003). It is of interest that the medial-most aspect of Heschl's gyrus is quite similar to the posterior-most aspect of the insula both in gross and fine anatomy (Musiek, 1986a).

The insula has a rather complex and wide variety of neural connections (see Bamiou et al., 2003). The focus here will be on auditory-related connections. The dorsal and medial segments of the MGB input to the insula. It appears that most of the input from the MGB to the insula terminates in the posterior third of the structure (Sudakov, McLean, Reeves, and Marino, 1971; Burton and Jones, 1976). However, there is some evidence that indicates that the MGB inputs to both the anterior and posterior insula as well (Mesulam and Mufson, 1985).

In primates the insula is well connected to both the primary auditory areas and the association areas (Mesulam and Mufson, 1985). Streitfeld (1980) identified connections from the STG to the insula in primates. It is believed that the arcuate fasciculus projecting from the posterior temporal lobe to the frontal lobe region may pick up from and input fibers to the insula (Carpenter and Sutin, 1983).

● Figure 12.7

This saggital view of the human brain exposes the lateral cortex of the insula. 1, 2, and 3 are the anterior, intermediate, and posterior short gyri, respectively, and 4 and 5 are the anterior and posterior long gyri. Each of these gyri has an associated sulcus (from Waddington, 1984, with permission).

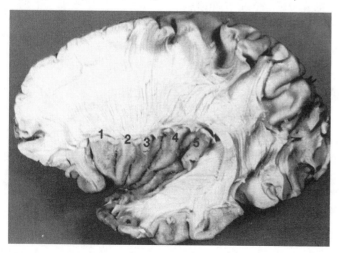

The insula also has interhemispheric connections. Pandya and Rosene (1985) demonstrated in primates that interhemispheric fibers from the insula are located in the inferior-anterior portion of the sulcus area of the corpus callosum (CC). This callosal region is in close proximity to where most of the auditory fibers from the temporal lobe are found in the CC.

A classic study by Colavita and associates revealed that if a cat's insula was ablated, the animal lost its ability to perform temporal pattern discrimination tasks (Colavita, Szeligo, and Zimmer, 1974). Functional imaging studies in humans have shown activation of the insula for a number of auditory functions. In general, such functions as sound detection and nonverbal processing, temporal processing, phonological processing, and visual–auditory integration all result in increased activation of the insula (see Bamiou et al., 2003 for review).

> ### CLINICAL CORRELATE
>
> One of the most compelling lines of evidence supporting the insula having a role in auditory processing is related to auditory test findings in patients with damage to the insula. Deficits in dichotic listening in the ear contralateral to the damaged insula have been reported by a number of investigators (Hyman and Tranel, 1989; Fifer, 1993; Gollegly and Musiek, 1993). Gollegly and Musiek (1993) reported a case of insular damage that yielded both abnormal middle latency evoked responses (MLRs) and abnormal performance on the dichotic rhyme test. The most compelling study to date, however, was a case study reported by Habib and colleagues (Habib, Daquin, Milandre, Royere, Ray, Lanteri, Salamon, and Khalil, 1995). This report was of a middle-aged woman who suffered strokes in each insula over the course of only a few days. After the second stroke, the patient was essentially centrally deaf. Although there was some recovery in function with time, severe auditory dysfunction continued with this patient. This patient demonstrated abnormal dichotic listening and evoked potentials (EPs)—even after several months of recovery. ●

Supramarginal Gyrus and Angular Gyrus

The supramarginal and angular gyri are important anatomical markers and although they are not often considered "key auditory" structures, there is evidence that they respond to or process acoustic stimuli in some form (Berry et al., 1995). It is fair to state that the supramarginal and angular gyri are generally considered under the category of "association auditory cortex." The supramarginal gyrus cups around the posterior termination point of the Sylvian fissure (Figure 12.4), while the angular gyrus is located posterior and superior to the supramarginal gyrus. However, if the Sylvian fissure has an ascending ramus, the angular gyrus may be located more inferiorally and posteriorly relative to the supramarginal gyrus (Figure 12.4) (see Rubens, 1977 for further discussion). More research (especially on humans) is needed to better define the role of these two gyri in audition.

> ### CLINICAL CORRELATE
>
> Hynd et al. (1990) reported that the size of the insula was smaller in children with learning disabilities than in a matched group of normal children. In another study, Corina and colleagues (2001) demonstrated that individuals with dyslexia had less fMRI activation in the region of the insula than normal controls for a phonological rhyming task. ●

PHYSIOLOGY OF THE AUDITORY CORTEX AND SUBCORTEX

Frequency Coding

Perhaps one of the most commonly studied areas related to the auditory cortex is frequency coding. This section will discuss tonotopic organization, tuning curves (TCs), and frequency discrimination. The tonotopic organization of the primary auditory cortex based on animal studies indicates that the low frequencies are located rostro-laterally and that the high frequencies are situated caudo-medially (Merzenich and Brugge, 1973). This tonotopic organization essentially courses along Heschl's gyrus in a relatively systematic manner, as this gyrus generally runs

● **Figure 12.8**

Looking down on the temporal plane of the right hemisphere of a human brain showing the tonotopic arrangement of Heschl's gyrus. L = low characteristic frequencies, H = high characteristic frequencies.

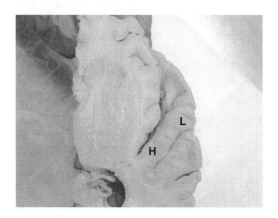

in a lateral to medial and a rostral to caudal manner (Figure 12.8). It has been suggested that the auditory cortex is arranged in iso-frequency columns, although the available data to support this is debatable (Pickles, 1988; Aitkin, 1990). More studies measuring the frequencies of fibers at various depths within the cortex need to be undertaken before a definitive statement regarding the columnar organization of frequency in the cortex can be rendered. It also has been shown that superficial layers of the auditory cortex may not be as responsive to tonal stimuli as the neurons in layers III and IV, which yield the most activity in regard to stimulation from various tones (see Aitkin, 1990).

Those investigators that support the core–belt organization of the auditory cortex suggest a different tonotopic arrangement at the cortex from what has been described above, at least for primates (Hackett et al., 2001). The core is divided into three segments (anterior, middle, and posterior). The anterior and posterior segments course from low- to high-frequency representations in a lateral to medial manner, and the middle segment courses from low to high frequencies in a posterior to anterior manner (Figure 12.9). The posterior field is considered to be the primary one. The belt (secondary areas) is usually divided into four fields with their own tonotopic maps, and the core and belt areas have their own cytoarchitecture and connections to the thalamus (see earlier discussion) (Hackett et al., 2001).

Functional imaging studies have permitted insights as to the human tonotopic organization at Heschl's gyrus (Lauter, Herscovitch, Formby, and Raichle, 1985; Le, Patel, and Roberts, 2001; Schonwieser, von Cramon, and Rubsamen, 2002). These studies have indicated that in the region of Heschl's gyrus the low frequencies are rostral and lateral while the high frequencies are caudal and medial—similar to the frequency representations noted in the early primate studies. However, functional imaging studies appear to show some variability in frequency representations within the cortex in terms of intersubject comparisons (Schonwieser et al., 2002). Intracerebral auditory EP recordings performed on humans have also provided insights as to the tonotopic

● **Figure 12.9**

A sketch showing the authors' impression of the tonotopic arrangement of the auditory cortex using the core–belt anatomical designations (for primates). In this sketch the tonotopy is only shown for the core area, which is segmented into rostral, medial, and caudal areas (from left to right), with each having its own frequency arrangement. L = low characteristic frequencies, H = high characteristic frequencies, R = rostral, C = caudal, M = medial, L = lateral.

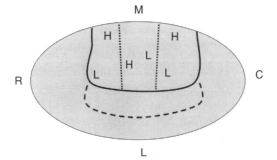

organization of the auditory cortex. Liegeois-Chauvel, Giraud, Badier, Marquis, and Chauvel (2001) showed that low and high frequencies were organized in a fashion similar to that noted in the functional imaging and primate studies. However, in the EP studies, the right hemisphere seemed better tonotopically organized than the left, with the left hemisphere demonstrating more variability than the right.

Insula Tonotopicity

The insula in the cat has been shown to be tonotopically organized (Woolsey, 1960). In the insula, the high frequencies are located dorsally and the low frequencies are found ventrally. The high-frequency region of the insula is in close proximity to the high-frequency region of Heschl's gyrus. It is not known whether this is the case in humans.

Tuning Curves

CLINICAL CORRELATE

Although there are not any clinical tests of frequency discrimination or selectivity that are commonly used to assess frequency coding in patients with auditory cortex lesions, there is evidence that suggests that such testing would be a valuable clinical tool. Thompson and Abel (1992a) showed significantly poorer performance on a frequency discrimination task by patients with temporal lobe lesions involving the left auditory cortex than for patients with acoustic tumors and normal controls. In this study, right temporal lobe lesions also affected difference limens for frequency but not to the extent that was noted for patients with left cortical lesions. Interestingly, in another investigation Robin, Tranel, and Damasio (1990) reported poor frequency discrimination for patients with right hemisphere lesions but normal results for those with left hemisphere involvement. This latter finding is consistent with an earlier study by Zatorre (1988), which reported similar findings. Although there is disagreement among the findings of these studies, which could be related to methodological differences, it is clear that auditory cortex lesions can compromise processing of spectral information in humans. •

(TCs) provide an indication of frequency selectivity. The TCs in the auditory cortex are V-shaped for the most part; however, broad TCs are also present (Calford, Webster, and Semple, 1983). In the cortex, there are broadly tuned high-frequency cells as well as broadly tuned low-frequency cells—irrespective of cochlear origin. This trend is similar to that noted for the TCs recorded at lower levels in the CANS. There is additional evidence that flatter TCs are found more superficially, while sharp, multipeaked TCs are found in the deeper layers of the auditory cortex, with the sharpest TCs usually recorded from layers III and IV (Oonishi and Katsuki, 1965, Aitkin, 1990).

There is a relationship between the TCs and intensity functions of the nerve fibers in the auditory cortex. Fibers that have monotonic intensity functions show TCs that change little with increases in intensity. However, the TCs for fibers that are nonmontonic are altered by changes in intensities and are different from monotonic fibers in their response patterns (Phillips, Judge, and Kelly, 1988).

As Aitkin (1990) pointed out, fibers with sharp TCs also have shorter response latencies compared to TCs that are relatively flat. This could be related to the concept that sharp TCs are high-frequency fibers originating from the basal part of the cochlea and flatter TCs are more apical in their peripheral origins.

Intensity Coding and the Auditory Cortex

The auditory cortex reflects increases in the intensity of an acoustic signal in a number of ways similar to those noted in other auditory areas of the brain. It has been known for some time that when the intensity of a sound is increased, two classes of neurons can be distinguished by the way they encode the amplitude of the stimulus (Pfingst and O'Connor, 1981; Phillips, Orman, Musicant, and Wilson, 1985). One class of neurons includes those that increase their firing rates as the stimulus intensity increases. This type of function is known as a monotonic function. The firing rate of the individual monotonic neuron continues to increase until additional increases in firing rate are no longer physiologically possible. Usually, at rather high intensity levels, the neuronal firing rate can no longer keep up with increases in the stimulus intensity and the firing rate levels off (see Pickles, 1988 for discussion).

Based on primate research, most auditory cortex neurons are monotonic from about 10 dB to 40 or 50 dB SPL (Pickles, 1988; Phillips, 1989), although Phillips (1989) relates that some cortical neurons may have a greater intensity dynamic range than 40 or 50 dB. Clearly, the threshold of the fiber is a factor. A neuron with a high threshold of response may increase firing rates for increases at high intensities but may have a rather small dynamic range.

The second type of nerve fiber in regard to intensity response is the one with a nonmonotonic response (Pfingst and O'Connor, 1981; Pickles, 1988; Phillips, 1989; de Ribaupierre, 1997). These are neurons that after small increases in intensity actually decrease in their firing rate, or "**roll over**." Phillips et al. (1985) provided examples of some cortical neurons that reached maximum firing rate with less than a 10 dB increase in intensity and then rolled over, decreasing their firing rate to nearly spontaneous levels with an additional increase in intensity of only 15 dB. These types of neurons have also been shown in the brainstem, as was discussed earlier.

It has been suggested that nonmonotonic fibers probably receive inhibitory input at frequencies adjacent to their characteristic frequencies (CF) (de Ribaupierre, 1997). This notion leads to an important consideration; that is, the establishment of an intensity function for a given neuron assumes that testing is being performed at the neuron's CF.

Another key concept in regard to the way cortical neurons respond to high intensities is the number of neurons involved. As expected, as the stimulus intensity increases, more neurons are activated as the threshold of the active monotonic neuron is exceeded. However, there are also some neurons that stop responding with increases in intensity because their dynamic intensity range has been exceeded (Phillips, 1989; Phillips, Semple, Calford, and Kitzes, 1994). The concept of increases in intensity yielding increases in the number of neurons firing has been demonstrated in humans with recent data from fMRI research. Lasota and colleagues showed that subjects had greater activation of the fibers in Heschl's gyrus at higher intensities than at lower intensities (Lasota, Ulmer, Firszt, Biswal, Daniels, and Prost, 2003). Specifically, these researchers found that there was a greater number of voxels activated at the higher intensities when compared to the number activated by less intense stimuli (indicating that a more neural substrate was involved at the higher intensities) and that greater bilateral activation was noted for high-intensity stimuli than for low-intensity stimuli. This interpretation, however, must be made with caution since the fMRI activation could perhaps be related to increased damping of inhibitory neurons at high intensities and not just more neurons responding.

The latency of the neuronal response is another index of auditory cortex function in regard to intensity. Near-field and far-field EPs derived from the auditory cortex show decrements in latency measurements as a function of increments in stimulus intensity. The MLR as well as the long latency and event-related potentials all show latency effects (i.e., shorter latencies) related to increases in intensity (Thornton, Mendel, and Anderson, 1977; Polich, 1989). Although all normal fibers demonstrate shorter latencies with increased intensity, Phillips (1989) has shown that nonmonotonic auditory cortex neurons generally have steeper latency–intensity functions than do monotonic neurons.

The concept of **tonotopicity** is well known in auditory neuroscience. There is a question, however, of whether intensity coding has a counterpart to tonotopicity. This may be a possibility, based on some recent fMRI data (Bilecen, Seifritz, Scheffler, Henning, and Schulte, 2002). In this study increases in intensity revealed systematic fMRI activations in a ventral to dorsal and lateral to medial direction in the primary auditory cortex. This activation trend is similar to tonotopic activations for increases in frequency at the primary auditory cortex (see Phillips et al., 1994).

Modulated Signals (FM and AM)

The new clinical interest in **auditory steady-state responses (ASSRs)** has resulted in increased interest in the responses of the auditory cortex to **amplitude-modulated (AM)** and **frequency-modulated (FM)** signals. Probably the key study in terms of how the auditory cortex handles these kinds of signals is the early work by Whitfield and Evans (1965). These investigators demonstrated that for FM signals the cortex yielded better (larger and more consistent) responses than for steady-state tones presented at the same frequency. This important finding was the basis for much basic, and more recently clinical, research on the application of modulated signals to assess hearing sensitivity. AM signals are also relevant stimuli in that most signals in our environment are signals that change in frequency and/or intensity over a short time period (e.g., speech and music).

The cortical response to FM signals is dependent on a host of stimulus characteristics such as excursion size, speed and direction of change, type of change (linear, logarithmic, or sinusoid), and signal frequency and signal intensity (see de Ribaupierre, 1997 for review). Cortical responses are strongest when the modulation direction is toward the CF of the neuron; however, this may not be the case with all cortical neurons. Responses for FM signals are also generally more robust if the frequency of the signal stays within the response area of the cortex (Phillips et al., 1985; Phillips, Reale, and Brugge, 1991). It appears that some cortical neurons are tuned to particular frequency modulation rates and that the best modulation rate for a given individual neuron is related to its particular CF (Whitfield and Evans, 1965; Schreiner and Urbas, 1986, 1988). For the most part, auditory cortex neurons respond to modulation rates of FM sinusoids in the range from about 5 to 15 Hz (Evans, 1974), and the size of the frequency modulation (range for excursion) determines the strength of the response noted, with greater excursions resulting in stronger neural responses (Moller, 2000). For linear frequency modulations, most of the neurons will respond to the ramps, both rising and falling (Moller, 2000).

AM signals and their neural responses within the cortex are influenced by the acoustic characteristics of the signal in a manner similar to that noted for FM signals. In general, AM rates from 1 to 50 Hz are best suited for cortical responses. At AM rates of 50 to 100 Hz, the cortex becomes less responsive, and responses from the brainstem pathways tend to dominate (Phillips et al., 1991). Hence, slow modulation rates are more effective in triggering responses from the cortical neurons, whereas fast modulation rates are better handled by neurons associated with auditory structures located lower within the auditory system. Individual amplitude modulation transfer functions of individual cells shift in shape from being predominantly low-pass at the AN to mostly high-band pass at the brainstem and cortex. As one progresses up the auditory system, the high-frequency cut-off drops. Therefore, there is a tendency for higher-frequency modulation transfer functions to be associated with neurons in the AN and low brainstem and lower-frequency modulation transfer functions to be associated with neurons in the auditory cortex (Phillips et al., 1991; Phillips and Hall, 1987). Interestingly, at carrier levels near threshold of signal detection with small excursion depths (6 dB), rapid AM rates (>50 Hz) result in higher firing rates from cats' auditory cortical neurons than do slow rates (Goldstein and Kiang, 1958). However, once the carrier level is increased and the modulation depth is greater, slow AMs become more effective than fast AMs for eliciting responses from the auditory cortex. This is probably related to the fact that at the higher intensities more neural units respond (Phillips and Hall, 1987). In addition, there may be auditory cortex neurons that selectively have a best modulation rate. These best modulation rates for the cortex are generally lower than the best modulation rates noted for brainstem neurons (Schreiner and Urbas, 1986).

CLINICAL CORRELATE

The ASSR procedure may differentiate what may be the best modulation rate for activation of cortical versus brainstem neurons. Slower modulation rates, usually less than 50 per second, are considered to be driven by the auditory cortex, whereas modulation rates greater than 50 may be best driven by brainstem structures (Phillips et al., 1991). Currently this general information drives the recommendations for clinical use of the ASSR. Interestingly, from a clinical perspective, the high modulation rates are less influenced by sleep compared to the low modulation rates. This is similar to the well-known effect of sleep on the late cortical EPs and the lack of it on the ABR. Recent data indicates that in humans, lesions of the auditory cortex influence threshold estimates made with ASSR (Shinn, 2005). •

Temporal Aspects of the Auditory Cortex

The auditory system can be highly sensitive to the timing characteristics of an acoustic stimulus. Because of this, the CANS has been considered an elegant time keeper. Two types of temporally based acoustic stimuli are relevant to this discussion of auditory cortex function. One is the periodic stimuli, such as pure tones or modulated tones, and the other is the transient or single-event stimuli, such as individual clicks. It is fairly well accepted that the majority of cortical neurons can only respond to periodicities in the 15 to 30 Hz range (Phillips and Hall, 1990), while brainstem neurons can respond to much higher periodicities. Therefore, discrimination of sounds that require fine periodic temporal processing is better handled by brainstem neurons. Interestingly, cortical neurons can respond extremely well to rapid individual acoustic stimuli like clicks. The temporal precision with which cortical neurons can encode individual acoustic events should allow them to temporally segregate responses to brief stimuli only 1 to 2 msec apart—an amazing degree of temporal precision for these kinds of neurons (see Phillips and Hall, 1990; Phillips et al., 1991).

Another procedure used to test temporal abilities is gap detection in noise (see Chapter 10 for additional discussion). Kelly, Rooney, and Phillips (1996) showed that gap detection thresholds were doubled for animals that had bilateral auditory cortex damage compared to control animals.

Speech and Complex Stimuli

It has been known for some time that auditory cortex areas in animals respond to vocalizations from other animals. Some fibers have been shown to be selective—only responding to certain elements of animal vocalizations—while other neurons respond to a variety of elements (Wollberg and Newman, 1972). Phillips et al. (1991)

CLINICAL CORRELATE

It is interesting to consider the results of some human studies using various temporal processing tasks. Lackner and Teuber (1973) used a click fusion paradigm to test temporal resolution in humans with temporal lobe injury. In their study, the threshold for discriminating two clicks was on the order of 2 to 3 msec in their normal subjects, whereas individuals with brain injury in either the left or right hemisphere needed larger gap thresholds to discern the presence of two clicks. Additionally, these researchers found that there were greater effects for subjects with left-sided involvement than for those with right-sided compromise. Robin et al. (1990) showed increased gap detection thresholds for individuals with left auditory cortex involvement but did not find similar temporal deficits in subjects with right auditory cortex lesions. These results were somewhat at odds with the results of an earlier study that showed gap detection abnormalities in subjects with both right and left temporal lobectomies (Efron, Yund, Nichols, and Crandall, 1985). Specifically, the deficits for the subjects in this study were noted in the ear opposite the damaged hemisphere.

These studies and others support the role that the cortex plays in certain temporal resolution paradigms. Given this information, it would seem as though a gap detection paradigm would work its way into the clinical domain. However, to date, this has not happened. It appears that most gap detection procedures require considerable administration time, which makes the clinical application of these tests difficult.

A new approach to measuring gap detection called the GIN (gaps-in-noise) test holds considerable promise for clinical use. This gap detection procedure is administratively feasible and shows good sensitivity to disorders of the central auditory system. (Musiek, Shinn, Virsa, Bamiou, Baran, Zaidan, in press). ●

reported that in animals, cortical neurons could respond to individual, as well as transient, elements in vocalizations. Steinschneider, Arezzo, and Vaughan (1982) showed multineuron responses from various depths of the auditory cortex in monkeys to consonant vowels (CVs) and clicks. These animals were trained to a level that allowed them to behaviorally discriminate different CVs and the CV stimuli from clicks. Neural responses were found to be markedly different for the CVs and the clicks. In addition, subtle differences in response patterns were noted across the different CVs.

In humans, auditory cortex responses to speech can be measured with functional imaging techniques. Zattore and colleagues demonstrated that various speech sounds activated areas immediately anterior to Heschl's gyrus in both hemispheres (Zatorre, Evans, Meyer, and Gjedde, 1992), while others have shown that words and syllables activated areas both immediately anterior and posterior to Heschl's gyrus but only in the left hemisphere (Giraud and Price, 2001). Mummery, Asburner, Scott, and Wise (1999) showed increasing activity in Heschl's gyrus in both hemispheres and also in an anterior-lateral direction of the superior temporal gyrus (STG) for words presented at increasing rates.

Dichotic listening studies using speech elements (CVs), and positron emission tomography (PET) procedures have shown activation in the mid to posterior segments of the STG with most activation in and around Heschl's gyrus in both hemispheres (Hugdahl, Bronnick, Kyllingsbaek, Law, Gade, and Paulson, 1999). When the extents of the activation in both hemispheres were compared, clearly more activation was noted in the left hemisphere, a finding consistent with behavioral findings for dichotic listening (Hugdahl et al., 1999). In addition, it appeared from this study that the activation area of the brain exceeded the core and possibly even the belt areas. Finally, it has been shown that directing attention to one ear or the other during dichotic listening for speech influences the amount of activation in the primary auditory cortex (Eslinger and Damasio, 1988; O'Leary, Andreasen, Hurtig, Hichwa, Watkins, Ponto, Rogers, and Kirchner, 1996; Hugdahl et al., 1999).

CLINICAL CORRELATE

There is a long and important history of dichotic listening for speech signals and how it is affected by lesions of the CANS (see Musiek and Pinheiro, 1985 and Hugdahl, 1988 for reviews). Dichotic listening essentially results in a suppression of the ipsilateral auditory pathways, making the system essentially a "crossed" system. Since most people can "speak" only out of their left hemisphere, one of the two crossed pathways has direct access to the dominant speech and language hemisphere, while the other pathway must take an indirect route to reach the dominant speech and language hemisphere. Speech stimuli directed to the right ear course directly to the (left) speech cortex, while speech materials presented to the left ear are routed first to the right auditory cortex and then across the CC to the left side for processing and a response (see also Chapter 13). In normal right-handed individuals and the majority of normal left-handed individuals, a slight right ear advantage (REA) is noted for dichotic testing, possibly related to the fact that the right ear has the more direct route to the left auditory/language cortex.

In contrast, patients with lesions of the auditory cortex may not show the expected REA but typically show deficits on dichotic tests in the ear contralateral to the involved hemisphere. If the right hemisphere is lesioned, then an REA may be evident, whereas if the left hemisphere is compromised, then a left ear advantage (LEA) may be evident. In either case, the performance of the ear contralateral to the lesioned hemisphere is typically noticeably depressed compared to normal expectations for performance, while the performance of the ipsilateral ear is normal or at least superior to that of the contralateral ear. Thus, if dichotic listening performance is measured for patients with lesions limited to one hemisphere, it is anticipated that the ear contralateral to the lesioned hemisphere will show scores that are lower than those observed for the ear ipsilateral to the lesion (Figure 12.10). Theoretically, since there are more contralateral than ipsilateral neurons, damage to the auditory areas of the brain generally results in greater compromise of contralateral neurons than ipsilateral neurons.

Some dichotic listening tests, such as the dichotic digits, have been shown to have good sensitivity (75%) and specificity (88%) in defining lesions of the auditory cortex or subcortex (see Musiek and Pinheiro, 1985 and Chermak and Musiek, 1997 for reviews). Although clinical research has not addressed the issue directly, it does appear that lesions closer to the primary auditory cortex result in greater deficits than those that are more distal. ●

● Figure 12.10

The effects of lesions involving the auditory cortex on three dichotic listening tests. Ipsilateral (ipsi) indicates scores for the ear on the same side as the lesion and contralateral (contra) designates the scores from the ear opposite the lesioned hemisphere. These mean scores reveal a contralateral ear deficit for all three dichotic tests. C.S. = competing sentences, S.S.W. = staggered spondaic words, D.D. = dichotic digits.

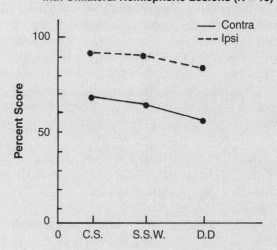

Contra and Ipsi Ear Mean Scores for Subjects with Unilateral Hemispheric Lesions (N = 15)

Acoustic patterns are another type of complex stimulus. The discrimination of acoustic patterns requires several types of processes including the (temporal) sequencing of the individual acoustic events as well as the discrimination of the individual acoustic elements. The classic studies of Neff, Butler, and Diamond, which are well summarized in Neff (1961), indicate that when the auditory cortex of the cat is ablated, accurate pattern perception cannot be accomplished.

CLINICAL CORRELATE

The application of pattern perception tasks was carried over to humans in the work by Pinheiro and Ptacek (1971), Musiek and Pinheiro (1987), and Musiek, Baran, and Pinheiro (1990). It is clear from these studies that pattern perception is compromised by lesions of the auditory cortex (see Figure 12.11). In studies examining pattern perception abilities wherein either the frequency or durational characteristics of the patterns were varied (frequency pattern sequences, duration pattern sequences), individuals with cortical lesions in either hemisphere tended to perform poorly in both ears (if asked to describe the pattern sequences). Interestingly, patients with lesions of the brainstem showed only mild deficits on pattern perception tasks. The sensitivity and specificity of pattern tests for cortical lesions has been reported to be above 80% for cortical and subcortical lesions.

In the majority of patients with a lesion limited to one hemisphere, test results for either the frequency or duration patterns commonly yield bilateral deficits. This has been interpreted to mean that auditory regions in both hemispheres need to be intact to decode the auditory pattern for proper perception and verbal report. It has been postulated that for frequency and duration patterns the contour and sequencing of the stimulus is mediated in the right hemisphere, whereas the linguistic labeling (and the necessary sequencing for this) and the initiation of the speech response take place in the left hemisphere (Pinheiro and Musiek, 1985).

Robin et al. (1990) showed deficits in temporal pattern perception for patients with left auditory cortex involvement. However, patients with right hemisphere involvement did not show temporal deficits. Although these results seem at odds with the pattern results earlier stated, it must be realized there were methodological differences between the Robin et al. study and these other studies. ●

● **Figure 12.11**

Mean duration pattern recognition scores for three groups of subjects (normals, N = 50; cochlear lesions, N = 42; lesions of the auditory cortex or subcortex, N = 21).

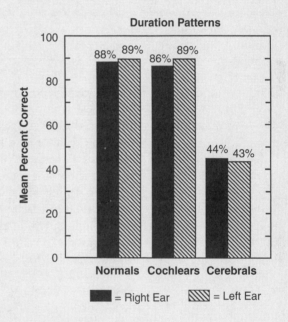

Auditory Cortex and Hearing in Noise

The ability to hear in noise is a phenomenon that is often associated with auditory cortex function but one that is poorly understood. One of the insights into the possible mechanisms that underlie hearing in noise was provided by a series of experiments by Phillips (1990), who described some interesting functions for some auditory cortex neurons when tones were presented in the presence of a broadband noise. The response thresholds of these neurons appear to be displaced to a higher level above the noise floor when background noise is present. However, what is unique about these neurons is that they have no sustained response to broadband noise; hence, the response to the tone presented in noise has a high signal-to-noise ratio. It also appears that the dynamic range of these neurons is preserved. These types of neurons do not seem to be present in lower areas of the CANS; hence they appear to be unique to the auditory cortex. At lower levels and for most other

CANS neurons, background noise compromises the response of the neurons to the primary acoustic signal. The cortical neurons that show a narrower dynamic range in noise are often those with large dynamic ranges in quiet. It would seem that the loudness growth functions of these neurons is steeper in noise than in quiet, which turns out to be the case (see Phillips and Hall, 1987).

Binaural Interactions and the Auditory Cortex

The focus of binaural interactions at the cortex relates primarily to functions associated with **localization** and **lateralization.** As with other regions of the auditory system, the auditory cortex plays an important role in the localization abilities of an individual. As was discussed in previous chapters, interaural intensity (IID) and interaural time differences (ITDs) serve as a basis for localization. These time and intensity factors relate to excitation and inhibition properties of cells in the auditory cortex (Middlebrooks, Dykes, and Merzenich, 1980). There are two main classes of cells in the cortex: excitation-excitation (EE) and excitation-inhibition (EI). The EE cells are related to stimulation at each ear being excitatory, and EI cells usually result in a response at the contralateral ear being excitatory while the response at the ipsilateral ear is inhibitory (Middlebrooks et al., 1980).

Although IID and ITD cues are used by the cortex, there does not seem to be distinct mapping for these cues on the auditory cortex (Reale and Brugge, 1990; de Ribaupierre, 1997). For ITD cues, certain cells appear to have an optimal interaural delay to which they respond (Reale and Brugge, 1990). In the auditory cortex, the majority of cells are responsive to IIDs when the intensity of the stimulus is greater in the contralateral hemifield compared to the situation in which the greater intensity is present in the ipsilateral hemifield. Overall, there is a contralateral bias for increased cortical activity related to cues originating from the contralateral side. This contralateral bias becomes most evident at stimulus intensity levels well above threshold. There are also some cells in the auditory cortex (considered binaural units) that only respond when both ears are stimulated at equal intensities (Aitkin, 1990).

Processing of acoustic cues for moving sound sources such as right to left, up and down, and near and far is different than the processing of acoustic cues for stationary sound sources (see de Ribaupierre, 1997). A relatively high number of cortical neurons are sensitive to moving sound sources, with multidirectional sensitive fibers playing a big role. It is important to note, however, that when the acoustic stimulus is near threshold, the sound reaching the contralateral ear may be at a level insufficient to stimulate the contralateral side; hence, only ipsilateral stimulation occurs. At suprathreshold levels (for a moving sound source) most cortical fibers are responsive to the contralateral hemifield. A smaller number of fibers respond to the ipsilateral hemifield, and even fewer fibers respond to a midline locus (0 to 20 degrees of midline) in space.

CLINICAL CORRELATE

There are not any commonly used tests of localization or lateralization in the clinic. Sanchez-Longo and Forester (1958) were among the first to use localization tasks to detect compromise of the auditory cortices. These researchers used a simple test of snapping their fingers at different locations on each side of the patient. The patient (with eyes closed) had to simply point to where he or she perceived the source of the sound was located. Interestingly, as crude as the measure was, it still revealed the same result that one sees today—poor localization in the auditory field opposite the involved hemisphere.

Perhaps one of the best potential clinical tests of sound localization is based on the **precedence effect**. The precedence effect requires the presentation of pairs of clicks through speakers on opposite sides of the sound room, with one speaker leading the other in time. Normal subjects perceive a fused image in space, with its location dependent on how much lead time one speaker has over the other. Changing the onset timing of the clicks at the two speakers results in the subject perceiving the sound image to move from one side to the other. Normal individuals can track this image with great accuracy; however, individuals with cortical lesions typically show poor tracking for the auditory field opposite the lesioned cortex (Moore, Cranford, and Rahn, 1990).

Intracranial lateralization is a procedure that has some strong clinical inferences but has never made its way into common clinical use. IIDs were discussed earlier as playing a key role in sound localization and lateralization. All things being equal, localization and lateralization of the perception of the sound stimulus will be to the ear that receives the greater intensity. Pinheiro and Tobin (1969) developed a simple test of intracranial lateralization that was aimed at clinical use. Two identical sound signals were initially presented to the ears at the same time, and a midline image was perceived. Then one of the signal's intensities was increased in 1-dB steps until the signal was localized to one side of the head. The same procedure was then repeated with the signal in the other ear adjusted in 1 dB steps and the results from the two procedures were compared. This test separated individuals with auditory cortical lesions from individuals without such lesions (e.g., controls and individuals with sensorineural loss) and as such proved to be a valuable test for the assessment of lateralization abilities in patients with lesions of the CANS. This simple but efficient test, however, still awaits further investigation and clinical application. ●

Evoked Potentials

A number of auditory EPs are presumably generated by the auditory cortex and/or subauditory cortex. Precise generator sites for certain EPs are difficult to determine; hence, there is continued debate about the generator site for many of these EPs. Given the limited scope of this section, it is difficult to even overview this topic because of the large amount of information in the literature about EPs and the auditory cortex. Therefore, we will offer only a few comments on EPs that have a relationship to auditory cortex structure and function.

The **middle latency response (MLR)** is likely generated by the primary auditory cortex, the thalamo-cortical pathway, and the reticular nuclei of the thalamus (see Kraus and McGee, 1995 for review; Musiek and Lee, 1999). The key waves of the MLR are the Na and Pa waves, which occur around 12 to 20 and 21 to 32 msec after the onset of a stimulus (of moderate intensity) in adult humans. The amplitude of the Na–Pa complex is around 1 μV depending on the intensity and other characteristics of the stimulus (Figure 12.12). Laterality effects are difficult to determine for middle and late potentials, although there does seem to be some indications that contralateral ear simulation may have more influence than ipsilateral ear stimulation—especially in cases of lesions limited to one hemisphere (Musiek, Charette, Kelly, Lee, and Musiek, 1999) (Figure 12.12).

Figure 12.12

Grand averages of the auditory middle latency response (MLR) for eight patients with cerebral vascular accidents involving the auditory areas of the cerebrum. Recordings were made over the left and right temporal-parietal region (C5, C6). When the electrode was over the lesioned hemisphere, the stimulated ear contralateral to the lesion yielded the poorer response. When the electrode was over the nonlesioned hemisphere, the contralateral ear provided a stronger response. All recordings of the Na–Pa waves in these patients were smaller in amplitude or greater in latency when compared to the MLR tracings obtained from normal subjects. Na and Nb = MLR negative waves, Pa and Pb = MLR positive waves, V = wave V of the auditory brainstem response.

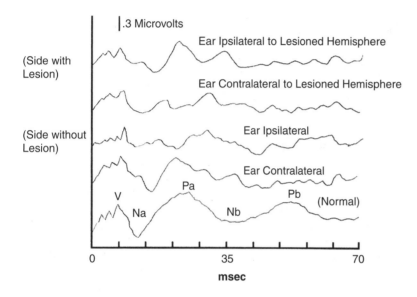

CLINICAL CORRELATE

The MLR has been shown to be compromised primarily in regard to amplitude and waveform morphology by damage to the auditory cortex and/or subcortex, including the thalamo-cortical pathways. These abnormal effects are best demonstrated by comparing the amplitudes of the Na–Pa responses for electrodes placed over the parietal areas for each hemisphere (C3, C4) (see Musiek et al., 1999). Major differences in the amplitudes when comparing these electrode sites can be indicative of pathology in the hemisphere yielding the smaller amplitude (an **electrode effect**). When one ear yields significantly smaller responses across all electrode sites than the other ear (an **ear effect**), this may also indicate pathology within the central auditory system (Figure 12.13). In this latter case, however, lateralization of the lesion is sometimes difficult to determine (Figure 12.12).

Interestingly, unlike ABRs, the MLR latency measures are not of great value diagnostically (Kileny, Paccioretti, and Wilson, 1987; Musiek et al., 1999). It has become increasingly clear that damage to thalamo-cortical auditory regions results in compromise of the MLR (see Musiek and Lee, 1999 for review). Based on these data, it is reasonable to believe that normal MLR responses are linked to a normal auditory cortex and thalamo-cortical pathway.

The MLR has a rather long and varied maturational course. In children under 10 years of age, the MLR is highly variable and therefore is difficult to use clinically. This variability may reflect maturational differences at the neural generation sites in younger children (Kraus, McGee, and Comperatore, 1989; Musiek and Lee, 1999). •

(continued)

● Figure 12.13

Schematic showing electrode and ear effects for the middle latency evoked responses (Na and Pa) derived from a patient with a lesion in the left hemisphere (stippled area). The arrows point to the lack of response for the C3 electrode for both ears (electrode effect) and to the right ear for all electrode sites (ear effect).

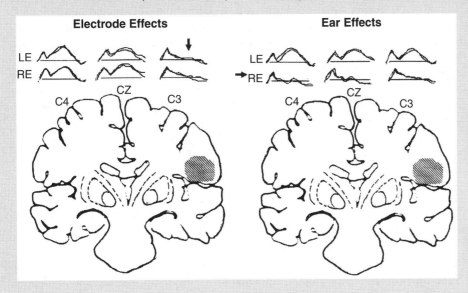

The **late potentials**, N1 and P2, sometimes referred to as the N1–P2 complex, is also likely generated by the primary auditory cortex (see Steinschneider et al., 1992 for review). These responses are larger than the MLR, with the N1 commonly being between 1 and 2 μV and the P2 being between 2 and 5 μV in size (see McPherson, 1996). The N1 usually occurs in the 80 to 100 msec latency range and the P2 in the 160 to 220 msec latency range (Figure 12.14).

● Figure 12.14

Late auditory-evoked potentials (N1, P2) and P300s in an adult patient with a right hemisphere stroke (top two sets of tracings) and an example of the same potentials in a subject with normal hearing (bottom two sets of waveforms). The upper tracings show the obliteration of the P300 in the patient with the right hemisphere stroke. Note that there is no laterality effect in this case (which is common) and there are no notable effects on the N1 and P2 in this case.

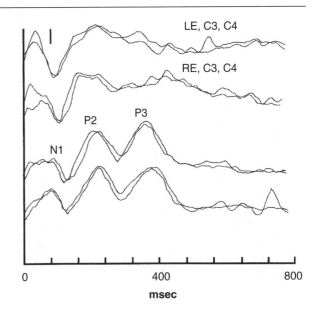

CLINICAL CORRELATE

Damage to the auditory cortex can compromise the N1–P2 waveform. Like the MLR, the N1–P2 complex has a rather long maturational course. Children of elementary school age may often have N1–P2 waveforms similar to those of adults, although some investigators claim the N1 and P2 continue to develop past the age of 10 years (see Kraus and McGee, 1994).

Knight, Hillyard, Woods, and Neville (1980) reported the N1 and P2 were compromised in adults with lesions in the tempero-parietal junction, but these potentials were essentially unaffected for lesions of the frontal lobe. In this study, electrode effects were clear.

These investigators also showed the N1 to be more sensitive than the P2 response to tempero-parietal lesions. Knight, Scabini, Woods, and Clayworth (1988) later compared N1 responses from control subjects to subjects with lesions of the STG and subjects with lesions of the inferior parietal lobe. The subjects with STG involvement demonstrated smaller amplitude N1 responses than did the other two groups. Interestingly, there were no significant differences among these three groups for the P2 response. The N1–P2 complex has also been shown to be abnormal in cases of suspected central auditory processing and language problems (Jirsa and Clontz, 1990; Tonnquist-Uhlen, 1996). ●

The **P300 or P3** probably has multiple contributors to its generation both intra-and interhemispherically. It is triggered by the subject attending to a targeted acoustic stimulus that occurs occasionally in a train of acoustic stimuli. This arrangement of acoustic stimuli is known as the odd-ball paradigm. Although most investigations have not yielded information strongly implicating the auditory cortex in the generation of the P300 (P3), damage to the auditory cortex and/or the temporal-parietal junction does seem to compromise the response (Knight, Scabini, Woods, and Clayworth, 1989; Obert and Cranford, 1990; see Musiek and Lee, 1999 for review). The P3 is greater in amplitude than the N1–P2 complex and usually occurs around 300 msec poststimulus. The P3 does not provide much laterality information. In fact, it is similar to pattern perception tests in that a lesion in one hemisphere seems to affect performance in both ears (see Figure 12.14).

The **mismatched negativity (MMN)** response is obtained by having subjects listen to standard and deviant sounds. The standard sound is a train of the same stimuli and the deviant sound is a stimulus that differs from the standard sound in some manner (i.e., frequency, intensity, duration, etc.). The deviant stimuli (if sufficiently different from the standard) will result in a negative shift in the time region after the P2. This negative shift is an indication that the subject's auditory system could discriminate the difference between standard and deviant sounds. The MMN

CLINICAL CORRELATE

Figure 12.14 demonstrates a case in which a right hemisphere lesion has had little effect on either the N1 or P2 waves but has essentially wiped out the P3 (P300) on all recordings. It has been shown in a number of studies that lesions in the region of the auditory cortex affect the amplitude and latency of the P3 response; however, in most cases there is no significant laterality information in regard to ear or electrode site for this potential (see Knight et al., 1989; and Musiek,

Baran, and Pinheiro, 1992 for a discussion of these issues). It is the impression of the authors (and others) that in cases with auditory cortex pathology, the P3 is probably a more sensitive measure of compromise than the N1 and P2 (Knight et al., 1989; Musiek et al., 1992; Musiek, Baran, and Pinheiro, 1994). Although the P300 is dependent on contributions from nonauditory areas of the brain, it seems clear that auditory cortex lesions compromise this EP. ●

is probably generated by or near the auditory cortex (Scherg, Vajar, and Picton, 1989). Unlike the P300, it is thought not to require attention (Naatanen, Paavilainen, Tiitinen, Jiang, and Alho, 1993). The MMN has been used experimentally to measure auditory discrimination for both speech and nonspeech sounds (see Musiek and Lee, 1999 for review). It has been measured in infants and is robust in school-aged children. However, because of the recording procedures and inconsistencies in responses (even in normal populations), this attractive technique has not been highly utilized clinically.

Ablation Studies of the Auditory Cortex

A number of studies have looked at ablation of the auditory cortex in animals to determine its effect on various parameters of hearing. Much of what we know regarding processes related to the CANS, such as threshold estimation, frequency discrimination, gap detection, and localization, has been accomplished through the use of ablation and lesion studies. Ablation studies provide a means for measuring the direct effect that impairment may have on specific auditory processes.

Behavioral ablation studies of the auditory cortex of the cat first began in the early 1940s (Kryter and Ades, 1943). This initial study investigated the effects of ablation on the auditory cortex with respect to intensity threshold estimation and discrimination. Although these authors reported no significant effect of intensity on absolute thresholds, later studies provided evidence to the contrary (Kavanagh and Kelly, 1988; Heffner and Heffner, 1989; Talwar, Musial, and Gerstein, 2001). Kavanagh and Kelly reported that following ablation to the primary auditory cortex of the ferret, the animal experienced a loss of sensitivity, particularly for frequencies above 32 kHz. A subsequent study of the effects of unilateral auditory cortex ablation in Japanese macaques also demonstrated hearing loss in the ear contralateral to the ablation (Heffner and Heffner, 1989). Although the performance of some of the macaques eventually returned to normal following the ablation, most of the experimental animals continued to exhibit elevated thresholds.

Many researchers have attempted to determine the effect of impairment to the auditory cortex on frequency discrimination (Meyer and Woolsey, 1952; Cranford, Igarashi, and Stamler, 1976; Cranford, 1979b; Heffner and Heffner, 1986; Ohl, Wetzel, Wagner, Rech, and Schiech, 1999). Cranford and colleagues (1976) studied the effects of auditory cortical ablation on frequency discrimination in the cat. Although most animals showed deficits in frequency discrimination immediately following the ablation, subsequent postoperative testing suggested that most animals relearned pitch discrimination for the task on which they were initially trained. Heffner and Heffner (1986) reported impairment of the macaques for discrimination of cooing vocalizations following unilateral ablation of the left auditory cortex; however, there was a return to normal performance during later test sessions that may be attributed to cortical reorganization. No significant effect was reported for right unilateral ablations. Only bilateral ablations of the auditory cortex in the macaques resulted in permanent impairment for discrimination among vocalizations.

Results among investigators still remain somewhat disparate; however, the more recent work by Talwar and colleagues (2001) has demonstrated some intriguing findings in support of the impact of auditory cortical damage on basic auditory functions. Although it was not an ablation study, these investigators examined the effects of a reversible inactivation of the rat auditory cortex through the use of γ-aminobutyric acid (GABA) agonist. Unlike many of the previous studies, this investigation followed a rapid time course to control for any reorganization at the cortical level. The animals exhibited a profound loss of sensitivity to tones, as well as impairment to their frequency discrimination immediately following the administration of the GABA agonist.

A significant number of studies have investigated the effects of ablation of the auditory cortex on sound localization (Jenkins and Merzenich, 1984; Altman and Kalmykova, 1986; Kelly and Kavanagh, 1986; Heffner and Heffner, 1990; Stepien, Stepien, and Lubinska, 1990; Beital and Kaas, 1993; Heffner, 1997; Zatorre and Penhune, 2001). It appears that there are differences among animal species with respect to sound localization abilities following impairment to the auditory cortex. The early work of Altman and Kalmykova (1986) suggests that unilateral ablation in the dog affects the animal's ability to localize on the side contralateral to the lesion. When a bilateral ablation was performed, it resulted in complete inability of the animal to localize source movement when changes in ITDs were initiated. However, results from this study were not supported in a study conducted with rats (Kelly and Kavanagh, 1986) that found only a slight reduction in localization performance following bilateral ablation of the auditory cortex. There remains continued debate as to the effects of these lesions on the localization performance in humans. The debate is not so much whether or not there is a compromise, but how much of a compromise is likely to result.

Temporal processing has also been shown to be impaired as a result of ablation to the auditory cortex. One of the initial studies to examine the effect of ablation on temporal processing, specifically pattern perception, was conducted in the cat (Diamond and Neff, 1957). These authors showed a correlation between the amount of impairment and the degree of deficit. Those animals with ablation restricted to primary AI showed no impairment to discrimination of tonal patterns, whereas those with partial ablation extending to secondary auditory cortex AII and associated auditory areas demonstrated loss of discrimination with recovery over time. However, those animals with complete ablation of these same areas exhibited complete loss of pattern perception with no recovery.

Temporal resolution has not received the same amount of attention as the previously mentioned processes, likely because of the difficulty in accurately measuring gap detection thresholds in both the human and animal model. Following complete ablation of the auditory cortex in the rat, a significant increase in gap detection thresholds was observed by Skya and colleagues (Syka, Rybalko, Mazelova, and Druga, 2002). Although some degree of recovery was observed in the first month following the ablations, the gap detection thresholds following recovery did not match those noted in a control group. The work of Cranford (1979a,b) demonstrated that brief tone thresholds were not impacted as a result of cortical ablation in the cat. However, this work also provided evidence that frequency difference limens for short-duration tones were significantly affected in the ear contralateral to the ablation. Cranford and colleagues subsequently studied the effects of temporal lobe lesions on humans and found results similar to those in the cat (Cranford, Stream, Rye, and Slade, 1982). In their investigation they demonstrated that although brief tone thresholds were not impaired in comparison to the threshold noted in a control group, the experimental subjects' difference limens for frequency were markedly poorer for signal durations less than 200 msec.

The effects of ablation on electrophysiological measures have generated objective support for the involvement of auditory cortical lesions in auditory evoked responses. These applications provide a measure of the direct impact an ablation or lesion at a particular location may have on auditory EPs (Harrison, Buchwald, and Kaga, 1986; Zhao and Wei, 1989; Talwar et al., 2001; Zappoli, et al., 2002; Zappoli, 2003). The Pa wave of the MLR is clearly affected in the ear contralateral to ablation in the guinea pig (Zhao and Wei, 1989). Diminished waveform morphology following ablation is also apparent in the rat (Talwar et al., 2001). Although this evidence suggests the primary component of the MLR (Pa) is generated by the auditory cortex, there is evidence that ablation does not impact on P300 in the cat (Harrison et al., 1986).

A significant body of evidence supports the notion that the auditory cortex has direct involvement in the processing of basic auditory information. However, as in any area of research, there remains some degree of controversy. This is likely a result of the debate regarding the implications of generalizing results of animal studies to the human model. In addition, this research also may be impacted by variables such as location of the ablation or lesion, age of the subject, and reorganization following insult, all of which can influence results.

Functional Imaging and the Auditory Cortex

At various places in this book functional imaging has been referred to in order to help support some of the functional or structural information being presented—especially in the human model. Herein lies the value of imaging techniques such as fMRI or PET: they allow the acquisition of structural and functional information on the human brain. Although imaging techniques have limitations, they remain one of the best ways to learn about the human brain.

The fMRI technique uses a strong magnetic field to align the body's protons, and then a brief radio signal is used to change this alignment. The protons resume their original alignment and give off energy that is measured. The blood acquires paramagnetic properties when the body is in a strong magnetic field, which permits blood flow to be visualized by fMRI. As blood flow increases, so does blood volume and oxygenation. When a certain part of the brain has to work hard, it requires more blood and oxygen, and this increased activity is noted in the MRI measurements (see Elliott, 1994). No radioactivity is involved in fMRI; however, the instrument emits high-intensity noise—a factor in auditory testing.

The PET technique is based on the decay of radioactive tracers that emit positrons. These positrons emit photons that are detected by the scanning equipment. The radioactive tracer is either injected into the blood or it is inhaled. As there is an increase in regional blood flow or metabolism (glucose) in the activated part of the brain, more photons are emitted, which are then measured by the instrument—reflecting greater activity (see Elliott, 1994).

Functional imaging has made many contributions to our understanding of the function and structure of the brain. To even briefly review this literature is beyond the scope of this chapter; however, a few examples of the contributions to auditory biology will be highlighted (Figure 12.15). One of the early contributions offered by Lauter et al. (1985) was a PET study that documented the tonotopicity of the human auditory cortex. Johnsrude et al. (2002) later published an excellent review of functional imaging of the auditory system. This publication reviewed lateralization studies for speech stimuli and tonal stimuli that showed a left hemisphere advantage for speech stimuli. Other significant findings reviewed included (1) that contralateral stimulation generally results in greater cortex activation than ipsilateral stimulation, (2) that larger activation areas are associated with greater intensity of the stimulus, (3) that attention versus nonattention paradigms confirmed the role that attention plays in activating regions of the brain, and (4) that certain areas of the brain are responsible for integration of information across different sensory modalities.

● Figure 12.15

fMRI showing transverse (a), left lateral (b), and coronal (c) views of the brain of a school-aged child listening to monosyllabic words presented to the right ear. Note the greater activity for the auditory regions of the left hemisphere compared to the right hemisphere, indicating contralateral enhancement (courtesy of Deborah Moncrieff, University of Connecticut).

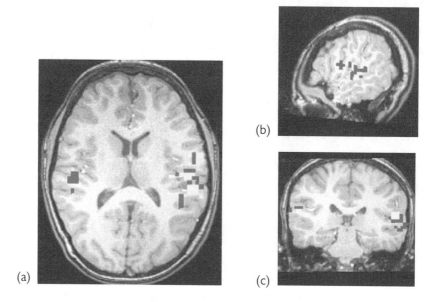

(a)   (b)   (c)

Neurotransmitters of the Auditory Cortex

In the cortex are some defined neurotransmitters that are involved in audition. Acetylcholine, GABA, glutamate, noradrenoline, and serotinin are now all receiving attention from investigators in regard to their role in hearing. Interactions between inhibitory chemicals like GABA and excitatory agents such as glutamate may govern receptive field properties in the cortex and thalamo-cortical pathways. These neurotransmitters may also be basic to plasticity in the cortex (Edeline, 2003).

SUMMARY

The auditory cortex and subcortex receive input from the MGB via the thalamo-cortical pathway, which courses at least in part through the internal capsule. The auditory cortex has six layers (in cat) and is located in the posterior two-thirds of the STP. Key structures in this region include Heschl's gyrus and the planum temporale. Recently the concept of the primary auditory region forming a core surrounded by belt and parabelt regions has gained much interest. It is clear that there is asymmetry in the size of Heschl's gyrus and the planum temporale for the left and right sides of the brain without neurologic compromise. Both of these structures are larger on the left side of the brain.

The insula is a major structure located medial to the temporal lobe. Gradually emerging evidence along several lines indicates that this structure is acoustically responsive and may play a major role in auditory processing.

The auditory cortex has numerous neurons with a 40 to 50 dB dynamic intensity range, with some reports claiming an even greater dynamic range for some select neurons. Heschl's gyrus is well organized tonotopically with low to high frequencies running posterio-medially. Tuning curves obtained from auditory cortex fibers are V-shaped, with sharpness increasing as a function of frequency. The auditory cortex responds best to AM and FM signals that modulate less than 50 times per second. While the cortex does not respond well to periodic stimuli, it does have great sensitivity to rapidly varying individual acoustic stimuli. The auditory cortex also responds well to speech stimuli and it plays an important role in the processing of speech stimuli that are dichotically presented. In humans, stronger responses to speech stimuli are generally noted for the left-sided auditory regions of the cortex than for the right-sided regions.

It appears that some special neurons in the auditory cortex play an interesting role in hearing in noise. These neurons only begin to fire at a level that is above the noise level, creating a very favorable signal-to-noise ratio. It also appears that the dynamic range of these neurons is preserved. The auditory cortex responds well to interaural intensity and timing cues, which provide a basis for localization and lateralization. Responses are generally stronger to stimuli presented in the contralateral auditory field. Evoked potentials that are generated at least in part by the auditory cortex are also more robust over the contralateral hemisphere. Evoked potentials, such as the MLR, N1-P2, P300, and mismatched negativity, can provide important information as to the integrity of the auditory cortex and its related structures. Other tests of cortical function also have the potential to advance clinical investigation of the auditory brain. Functional imaging techniques such as PET and fMRI will continue to advance our knowledge of the human auditory cortex.

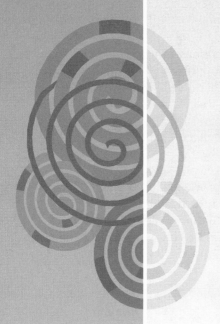

13

The Corpus Callosum and Auditory Interhemispheric Function

Introduction

The corpus callosum (CC) is a major structure within the central nervous system that connects the two hemispheres of the brain by transferring information from one side of the cerebrum to the other. The CC has received considerable attention in the recent past as the neuropsychological literature has begun to focus on its many functional aspects. The CC has been shown to be relevant to studies on maturation and aging and it appears to be an important factor in studies on attention. Perhaps the biggest force behind the increasing interest in the CC is the information that has emerged from split-brain studies. These human studies have allowed great insights into how the CC functions and they have provided important knowledge as to the ways in which the two hemispheres of the brain interact. Of particular significance to this discussion is the split-brain research that has addressed the role of the CC in the processing of auditory information. Much of what is currently known about the role of the CC in audition has been gleaned from the study of split-brain patients, and this knowledge has led to a number of clinical spin-offs that will be discussed in this chapter.

CLINICAL CORRELATE

The study of auditory function in split-brain patients has elucidated the critical role that the CC plays in the processing and transfer of auditory information in the brain. Split-brain patients include those individuals who have undergone a specialized neurosurgical procedure, which is usually performed in an effort to help control intractable seizures. The medical terminology for this type of surgery is *corpus callosotomy;* however, the term *corpus commissurotomy* is often used as an alternative. This neurosurgical procedure involves cutting all or a portion of the CC to stop the spread of epileptic seizure activity across the CC to structures in the other half of the brain. This surgery was first done in the 1940s by Van Wagenen (Van Wagenen and Herren, 1940). Interestingly, few auditory (or neuropsychological) deficits were documented in these patients after this major surgical operation. However, as was learned later, the right kinds of questions were not asked of Van Wagenen's patients. Therefore, the function of the CC in audition was not discovered for a number of years.

(continued)

Commissurotomy failed to become an accepted surgical procedure after its introduction by Van Wagenen in 1940. It wasn't until the 1960s when this surgical procedure was reintroduced by Joseph Bogen that any additional surgeries were performed. At this time, two investigators (Roger Sperry and Michael Gazzaniga) studied the performance of Bogen's split-brain patients following surgical intervention and uncovered some important information about the role of the CC in processing sensory information. However, in spite of these important initial findings, further study of the function of this important structure was delayed by a number of years since the surgical procedure remained poorly accepted. Some acceptance of commissurotomy as a neurosurgical procedure came in the 1970s when

Donald Wilson began using microsurgical techniques to perform the surgical procedure. At this time it became clear that some patients with intractable seizures profited from this surgery in regard to their quality of life and the procedure became more commonly accepted in the medical community.

Two important clinical spin-offs from the research into auditory function in split-brain patients have occurred. These include (1) the establishment of diagnostic trends or profiles for various audiological tests that are linked to abnormal CC function and (2) new schemes for rehabilitation of auditory deficits related to interhemispheric dysfunction. The interest in these diagnostic trends and treatment approaches is currently gaining momentum in the field of (central) auditory processing disorders. ●

ANATOMY OF THE CORPUS CALLOSUM AND INTERHEMISPHERIC NEURONAL PATHWAYS

The CC is large fiber tract that connects the two hemispheres of the brain. It can be observed from a superior view by separating the two hemispheres of the brain and looking down toward the base of the brain. Inferior to the CC is the **septum pellucidum** and the lateral ventricles. Laterally, the CC reaches out to the cortex, while in the anterior to posterior plane the CC extends from the posterior region of the frontal lobe to the anterior region of the occipital lobe (Figure 13.1).

Viewing the CC in an anterior to posterior plane along the midline of the brain reveals a structure that is banana shaped. In adult humans, the length of the CC is

● **Figure 13.1**

A midsaggital section of the human corpus callosum (arrows outlining the superior surface).

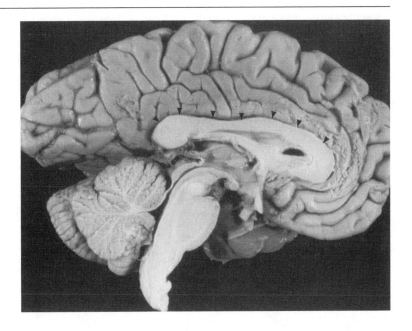

● **Figure 13.2**

(a) Sketch of the human brain (coronal view) depicting homolateral fibers running from the cortex (stippled area) in one hemisphere to essentially the same area in the cortex of the opposite hemisphere. (b) A coronal section of a human brain with arrows showing the interhemispheric pathway. Note how this pathway courses around the lateral ventricles (shown by lines connected to #1) (from Waddington, 1984, with permission).

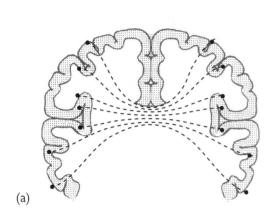

(a)

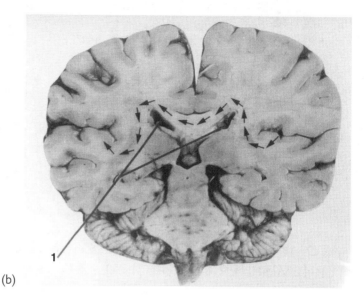

(b)

● **Figure 13.3**

Sketch of the human brain (horizontal view) depicting homolateral fibers, some of which branch into heterolateral fibers (dotted line to open circles), and regular heterolateral fibers (filled circles) connecting one hemisphere to the other.

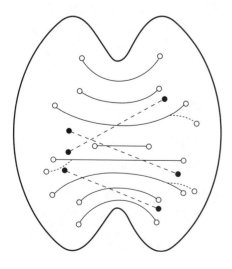

approximately 6.5 cm from the anterior-most to posterior-most point, and the thickness ranges from about 0.5 cm to slightly over 1 cm. Generally, the thickest region is in the posterior-most area of the CC, called the splenium. The total area of the CC is around 700 mm² (Jancke and Steinmetz, 2003). It is estimated that some 200 to 350 million fibers course through the CC in the adult human (Jancke and Steinmetz, 2003). These fibers are heavily myelinated and are among the largest fibers in the brain. In fact, in primates it has been estimated that 94% of the fibers are myelinated (LaMantia and Rakic, 1984). The smaller unmyelinated fibers tend to be found in the anterior one-third of the CC, while the larger myelinated fibers are typically found in the posterior two-thirds of the CC. In addition, it has been reported that some of the largest fibers in this structure are found in the auditory and visual areas of the CC, which are located in the posterior regions of the CC (Aboitiz, Ide, and Olivares, 2003).

The CC has two types of fibers, **homolateral** and **heterolateral** (also termed homotopic and heterotopic). Homolateral fibers are those that connect one site in one hemisphere to essentially the same site in the opposite hemisphere via the CC (Figure 13.2). Heterolateral fibers are those fibers that connect to different sites in each hemisphere after running through the CC (Figure 13.3). It had been assumed initially that most callosal fibers were homolateral in nature, with only a few heterolateral fibers being represented in the CC population of neural fibers. However, recent data shows heavy networks of heterolateral fibers in the occipital areas and temporal areas of the brain (Clarke, 2003). It is also possible that by processes of bifurcation, a homolateral fiber could send off a heterolateral collateral branch (Innocenti and Bressoud, 2003) (Figure 13.3). The branched fiber could then connect to a different area of the brain than the original homolateral fiber. Therefore, one fiber could have a both a homolateral and a heterolateral connection.

The midsaggital portion of the CC is divided into several anatomical segments that reflect the origin of the fibers running through the CC. As mentioned earlier, this part of the CC is banana shaped. The neuroanatomy of this section of the CC will be defined as proceeding from the posterior-most portion to the anterior and inferior portions (Figure 13.4).

The most posterior segment of the CC is the **splenium,** which makes up about one-fifth of the total area of the CC. In the primate, and most likely in the human as well, the splenium is where the occipital fibers cross from one visual cortex to the other (Pandya and Rosene, 1985). These visual fibers are referred to as the occipital forceps. Therefore, the splenium is considered the visual part of the CC. Some data, however, indicate that there are some auditory fibers in the anterior part of the splenium (Pollmann, Maertens, von Cramon, Lepsien, and Hugdahl, 2002). Immediately anterior to the splenium is an area of the CC where the structure becomes thinner. This somewhat anatomically restricted area of the CC has been labeled the **isthmus,** or **sulcus,** and is the area where the majority of the auditory fibers cross. Fibers traveling through this part of the CC arise from the frontal lobe (Pandya and Rosene, 1985). As one proceeds in an anterior direction beyond the sulcus, the CC begins to thicken and the middle one-third of the CC is observed. This segment is called the **body,** or the **trunk,** and this is where the somatosensory and motor fibers originating from the parietal lobe cross the midline. In the posterior aspect of this superior temporal plane (posterior half) and gyrus, the posterior insula, the posterior-inferior parietal lobe, and the posterior segment of the CC, there could also be some auditory fibers (Aboitiz et al., 2003). The anterior one-third of the CC is termed the **genu,** and this is the locus where most of the fibers originating from the frontal lobe cross the midline. The **rostrum,** which is located inferior and posterior to the genu, carries fibers from the medial prefrontal cortex, and for the most part, these neurons have olfactory functions. The **anterior commissure** (AC) is located inferior to the anterior one-third of the CC. It carries neurons from the orbital frontal cortex and anterior superior and inferior temporal cortex (Pandya and

● **Figure 13.4**

Sketch (midsaggital view) depicting the major segments of the corpus callosum. Also shown is the anterior commissure.

Anatomical Areas of the Corpus Callosum

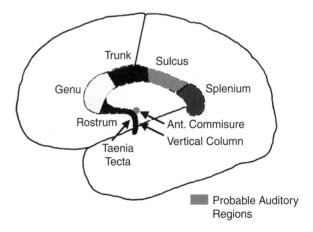

● **Figure 13.5**

Three sketches of the corpus callosum showing the variance in shape of this structure (midsaggital views) (based on Bookstein, 2003).

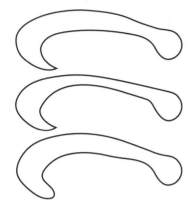

CLINICAL CORRELATE

Since the midsaggital section of the CC has a topography that is related to distinct areas of the cortex, damage to specific regions of the CC is likely to result in specific types of deficits. For example, if the sulcus or isthmus area is damaged, then interhemispheric auditory processing would likely be compromised. ●

Rosene, 1985). Recent work by Bamiou and colleagues (2004) indicates that some auditory fibers may be present in the AC. However, the specific fiber types that cross the AC are not well defined at this time and additional research is needed before a definitive determination of the neuronal types within the AC can be made.

Although the midsaggital section of the CC has been defined as banana shaped for the adult human, there is some variability in its shape across the species. It is difficult to know if these varying shapes of the CC have functional relevancy. For example, it is of interest to note that the shape of the CC in schizophrenics has been found to be structurally different from the shape of the CC in control subjects (Cowell, Denenberg, Boehm, Kertesz, and Nasrallah, 2003). However, it should be noted that even in control groups, there is some variability in the shape of the CC (Figure 13.5). Therefore, it may be difficult, if not impossible, to link these structural differences to physiological differences in brain functioning.

The pathway of the callosal fibers that connects the hemispheres is referred to as the **transcallosal pathway.** This pathway is composed of (1) transverse fibers that at the anterior and posterior ends of the CC arch around to reach the posterior and anterior poles of the cortex—hence, the name forceps—and (2) other transverse fibers (those in the remainder of the CC), which radiate outward in a more direct route to connect to the various lobes of the brain. Of interest to this discussion is the portion of the transcallosal pathway that carries auditory information. This pathway is known as the **transcallosal auditory pathway** (TCAP) and it will be the focus of the anatomical description that follows.

Based on information provided by Pandya and Rosene (1985) and Ptito and Boire (2003), the origins of the TCAP are in the primary auditory cortex and the association auditory cortex. It is speculated, however, that most callosal fibers arise from higher-order association areas and that they transfer rather complex, but subtle, information (Ptito and Boire, 2003). These fibers are believed to travel from their origins in the auditory cortex by traveling posteriorly and superiorly through the white matter of the parietal lobe before running around the lateral and superior aspect of the lateral ventricle (in a region known as the **trigone**) and then crossing the midline to connect to the opposite side. This pathway has been primarily defined by careful study of the effect of lesions in the subcortical white matter on the interhemispheric transfer of auditory information (Damasio and Damasio, 1979).

CLINICAL CORRELATE

It is important to realize that the CC fibers (white matter) extend from the gray matter area in one cortex to the gray matter area in the other cortex. Hence, the CC fibers make up a large portion of the subcortical white matter. For this reason, it is likely that a lesion anywhere along the TCAP will result in a deficit of interhemispheric transfer. Of particular interest here is the trigone area. This area, which is situated around the lateral ventricles, seems to have a tendency toward early involvement in patients with multiple sclerosis (Damasio and Damasio, 1979). It has been shown that many patients with multiple sclerosis demonstrate left ear deficits on dichotic listening tests, secondary to involvement of the CC (Gadea, Marti-Bonmati, Arana, Espert, Casanova, and Pascual, 2002). ●

● Figure 13.6

The midsaggital corpus callosum region. The dark to light progression is from the posterior to anterior regions of the CC. This progression corresponds to the direction of maturation of the corpus callosum (i.e., myelination), as well as the progression from regions of larger to smaller fibers in this structure.

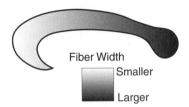

Maturation, Age, and Gender Effects on Corpus Callosum Anatomy

The key anatomical components and neuronal differentiation of the CC are established before birth. However, the maturation of the CC is far from complete at the time of birth since the CC is composed primarily of myelinated fibers, and **myelin maturation** of the brain is not usually achieved until the teen years or later (Thompson, Narr, Blanton, and Toga, 2003). The course of maturation of the CC is quite long, with developmental changes in the size of this structure related to increased size of the brain and increased amounts of myelination of the callosal fibers. It has been shown that the CC doubles in size from birth to two years of age (Rakic and Yakovlev, 1968) and that further increases occur up through the teenage years and beyond (Thompson et al., 2003). The myelination of the CC, which is also related to increases in size, appears to progress from the posterior to the anterior portion of the CC, with the splenium becoming myelinated first (Kier and Truwit, 1996) (Figure 13.6). It is interesting to note that the larger fibers of the CC are located in the posterior region, while smaller fibers are located in the more anterior regions of the CC (Figure 13.6).

Reports have clearly shown increases in the size of the CC resulting from increases in myelination of the callosal fibers up to adulthood (Schaefer, Thompson, Bodensteiner, Hamza, Tucker, Marks, Gay, and Wilson, 1990; see Thompson et al., 2003 for review). However, most of the later maturational changes in the CC involve only the splenium and the isthmus (sulcus) (Giedd et al., 1996). These areas correspond to primarily the visual and auditory areas of the CC. Giedd et al. (1999), using a longitudinal MRI study, showed white matter increasing in volume in the cerebrum from ages 4 through 22 years (Figure 13.7). This is consistent with earlier information provided by Yakovlev and LeCours (1967), who were among

● Figure 13.7

Graph showing white matter maturation in the (human) cerebrum (based on data from Giedd et al., 1996).

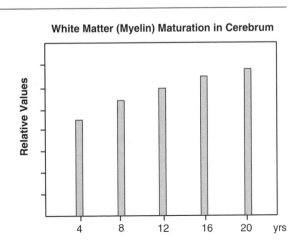

CLINICAL CORRELATE

Audiological tests, such as dichotic speech procedures, that require normal and efficient callosal functioning typically demonstrate an extended maturational course that parallels the maturational development of the myelin sheaths lining the CC fibers. For example, performance on dichotic tests such as dichotic digits and competing sentences does not reach adult values for left ear performance until 11 years of age (Musiek, Kibbe, and Baran, 1984b). ●

the first to draw attention to the fact that myelination of the CC requires many years to reach adult stages. This observation had profound implications in regard to the understanding of interhemispheric function in humans.

Gender effects on the morphology of the CC are highly controversial. Extensive bodies of literature argue for and against a gender effect on the anatomy of the CC. These arguments will not be detailed here, but the reader who is interested in this topic can find an excellent review of this topic in Thompson et al. (2003). The following discussion provides a brief account of the information taken from this source along with some personal interpretations of this data. It appears, based upon the prevailing evidence, that there is little difference in the size of the CC of men and women when normalizing is done—except possibly in the area of the splenium. It does seem that the preponderance of evidence supports the notion that the splenium is larger in females than in males and that this difference continues throughout the normal lifespan and may actually increase with advancing age.

As people age, there may be associated effects on the size and shape of the CC (Pujol, Vendrell, Junque, Marti-Vilalta, and Capdevila, 1993; Thompson et al., 2003). It has been reported that the CC maintains its size and shape in individuals up to the age of approximately 50 years, but after that age it begins to undergo a gradual process of thinning, which is most likely secondary to a reduction in myelin (Pujol et al., 1993; Aboitiz, Rodriquez, Olivares, and Zaidel, 1996). There is some disagreement as to whether regional changes occur in the CC with increasing age. Some reports indicate that aging effects are most often noted in the anterior region, while others have reported posterior CC aging effects (see Thompson et al., 2003 for review). Clearly, the thinning of the CC has functional consequences (interhemispheric transfer), which will be discussed later in this chapter.

Some specific information exists as to how different regions of the CC change with age. Takeda and colleagues showed that the widths of the rostrum, body (including the isthmus), and splenium become thinner with increasing age (Takeda, Hirashima, Ikeda, Yamamoto, Sugino, and Endo, 2003). It appears from their findings that the effects became most evident at the ages of 40 to 50 years and older. Interestingly, these same researchers found that the height and anterior to posterior length of the CC actually become larger with age.

In summary, it appears that the CC requires many years to fully develop, as maturation of this structure is highly dependent on the myelination of the callosal fibers, especially the large callosal fibers. In normally developing individuals, this process may not be complete until the teenage or early adult years. On the other end of the age continuum, there appears to be a reversal of this process; that is, as people age (become elderly) a progressive thinning of the CC occurs. This thinning process is most likely secondary to the gradual loss of myelin within the CC (i.e., a demyelination of the callosal fibers). These maturational and degenerative changes have many interesting consequences for the young and the elderly, as both of these processes can affect a number of auditory functions that are callosal dependent.

PHYSIOLOGY OF THE CORPUS CALLOSUM AND INTERHEMISPHERIC NEURONAL PATHWAYS

Less is known about the physiology of the CC than about the anatomy of the CC, especially in the human model. Perhaps the most popular physiologic measure involving the CC is the **interhemispheric transfer time** (IHTT), also known as the

transcallosal transfer time (TCTT). This measurement is made to determine the latency of the impulses that travel from a site within the cortex of one hemisphere to its counterpart in the cortex of the other hemisphere (via the CC). The measurement is typically derived by measuring the difference in reaction time of a manual response to a stimulus that is delivered via a crossed pathway to that noted when the stimulus is delivered in an uncrossed mode. For example, latency measures can be derived when a lateralized visual or somatosensory stimulus is presented ipsilateral to the hand generating a response and when the stimulus is presented contralateral to the hand creating the response. The time difference between the two measures is considered the callosal transfer time or the crossed-uncrossed difference (CUD). Simple tasks involving simple decisions are important in setting up this paradigm, and visual and somatosensory stimuli are routinely used. Auditory stimuli are not used because the auditory system has both ipsilateral and contralateral inputs to the cerebral hemispheres. Evoked potentials (EPs) can also be used to determine IHTTs. Electrodes are placed over the cortical region that is stimulated by a lateralized stimulus (left or right) and latencies are measured ipsilaterally and contralaterally, with the difference being the IHTT.

The IHTT may vary depending on which site within the central system is being assessed and which system is being stimulated (Milner and Rugg, 1989). IHTTs derived from occipital sites have been reported to range from about 12 to 19 msec, while those derived from more central sites tend to be shorter (i.e., around 3 msec) (Chang, 1953; Jeeves and Moes, 1996). On the other hand, IHTTs of over 100 msec have been reported for complex test conditions (Bremer, Brihaye, and Andre-Balisaux, 1956). Consistent with many of the earlier findings on IHTT, Aboitiz and colleagues (2003) reported that small fibers showed slower conduction times and increased IHTTs, while larger fibers conducted impulses more rapidly and yielded shorter IHTTs. These investigators found interhemispheric transmission delays ranging from 19 to 25 msec for the smaller (and more abundant) fibers studied, whereas the larger fibers tended to yield the shortest IHTTs (3 msec). The transfer times reported by Aboitiz et al. (2003) were derived with simple motor reaction and EP measures. These researchers suggest that more complex tasks (e.g., such as those that may involve association areas and/or smaller myelinated fibers) may require as long as a 45 msec transfer time. These longer IHTTs would be consistent with those reported by Bremer et al. (1956). It appears that longer IHTTs may be more commonly observed for heterotopic than homotopic fibers (Innocenti and Bressoud, 2003). However, this observation may be somewhat tenuous in that increased IHTTs are dependent on a number of other factors such as the amount of myelin in the fiber and whether the fiber is inhibitory or excitatory. Some neurons in the CC create inhibitory and excitatory influences on the cortex (Berlucchi, 2003). Exactly how the callosal fibers play a role in this inhibition or excitation is not well understood. It could be that one cortex mediates the excitation and inhibition and the callosal fibers simply transfer the patterns. On the other hand, it is possible that the callosal fibers directly mediate or contribute to the excitation and inhibition patterns in the cortex. It is known that when the CC is sectioned there can be a release in one hemisphere from the influences of neural impulses arising from the other hemisphere. Therefore, functions in the released hemisphere can be either enhanced or decreased depending upon whether the neural impulses traveling from the opposite half of the brain are excitatory or inhibitory in nature (Berlucchi, 2003). For example, it has been demonstrated that for dichotic tasks there can be an increase in right ear scores after **commissurotomy** (Musiek, Reeves, and Baran, 1985). This increase has been attributed to the fact the left hemisphere no longer has to manipulate impulse patterns coming from the left ear to the right hemisphere and to the left hemisphere via the CC. Without this competition for processing of speech materials coming from the right hemisphere, more neural substrate within the left hemisphere can be dedicated to processing the information arising from the right ear (left hemisphere); hence, performance for the right ear improves.

Physiological evidence for the observations of inhibition and excitation within the CC is quite limited. It appears that most CC fibers, at least those that have been tested in animals, are directly excitatory. Some inhibitory responses are also believed to exist, but these responses are likely to be indirect and possibly postsynaptic. In animals, γ-aminobutyric acid (GABA)-sensitive neurons have been shown to be present in the CC and GABA is generally considered to be an inhibitory neurotransmitter (Gonchar, Johnson, and Weinberg, 1995). Based upon a review provided by Berlucchi (2003), it appears that excitatory CC neurons are monosynaptic fibers, while those that are inhibitory in nature are polysynaptic. There are also CC neurons that are corticofugal. These neurons can provide for various feedback loops that are often associated with either an enhancement or a decrease in activity.

One of the key outcomes of callosal inhibition and excitation is the equalization of activity arising from the two hemispheres, which may be the basis for optimal integration of cortical activity (Berlucchi, 1983). Lassonde (1986) relates that the CC serves as a modulator of cortical activity, probably secondary to inhibitory and excitatory influences created by fibers of the CC for cortical responses. The modulation of cortical activity permits a balance of inhibitory and excitatory activity in the brain. This concept has become an important notion in brain physiology that has far-reaching implications (see Chapter 1).

Impulse conduction time for CC axons has been studied in animals. Swadlow (1986) has reported on the velocity of CC impulse conduction in primates and rabbits. Generally, the primates' conduction times were faster than those for the rabbits. For example, the primates' conduction velocity ranged from 4.7 to 27 m per second. These values were more than twice those noted for the rabbit. Refractory periods for CC fibers that were slow conductors were greater than for those fibers that were fast conductors. Refractory periods varied from 0.55 to 1.3 msec for the primates. Our interpretation of this data is as follows: (1) primates may have more heavily myelinated neurons in the CC, or (2) since the rabbits' brains are smaller, faster conduction times may not be required.

Maturation and Age Effects on Callosal Transfer Time

The IHTT is likely a function of the extent of myelination of the callosal fibers. The more heavily myelinated the fibers, the faster the impulses will travel between the hemispheres. Unlike the peripheral auditory system, the CC is not mature at birth. Rather its maturational course lasts a significant portion of an animal's life and for many years in the case of humans. Numerous animal studies that have recorded transcallosal EPs have shown a definite decrease in the latencies of these measures as the animal matures (Chang, 1953; Grafstein, 1963; Seggie and Berry, 1972). Perhaps one of the most frequently cited articles on the maturation of IHTT in humans is that authored by Salamy (1978). Salamy used somatosensory EPs to measure IHTTs in subjects ranging in age from 4 to 20 years of age. He recorded responses from electrodes placed over the temporal areas of the scalp and compared the latencies of the EPs from ipsilateral and contralateral sites that were triggered by electrical stimulation of the index finger (Figure 13.8). His results showed a decrease in

IHTTs with increasing age. Of interest, however, was the fact that 9-year-olds showed IHTTs that were longer than those of 20-year-olds, indicating that maturation of this response was not achieved in normally developing subjects until some time between the ages of 9 and 20 years. This finding was consistent with the earlier anatomical data reviewed, which showed myelin maturation to continue to the teenage years and possibly beyond (Yakovlev and LeCours, 1967). A potential consequence of such an extended maturational course of development is that complex auditory tasks that place increased processing demands on the CC may yield ear differences in young children. In fact, ear differences are common among young children for a number of audiological tests, such as those that involve dichotic listening, which by their very nature place heavy demands on efficient interhemispheric transfer.

Human Psychophysics and Function of the Corpus Callosum

A great deal of our basic understanding of the CC has been a result of the study of split-brain patients. The human model has done much to advance

● **Figure 13.8**

Graph showing interhemispheric transfer time (IHTT) as a function of age in humans using stimulation of the somatosensory system (based on data from Salamy, 1978).

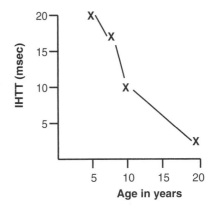

CLINICAL CORRELATE

The fact that in humans the CC has a long maturational course has profound implications for audiological tests that are dependent on efficient interhemispheric transfer, as is the case for dichotic listening tests. As alluded to earlier, it is clear from maturational information on dichotic listening that performance in children improves until approximately the age of 11 years. This timeline correlates well with the documented course of CC myelin maturation in children and also with the available information for IHTT maturation in younger individuals. Moreover, the pattern of improvement in dichotic listening performance that is observed for young children strongly suggests that the developmental changes in the CC are responsible for the behavioral changes noted; that is, improvements in performance are noted primarily for the left ear as the child matures, while little or no change is observed for the right ear. The left ear improvements would be expected since as the neurological system matures, the information traveling from the left ear to the right hemisphere is able to cross to the left hemisphere (i.e., the dominant hemisphere for language) via the CC more efficiently. In the right ear little or no change is noted on dichotic tests since the contralateral pathway is preeminent in dichotic speech testing, and the information being delivered to the right ear travels directly to the left hemisphere for processing (Musiek and Gollegly, 1988; Whiteside and Cowell, 2001). ●

our knowledge about what the CC does and how the hemispheres interact via the CC. The main approach to testing patients with commissurotomy lies in the use of psychophysical procedures. Visual, somatosensory, and auditory psychophysical procedures have all been used extensively in studying the CC and its relationship to the hemispheres of the brain. In the study of human patients with commissurotomy, a key question has been, what is the role of the CC in regard to brain function? This in turn has led to an interest in determining how the CC works with the other parts of the brain to achieve normal information processing.

It is well known that each hemisphere in its normal state is dominant, or specialized, for certain kinds of tasks (see Musiek, 1986a for review). Because one hemisphere can handle certain tasks better than the other and yet the other hemisphere requires or may require this information, there is a need for information to be transferred from one side of the brain to the other. This is achieved via the CC. In this way the brain as a whole can profit from the specialization of each hemisphere. One of the major and more generalized differences between the right and left hemispheres lies in the nature of the processing that each hemisphere is best equipped to provide, that is, an analytic versus a gestalt type of processing. It is well known that the left hemisphere is dominant for analytic, or very detailed, functions, whereas the right hemisphere is dominant for gestalt, or very generalized, processing. (Table 13.1 provides a list of some of the dominant functions for each hemisphere.) For overall optimum perception, however, the brain needs information from both hemispheres to be combined and integrated. The mechanism by which this integration occurs is through an exchange of information between the hemispheres via the CC.

● **Table 13.1**

Word descriptions of the dominant functions associated with each hemisphere.

Left Hemisphere	**Right Hemisphere**
Analytic	Gestalt
Detailed	General
Word recognition	Figure recognition
Concrete	Abstract
Controlled	Emotional
Letters	Numbers
Speech	Rhythm, prosody

It is important to realize that just because one hemisphere is dominant for a certain function, it does not mean that the other hemisphere cannot perform that function at all. Often, in cases of injury, the nondominant hemisphere takes over handling the function for which the damaged hemisphere was dominant. As a result, the individual with injury to one hemisphere may be able to perform functions that he or she otherwise would be incapable of performing if the processing of the information could not be assumed by the nondominant hemisphere (Springer and Deutsch, 1978).

Dichotic listening has proven to be a valuable measure of callosal transfer of auditory information. Much of the early interest in the application of dichotic listening as a measure of CC function can be traced back to the early theories of Kimura (1961), as well as to a number of studies with split-brain patients. Dichotic listening will be used here to show the underlying function of the CC for this particular kind of auditory task.

Dichotic speech listening requires that two (or more) different words, numbers, consonant–vowel combinations (CVs), or other type of speech material be presented to the two ears in a simultaneous and overlapping manner. For example, the word *dog* may be presented to the right ear at the same time that the word *cat* is presented to the left ear. The subject is then asked to repeat both words (other response paradigms can also be used, but verbal reporting is probably the most common).

In a nondichotic listening paradigm, speech stimuli can reach the auditory cortices by an ipsilateral route and a contralateral route (Figure 13.9). For left ear stimuli, one neural pathway courses ipsilaterally from the left ear directly to the left hemisphere (i.e., the hemisphere dominant for language functions). At the same time, the signal also travels contralaterally from the left ear to the right hemisphere (i.e., the hemisphere that is dominant for other auditory functions). In nondichotic listening situations, the information from the right hemisphere can then cross over to the dominant left hemisphere via the CC. Right ear stimuli travel in a similar manner, making use of both ipsilateral and contralateral pathways. Here again, one pathway connects one ear to the dominant hemisphere (in this case, the contralateral pathway from the right ear to left hemisphere), while the other pathway connects the right ear to the nondominant hemisphere (i.e., the ipsilateral pathway from the right ear to right hemisphere). As was the case above, under nondichotic listen conditions, the information from the right hemisphere can travel across the CC to reach the dominant left hemisphere for processing. However, under nondichotic listening conditions, it is not essential that normal function of the CC exist since a signal presented to either ear can reach the dominant left hemisphere by one of the two available pathways, that is the ipsilateral pathway for left ear stimuli and the contralateral pathway for the right ear stimuli.

In dichotic speech testing conditions, the ipsilateral pathways are suppressed and the auditory system becomes essentially a crossed system (Kimura, 1961). This means that only the contralateral routes are effective in transferring the neural representations of the auditory signals, as the ipsilateral pathways have been rendered ineffective at transferring auditory information to the cerebrum. Under these conditions, the left ear stimulus travels to the right hemisphere via the contralateral pathway, and since this hemisphere is not the dominant hemisphere for speech, the stimulus must cross the CC to reach the left hemisphere for processing and a speech response. The right ear stimulus travels directly to the left hemisphere (the speech hemisphere). Therefore, transferring of neural information across the CC is not needed since the right ear stimulus has reached the dominant hemisphere for speech and language.

If the CC is compromised, such as in the extreme case of the split-brain patient, then deficits in dichotic listening are expected. In these cases (at least those who have had the auditory areas of the CC sectioned), there will be a marked left ear deficit and normal performance in the right ear. This pattern of performance occurs because the speech stimuli presented to the left ear travel to the right hemisphere via the contralateral pathway, and since the ipsilateral route is suppressed during dichotic testing, the only route to the left hemisphere is from the right hemisphere via the CC. In the split-brain patient, this transfer cannot happen since sectioning of the CC preempts transcallosal transfer of the neural information; hence, processing of left ear stimuli is not achieved and verbal responses are not possible. The right ear scores are normal because the right ear stimuli travel directly to the left hemisphere for processing and a speech response; therefore, the CC is not needed.

Most other types of auditory tests that are used clinically are not dependent on the transfer of neural information across the CC for accurate perception. Therefore, deficits on most of the nondichotic tests used to assess auditory function are not common among split-brain patients, with the possible exception of some pattern perception tests. It has been postulated that pattern perception tasks that require a

Figure 13.9

The auditory afferent pathways to the auditory cortices and the callosal fiber pathway that connect the two hemispheres of the brain. The dashed arrows indicate the weaker ipsilateral tracts to the cortices, and the crossed arrows indicate the stronger contralateral pathways. The curved arrow at the top of the figure indicates the callosal pathway from right to left hemisphere.

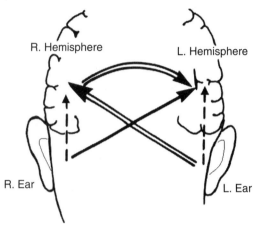

verbal report do require interaction of both hemispheres (Musiek, Pinheiro, and Wilson, 1980). For these types of tasks it is theorized that the right hemisphere recognizes the pattern contour (gestalt) of the test stimuli and that the left hemisphere is needed for linguistically labeling the patterns perceived. Therefore, the two hemispheres must exchange information for these types of pattern perception tasks, even if the stimulus is presented to one ear at a time. It has been shown that split-brain patients tend to exhibit bilateral deficits on such tests as **frequency (pitch) pattern perception** with verbal report (Musiek et al., 1980). This bilateral deficit is expected since each hemisphere requires information from the other for normal performance on this type of auditory task, and when this exchange is disallowed, neither hemisphere alone can make sense of the stimuli and a pattern is not perceived and labeled—hence, bilateral deficits are seen (Musiek et al., 1980). Further, it has been shown that split-brain patients can correctly hum the patterns even if they cannot verbally report them correctly. This probably means that the right hemisphere can mediate the humming response so that accurate processing of the acoustic envelope of the auditory signal has occurred. This is similar to patients with aphasia who can whistle a response but cannot talk.

The application of psychophysical test procedures with human subjects has contributed to our understanding of the specific functional anatomy of the CC. Specific visual, auditory, and somatosensory areas of the CC have been delineated by anatomical studies. Also contributing to this knowledge are studies involving human psychophysics. Psychophysics performed on patients with specific lesions of

CLINICAL CORRELATE

Individuals who have had commissurotomies or neurological compromise of the CC yield a unique pattern of audiological test results if the auditory fibers of the CC are involved. Certainly this would be the case in complete sectioning of the CC. In these cases, the pure-tone audiogram and speech recognition scores are typically normal (or unaffected). However, results of dichotic testing generally reveal major left ear deficits and normal right ear performance. In addition, pattern perception tasks (with verbal report) yield bilateral deficits, but other central auditory tests that are not dichotic in nature and do not require action of the CC (e.g., filtered speech) are essentially normal (Figure 13.10). The audiological pattern demonstrated by split-brain subjects has been termed the auditory disconnection profile and includes the following performance trends: (1) severe left ear deficits and normal performance for the right ear on dichotic listening tests, (2) bilateral deficits on verbally reported pattern sequence tests with preservation of the ability to hum the patterns without difficulty, and (3) normal performance on all other peripheral and central auditory tests (Musiek et al., 1984b). Interestingly, a similar auditory profile has also been shown to exist in a number of children with

learning disabilities and auditory symptoms (Musiek, Gollegly, and Baran, 1984a). Based upon the similarity of the profiles for these two groups of subjects, Musiek et al. (1984a) postulated that these children may have delayed maturation of the myelin sheaths lining the callosal fibers and that this may be why these individuals show this type of auditory disconnection profile.

Another clinical population that shows a left ear deficit on dichotic listening tests is the elderly. Bellis and Wilbur (2001) documented a decrease in left ear performance on a dichotic listening task (dichotic digits) in older individuals. In testing subjects between the ages of 20 and 75 years, it was noted that left ear decrements were first noted in the 40- to 55-year-old group and that the deficits continued to increase with increasing age. This finding is consistent with the anatomical and physiologic data presented earlier, indicating that a loss or a deterioration in the myelin sheaths of the callosal fibers (a process called demyelination) may occur with age. If this is the case, then the left ear deficits are expected since the speech information arriving at the right hemisphere via the contralateral pathway from the left ear will not be transmitted efficiently across the CC to the left hemisphere. Cowell

(continued)

● **Figure 13.10**

Mean central auditory test results for four adult patients before and after commissurotomy. Note the deficits for the left ear on the dichotic listening tests (C. Sent., D. Digits, and SSW) and for both ears on the pattern perception (FP) test. sp. Rec. = speech recognition, C. Sent. = competing sentences, D. Digits = dichotic digits, SSW = staggered spondaic words, FP = frequency patterns, LPFS = low-pass filtered speech.

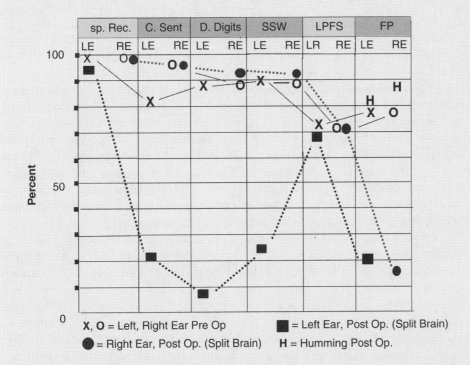

and Hugdahl (2000) also showed a tendency toward increased left ear deficits with increasing age under certain dichotic listening conditions. In addition, these researchers found that this left ear deficit was more pronounced in men than in women. This study, however, did show great variability in performance across the ages tested. These findings may suggest that chronological age is not a good predictor of physiological aging.

A number of disorders can affect the CC and result in abnormal auditory function, such as tumors, strokes, and degenerative diseases. Perhaps one of the most common and interesting disorders that affects the CC is multiple sclerosis (MS). Since the neural fibers of the CC are heavily myelinated and MS is a demyelinating disease, the CC is a likely site (specifically the trigone) for MS plaques. It has been shown that individuals with MS often show left ear deficits on dichotic listening. Such findings would implicate the CC, as strong correlations have been drawn between MRIs showing MS plaques in the CC and left ear deficits on

● **Table 13.2**

Performance of a patient with multiple sclerosis on two dichotic listening tests.

Dichotic Digits Test		Dichotic Rhyme Test	
Left Ear	Right Ear	Left Ear	Right Ear
80%	100%	25%	72%

(continued)

dichotic listening tasks (Damasio and Damasio, 1979; Rao, Bernardin, Leo, Ellington, Ryan, and Burg, 1989).

The dichotic listening scores for a young adult with definite MS are shown in Table 13.2. An inspection of this data reveals a clear left ear deficit on both dichotic listening tests. This patient had normal hearing sensitivity, normal acoustic reflex thresholds (contralateral stimulation), and normal auditory brainstem responses (ABRs) bilaterally. This constellation of auditory test results is consistent with involvement of the callosal fibers, since the other tests administered failed to identify a potential peripheral basis for the observed deficits. ●

the CC, as well as on patients with commissurotomies, have been a major factor in advancing our understanding of this anatomy. Much of the research on patients with commissurotomies has been done with subjects who have had complete commissurotomies. However, a small number of studies have used psychophysical tests to assess auditory function in patients with partial commissurotomies. The specification of the surgical procedures in these studies allow detailed information as to what areas of the CC have been cut and what aspects remain intact. Additionally, they allow the investigators to correlate test results with specific areas of CC compromise (i.e., the areas sectioned during the surgical procedure).

Patients with partial sectioning of the CC are rare. Springer and Gazzaniga (1975) reported on a patient whose surgical section was limited to the anterior one-third of the CC, and no left ear deficits were noted for this patient. These same investigators reported the absence of left ear deficits in another patient, whose section was limited to the area of the splenium (Springer and Gazzaniga, 1975). However, in a more recent investigation, Pollmann and colleagues (2002) showed left ear deficits on dichotic listening tests in a group of patients with lesions of the splenium. These latter findings were in agreement with data from an earlier investigation (Sugishita, Otomo, Yamazaki, Shimizu, Yoshioka, and Shinohara, 1995) that indicated that lesions in the posterior 20 to 25% of the CC resulted in left ear deficits on dichotic listening tests. These last two studies argue for the presence of auditory fibers in the splenium area (which based upon anatomical data was considered to be primarily a visual area of the CC). Alexander and Warren (1988) reported a marked left ear deficit on dichotic listening for a patient who had a lesion in the posterior part of the body, or trunk, of the CC (this area is also called the isthmus or sulcus and is considered the auditory area of the CC).

Baran, Musiek, and Reeves (1986) tested eight patients before and after the anterior half (just anterior to the isthmus, or sulcus) of the CC was surgically sectioned. These researchers found little or no change in the performance of their subjects on three dichotic listening tests when pre- and postsurgical results were compared. The slight change noted in the averaged results of this study was attributable to the fact that one patient did show a marked, unexplained change in dichotic listening on one dichotic test (Figure 13.11). These findings, when considered in tandem with the results of the studies discussed earlier that looked at dichotic test performance in patients with lesions of the posterior portions of the CC (Alexander and Warren, 1988; Sugishita et al., 1995; Pollmann et al., 2002) indicate that in humans the auditory regions of the CC are located in the posterior half of the structure, a finding consistent with the anatomical data on primates (Pandya and Rosene, 1985).

The application of EPs in humans with reference to CC function has not been a popular research effort. As discussed earlier in this chapter, nonauditory EPs have been used to measure IHTTs in humans. However, this section will focus on some

● Figure 13.11

(a) Bar graphs showing mean dichotic listening performance before and after anterior commissurotomy (n = 8). (b) Sketch showing the anatomical correlate to the anterior commissurotomy. The black area was the portion surgically sectioned.

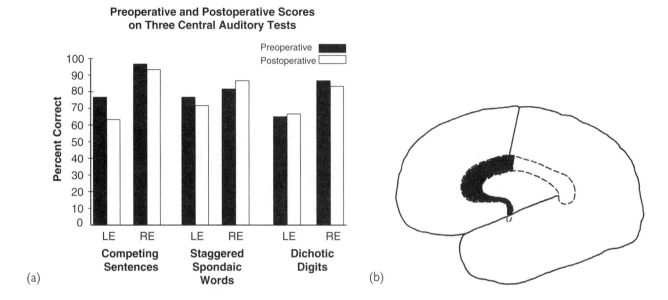

(a)

(b)

of the EPs that have not been exclusively employed for IHTT measurements. Moreover, the emphasis will be on those auditory EPs that have been used for the assessment of callosal function and dysfunction.

Again, as for psychophysics, the split-brain patient has been the main target for measuring CC function or lack of it. Gazzaniga and Hillyard (1973), using the contingent negative variation (CNV) procedure, showed no difference between split-brain subjects and controls. Kutas, Hillyard, Volpe, and Gazzaniga (1990) tested a control group and five split-brain patients using a standard and an odd-ball paradigm for the late potentials (N1 and P2) and the P300 for visual and auditory stimuli. The N1 and P2 components did not show any significant differences between the split-brain and control subjects for either the visual or auditory stimuli. However, for both the visual and auditory stimuli there was a larger P300 response over the right hemisphere compared to the left hemisphere for the split-brain subjects compared to controls. Kutus and colleagues (1990) speculated that attention may be asymmetrical in its cortical distribution and this is why the EPs were greater over the right hemisphere. However, this asymmetrical finding could also be related to the notion that when the CC is sectioned, a normal inhibitory–excitatory balance cannot be achieved (as was discussed earlier). This finding could also be related to the concept that sensory information is activated in the right hemisphere but it cannot cross the CC to activate the left hemisphere.

Anterior Commissure

The anterior commissure (AC) is generally considered as part of the CC. However, its functional significance is controversial. The AC is located beneath the body of the CC, immediately anterior to the lateral columns of the fornix, posterior to the taenia tecta, and superior to the vertical limb (Figure 13.4). The AC is a tightly organized

CLINICAL CORRELATE

It may be necessary to use speech stimuli in an EP paradigm to demonstrate the same kinds of auditory deficits for electrophysiological measures as have been shown for psychophysical test measures in split-brain patients. Jerger and colleagues have documented a lack of transfer of auditory information from the right to the left hemisphere for speech stimuli in an elderly individual by using topographic mapping techniques (Jerger, Alford, Lew, Rivera, and Chmiel, 1995). This subject also showed left ear deficits on dichotic listening. ●

fiber tract that connects loci in each hemisphere in a manner similar to that noted for the CC. This is perhaps one of the reasons that AC is considered by some to be part of the CC anatomy (Nauta and Feirtag, 1986). Pandya and Rosene (1985) have shown that fibers from the temporal pole, the superior temporal gyrus, the superior temporal plane (anterior one-half), and the middle temporal gyrus course through the AC. Because of its location, it is likely that the AC does have auditory neurons passing through it. In addition to the fibers from various sites in the temporal cortex, other fibers passing through the AC originate from the anterior frontal cortex and the amygdala (Demeter, Rosene, and Van Hoesen, 1990). Thus, it appears that numerous areas of the cortex could be represented in the AC; however, it should be noted that these findings are considered preliminary and that further research is needed before a definitive determination can be made as to which type (or types) of neurons are represented in the AC.

Little psychophysical or electrophysiological data has come from examination of AC function. It has been speculated that if the CC is sectioned and the AC is left intact, the AC may take over some of the CC functions (McKeever, Sullivan, Ferguson, and Rayport, 1985). This assumption is supported, at least in part, by a controversial paper by Risse, LeDoux, Springer, Wilson, and Gazzaniga (1978). Risse and colleagues reported that three out of four subjects with CC sections that spared the AC showed good visual interhemispheric transfer. Since the visual areas of the CC were sectioned, it was argued that the interhemispheric transfer of the visual information had to occur through the AC. Also reported in the literature was a case of a patient who had the anterior one-third of the CC and the AC sectioned and this patient showed a left ear deficit for dichotic listening (Springer and Gazzaniga, 1975). Since the anterior one-third of the CC is believed to connect the somatosensory and motor areas of the brain, it could be argued that the auditory deficits noted in this patient were not likely the result of the sectioning of the CC. In light of this line of reasoning, the results could be interpreted to indicate that the AC may contain auditory fibers and that the left ear deficits were the result of the surgical compromise of this structure; however, other interpretations of the data may also be possible.

More recently, a study by Bamiou et al. (2004) on patients with the PAX 6 mutation (a condition that results in absent or hypoplastic ACs) showed these individuals to have abnormal function on tests of interhemispheric transfer. Although in many of the cases, the researchers were not able to document central compromise limited to the AC, there did appear to be some patients in their subject pool with anatomically normal CCs but absent ACs as determined by MRI. These patients showed abnormal dichotic listening scores for the left ear. The implication, similar to that of the Springer and Gazzaniga (1975) study, is that the AC is likely to play a role in auditory transfer.

Agenesis of the Corpus Callosum

Agenesis of the CC is considered a congenital malformation of the midline structures of the brain (Lassonde, Sauerwein, and Lepore, 2003). The presentation of this disorder is somewhat variable and may include involvement of only the CC or it may involve compromise of the CC along with other midline or near midline structures of the brain. Generally, the extent of damage to structures other than the CC dictates the degree and types of behavioral deficits noted for patients with this disorder. Individuals with involvement limited to the CC often do quite well in their daily activities and many of them are not likely to be aware that they have this condition unless they undergo radiologic testing for some other reason. However, many individuals with agenesis of the CC also have incomplete development of other areas of the brain. This concomitant lack of development is often manifested by a reduced intelligence score. Sauerwein and Lassonde (1994) reported that 42.5% of their series of patients with agenesis had IQ scores in the low average range, while 20% showed performance in the high to superior IQ range. The findings for the group with scores in the low average range are likely to reflect involvement of central structures beyond just the CC.

Quite early on it was known that patients with agenesis of the CC (especially those with involvement limited to the CC) perform differently than patients with other types of CC compromise. These individuals do not show the disconnection syndrome that is generally observed for patients who have undergone surgical sectioning of the commissure (see Lassonde et al., 2003, for review). The lack of deficits in the agenesis patients is generally attributed to the high degree of neural plasticity that is present in early life. This neural plasticity is believed to play a key role in the compensation of impaired interhemispheric interaction in individuals who have had CC compromise since birth. One potential compensation includes the bilateral representation of speech in the brains of individuals with agenesis. This may be why these individuals can name items presented to the left visual field or repeat words presented to the left ear in the dichotic mode, while other patients with CC compromise cannot perform these left-sided tasks (see Lassonde et al., 2003). It may be that each hemisphere develops more capabilities during the early developmental years when there is an agenesis of the CC than when there is not, the end result being that both hemispheres become efficient at processing various types of stimuli and each can function independently. This independent development of each hemisphere has an opportunity to start early in life, possibly even in utero, thus allowing individuals with agenesis of the CC ample opportunity to take full advantage of neural or brain plasticity.

Another possible compensation for the agenesis of the CC might be increased reliance on the AC for interhemispheric communication. It has been reported that in acallosal patients, the AC is usually present and it may even be enlarged (Jeeves, 1994). Although it seems possible that the AC could play a role in compensating for the lack of the CC, it is doubtful that this structure can fully take over the CC's functions. Among other things, the anatomy argues against reasonable compensation of the AC for the CC—specifically, it is too small (even when it is enlarged). In addition, the speed of interhemispheric transfer in acallosal patients is much slower than in controls. This would argue against the ability of the AC to fully compensate for impaired CC function (Jeeves, 1969).

Although it is difficult to know exactly what the compensatory mechanisms are for individuals with agenesis of the CC, it seems clear that they do not experience as many deficits and/or the degree of deficits as are noted in commissurotomized patients. In our experience we have tested one patient with callosal agenesis. This was the case of a 19-year-old male who had had a CT scan because of a slight head injury. It was discovered at the time of his radiologic study that he had agenesis of the CC. This was a surprise to the patient and his family, as this patient had essentially normal developmental milestones. The only indication of any potential deficit was a comment in his medical/educational history of some mild language delays when he was young. This patient's performance on dichotic listening following the radiologic study was within the normal range bilaterally, consistent with the typical findings for individuals with CC agenesis. Certainly these findings argue for some type of compensation for the compromised CC.

SUMMARY

The CC is a large fiber tract composed of 2 million or more fibers that connect the two halves of the brain. It has been estimated that 94% of the callosal fibers are myelinated and that there is a greater concentration of myelinated fibers in the posterior portion of the CC than in the anterior segment. The CC, in general, has two types of fibers: homolateral and heterolateral (also termed homotopic and heterotopic). Homolateral fibers connect one site in one hemisphere to essentially the same site in the opposite hemisphere via the CC. Heterolateral fibers connect to different sites in each hemisphere after running through the CC.

The CC has been divided into several segments. The posterior one-fifth is the splenium, which connects the occipital lobes (vision). Just anterior to the splenium is the sulcus, or isthmus, which connects the temporal lobes and insula (auditory). The body, or trunk, of the CC connects the parietal lobes (motor, somatosensory) and is anterior to the sulcus but posterior to the genu, which connects the frontal lobes. The genu curves downward and then runs posteriorly where the rostrum is found. The rostrum contains olfactory fibers.

The most popular physiologic measure involving the CC is the IHTT, or TCTT. This measurement is made to determine the latency of impulses traveling from one site on the cortex to its counterpart in the other cortex via the CC. Investigators report that IHTTs range from 19 to 25 msec for the smaller (and more abundant) fibers and that the larger fibers yield shorter IHTTs, generally on the order of 3 msec. The IHTT is likely a function of the extent of myelination within the CC. The amount of myelination is influenced by age, with very young and very old people demonstrating smaller amounts and hence increased IHTTs.

The application of psychophysical tests to the assessment of auditory performance in split-brain patients has done much to inform us about the function of the CC. If the CC is compromised, such as in the extreme case of the split-brain patient, then deficits in dichotic listening are likely to occur, that is, unless the auditory areas of the CC have been spared by the surgical procedure. Specifically, if the auditory areas of the CC have been compromised, then marked left ear deficits for dichotic speech materials and normal right ear performance will be the norm. This pattern of results occurs because stimuli presented to the left ear in the dichotic condition are limited to the contralateral pathway (left ear to right hemisphere) since the ipsilateral route is suppressed during dichotic presentations. Hence, the only avenue to the left hemisphere for stimuli presented to the left ear is from the left ear to the right hemisphere and then to the left hemisphere via the CC. If the dichotic task requires a verbal response, then it is imperative that the auditory information be transferred from the right to the left hemisphere. In split-brain patients this transfer cannot happen; hence, there is no appreciable response to left ear stimuli. The right ear scores are normal because the right ear stimuli travel directly to the left hemisphere. Therefore, the CC is not needed for the processing of speech stimuli directed to the right ear.

The AC remains something of a mystery in regard to its function. It seems that fibers from the anterior-superior temporal lobe cross at the AC, and there is an accumulating body of evidence that suggests that the AC may play a role in audition. However, many investigators argue that fibers from most of the areas of the brain are found in the AC. Given the size of this structure and the emergent evidence that it may contain fibers from many, if not most, areas of the brain, it appears unlikely that the AC plays a major role in the interhemispheric transfer of auditory information. This, however, is an area that is in need of further investigation before a definitive determination regarding the role of the AC in the transfer of auditory information across the midline of the brain can be made.

Agenesis of the CC is considered a congenital malformation of the midline structures of the brain. Patients with agenesis of the CC (especially those with involvement limited to the CC) function differently than those patients who have lesions of the CC or who have had commissurotomies. Individuals with agenesis do not show the auditory disconnection syndrome that is generally observed in patients who have undergone surgical sectioning of the auditory areas of the CC. In general, agenesis patients do not demonstrate any obvious deficits on dichotic listening tasks.

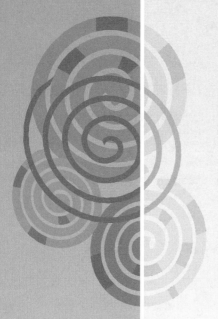

14

Vascular Anatomy of the Auditory System

Introduction

Vascular anatomy is key information for both the scientist and the clinician interested in auditory function. The blood supplies to the various structures within the auditory system are responsible for cell metabolism within these structures, and therefore are closely linked to the appropriate physiology of the various portions of the system. When there is a disruption or some type of alteration in blood supply to one of these structures, the tissue dependent on this blood supply is likely to be damaged and its function compromised. Many of the vascular disorders, such as hemorrhage, aneurysms, atherosclerosis, and various occlusive problems, affect the central auditory system, and the effects of these types of disorders can be subtle or major and chronic or acute. Interestingly, many publications on the anatomy and physiology of the auditory system include little or no information on the vascular system.

VASCULAR ANATOMY OF THE AUDITORY PERIPHERY

The vascular (functional) anatomy of the peripheral auditory system will be presented in two sections. First, the vascular anatomy of the outer ear (OE) and the middle ear (ME) will be covered. This will be followed by a discussion of the vascular anatomy of the cochlea and auditory nerve (AN). The reason for the division of the vascular anatomy into two segments is that these two main regions of the peripheral auditory system (OE/ME and cochlea/AN) have distinctly different origins of their blood supplies.

The Outer Ear and the Middle Ear

The outer, or external, ear (auricle and external auditory meatus) receives its blood supply primarily from the **external carotid** artery through two key branches of this artery, the **superficial temporal artery** (STA) and **the posterior auricular artery** (PAA). The STA supplies the more anterior portion of the auricle or pinna via three branches that provide blood to the anterior helix, the tragus, and the ear lobe. The STA crosses the zygomatic process of the temporal bone before it divides into frontal and parietal branches. The PAA courses inferior to the posterior auricular muscle and to the postero-medial regions of the ear, where it supplies this tissue with a rich blood supply (Anson and Donaldson, 1967; Davis, 1987).

The venous system for the auricle and the postero-medial region of the ear includes the veins that are the counterparts to the STA and PAA and the mastoid emissary veins. These veins empty into the external and internal jugular veins (Davis, 1987).

The external auditory meatus (EAM) is supplied by additional branches of the PAA and STA. In addition, the deep auricular and maxillary arteries make significant contributions to the EAM. This area has venous drainage to the external jugular and pterygoid venous complex (Polyak, McHugh, and Judd, 1946; Gulya, 1997).

The tympanic membrane (TM) and the ME's blood supplies are not well established and remain somewhat controversial at this time. This chapter will present the most commonly accepted descriptions.

The TM's blood supply comes mainly from branches of the deep auricular and maxillary arteries. The latter descends from the superior aspect of the EAM toward the umbo and then sends branches that radiate outward to supply the perimeter of the TM and the annulus. The tympanic branch (from the maxillary artery) and the stylomastoid branch of the PAA supply the rim of the TM (Saini, 1964). Saini (1964) used the analogy of a wheel to describe the vascular supply to the TM, with fine branches from the deep auricular and maxillary arteries forming the spokes of the vascular supply to the TM and branches from the tympanic and stylomastoid arteries forming the rim (Figure 14.1).

The ME region derives its blood supply from branches of the internal carotid, external carotid, and in some instances the subclavian arteries. It may be best to view the ME's vascular system as including vessels that supply the bony aspects (temporal bone) and vessels that supply the soft tissue. The bony portion of the ME is supplied by the superficial temporal, postauricular, occipital, and middle temporal arteries. These arteries are all branches of the external carotid. The ossicular chain derives its blood supply from the anterior and posterior tympanic arteries that are often branches of the internal carotid artery and the stylomastoid artery, which comes from the external carotid artery (Anson and Donaldson, 1967; Maher, 1988; Gulya, 1997). The mucous membrane and other soft tissues of the

● **Figure 14.1**

The vascular network of the tympanic membrane.

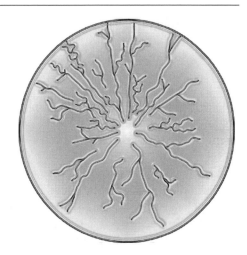

ME have as their vascular basis the anterior tympanic branch of the maxillary artery (a branch of the external carotid artery) for its lateral aspect. Also contributing to the ME tissue's vascular supply are the tympanic, deep auricular, mastoid, stylomastoid, superficial petrosal, and tubal arteries (external carotid) (Gulya, 1997). The more internal surface of the ME is supplied by the cariticitympanic artery, which evolves from the internal carotid artery, and in some cases it may also receive a blood supply from the subclavian artery (Anson and Donaldson, 1967).

An important vascular structure that is not located in the ME itself is the **jugular bulb**. It arises from the internal jugular vein and is continuous with the sigmoid venous sinus (Polyak et al., 1946). It is mentioned here because this structure is located immediately inferior to the ME, and because of this close proximity to the ME, any tumors arising from this structure would have the potential of invading the ME space (see the clinical correlate that follows for additional information on this topic).

The Cochlea and the Auditory Nerve

The basis of the blood supply in the cochlea and AN is the **vertebro-basilar vascular system** (Portmann, Sterkers, Charachon, and Chouard, 1975; Moller, 2000). The vertebro-basilar system can be traced back to the vertebral arteries, which course up each side of the vertebral column. These vessels enter the cranium at the foramen magnum and course anteriorly to the ventral aspect of the medulla. Usually a few millimeters below the ponto-medullary junction (the anatomical demarcation separating the pons and medulla), the two vertebral arteries join to form the basilar artery. The basilar artery, which is the main artery in the brainstem, courses midline up most of the length of the ventral pons. An extensive distribution of the basilar artery within the brainstem provides the blood supply to many of the auditory structures within the central auditory nervous system (CANS). This information will be covered in the section on the vascular supply of the CANS.

Key to the peripheral vascular anatomy is that the basilar artery gives rise to the **internal auditory artery (IAA)** (often termed the **labyrinthine artery**) in two possible ways. One way is that the IAA branches directly from the basilar artery and the other is that the IAA arises from the **anterior inferior cerebellar artery (AICA)** (Waddington, 1974; Portmann et al., 1975). Whether originating from the AICA or the basilar artery, the IAA branches in the inferior (caudal) half of the pons and courses laterally across the cerebellopontine angle (CPA) and into the internal auditory meatus (IAM) to supply the facial nerve, the vestibular nerves, and the AN (Waddington, 1974; Axelsson and Ryan, 2001). In the IAM, the IAA branches into a cochlear branch and a vestibular branch at a minimum. However, there may be additional branches from the IAA to both the vestibular and auditory end organs (Portmann et al., 1975; Moller, 2000; Axelsson and Ryan, 2001). The cochlear artery branches into two important vessels, the spiral modiolar artery and the cochlear-vestibular artery. The spiral modiolar vessel spirals around the modiolus and supplies the apical portion of the cochlea (Figures 14.2 and 14.3). The **cochlear–vestibular artery** supplies the basal turns of the cochlea (see Axelsson and Ryan, 2001 for review).

As Smith (1973) describes, a branching of the cochlear vessels (radiating arterioles) in the cochlea eventually forms a network of **arterioles** that supply most of the cochlear regions (Figures 14.4 and 14.5). The main **radiating arterioles** emerge from the area of Rosenthal's canal, with the more obvious branches in the region supplying the limbus, the tectorial membrane, and the organ of Corti (beneath the

Figure 14.2

A transverse section of the cochlea showing the main vascular anatomy (from Axelsson and Ryan, 2001, reprinted with permission).

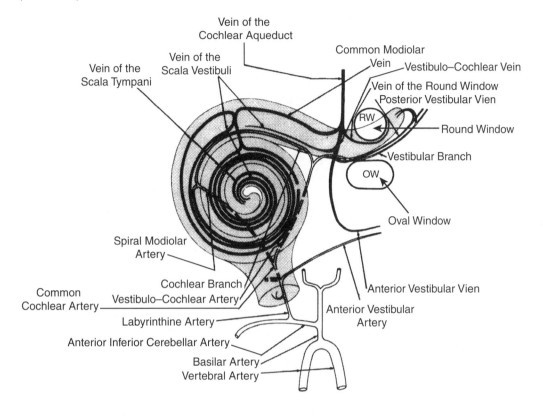

Figure 14.3

A longitudinal view of the cochlea emphasizing the spiral modiolar artery and vein and their branches (from Axelsson and Ryan, 2001, reprinted with permission).

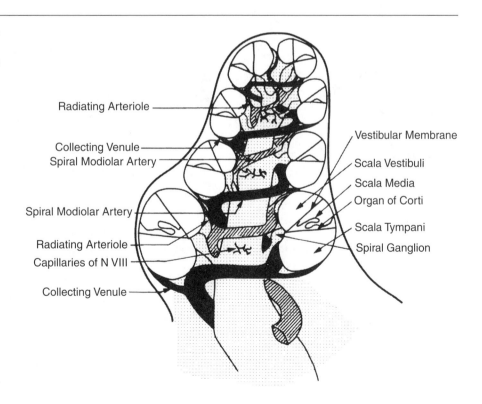

● **Figure 14.4**

Cross-section of the cochlea showing the spiral artery and vein branches as they encompass the end organ of hearing. SA = spiral artery, SV = spiral vein, CV = collecting venule, Sc. V = scala vestibuli, Sc. T = scala tympani, Sc. M = scala media, St. V = stria vascularis, SL = spiral ligament, BM = basilar membrane, OC = organ of Corti.

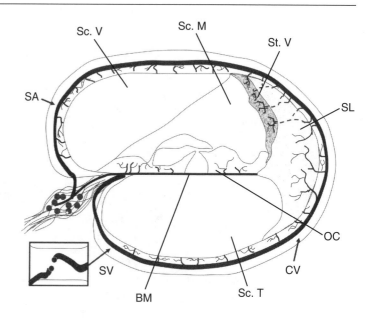

● **Figure 14.5**

The radiating arterioles of (a) the gerbil and (b) the guinea pig and the regions of the membranous cochlea that they serve. RAL = radiating arterioles, OW = level of the oval window, VRW = vein of the round window area, SVS = stria vascularis capillary area, VSSP = vessel of the spiral prominence, SL = spiral lamina (from Axelsson and Ryan, 2001, reprinted with permission).

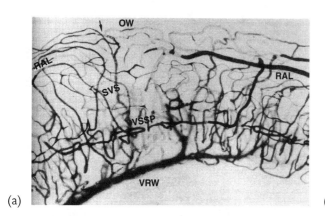

(a)

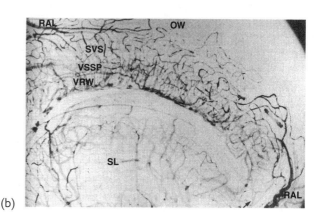

(b)

tunnel of Corti). There are also branches that course over the scala vestibuli and form a network of arterioles on the far wall of the cochlea. This latter vascular network is in the proximity of the spiral ligament and the stria vascularis and it supplies these structures with blood (Figures 14.4, 14.5, and 14.6).

In the cochlea there is a venous network that is the anatomical counterpart of the arteriole network (i.e., the arteries and arterioles) just described. The venous network communicates with the arteriole network on the back wall of the cochlea, and beneath the scala tympani there are larger collecting venules (Smith, 1973; Axelsson and Ryan, 2001).

Axelsson and Ryan (2001) discuss some interesting observations regarding the vascularization of the cochlea. The amount of vascularization tends to decrease as one progresses from the base to the apex of the cochlea. This is consistent with the concept that there is greater physiological activity of the cochlea at the base than at the apex. In addition, some structures in the cochlea require considerable vascular supply (e.g., the stria vascularis) and some require little or none (e.g., Reissner's membrane).

Perhaps one of the more important concepts to evolve recently is the relationship between the amount of blood flow (i.e., blood supply) and the level of metabolism of the cells in the region of that blood supply. Glucose, a substance supplied by the vascular system, is critical to cell metabolism and can be quantified through radiographic procedures. Researchers have been able to establish correlations between rates of glucose uptake and level of blood flow (see Sokoloff et al., 1977). This correlation is quite logical and provides a manner of measuring metabolic activity. By adding a radiologic tracer to 2-deoxyglucose, radiographic techniques can be used to measure glucose uptake and hence provide insights to local metabolism.

● **Figure 14.6**

Photomicrograph of the stria vascularis showing blood cells in the vessels of this highly vascular structure (courtesy of M. Pinheiro).

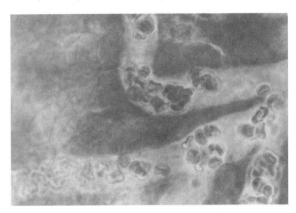

Ryan (2001) used 2-deoxyglucose and **autoradiography** to study blood circulation in the cochlea of gerbils. When the animals were in quiet conditions, deoxyglucose uptake was high in the stria vascularis, spiral prominence, and spiral ligament, but there was little uptake of glucose in the organ of Corti, spiral ganglion, and eighth nerve. When the animals were exposed to relatively high-intensity broadband noise, there was little change in deoxyglucose uptake for the structures on the external wall of the cochlea; however, noticeable increases were evident for the spiral ganglion and eighth nerve. In addition, it was noted that the inner hair cells (IHCs) but not the outer hair cells (OHCs) showed an increase in glucose uptake under these conditions. The greater glucose uptake for the IHCs than the OHCs is consistent with a number of other auditory functions that are believed to be different for these two types of cells. For example, as was discussed in Chapters 5 and 6, the IHCs are key in handling high-intensity acoustic stimuli. It is logical to assume that this function of the IHCs is likely to require more energy than would be required by the OHCs since the latter cells are involved primarily with lower-intensity stimuli.

The work of Ryan (2001), showing increased blood flow during acoustic stimulation, follows a concept that Johnsson (1972) introduced a number of years ago regarding the regulation of blood flow. This concept relates that local capillaries open and close depending on the metabolic requirements of the activated tissue (Johnsson, 1972). For example, if the cochlea is presented with high-intensity signals at high frequencies, then it is predicted that the metabolic requirements will increase in the basal area of the cochlea (where the high frequencies are represented) and that the blood vessels supplying this region will open to supply more blood to this particular area of the cochlea. Such regional increases in blood flow associated with differences in frequency of an acoustic stimulus were documented clearly by Ryan (2001).

The expansion and contraction of blood vessels also relates to the vascular tone of the vessels, which has as its base adrenergic and cholinergic responsive nerve fibers. First described by Lorente de No in 1937, these nerves branch from the AN and course to the vessels of the cochlea, with the adrenergic nerve fibers more prominent than the cholinergic (Snow and Suga, 1973).

CLINICAL CORRELATE

General circulatory problems that are systemic in nature can affect the peripheral auditory system. Atherosclerosis, vasculitis, vessel trauma, and vascular aging can all affect the auditory system indirectly.

Vascular Abnormalities Affecting the Middle Ear Perhaps one of the key vascular abnormalities affecting the ME is the glomus jugulare tumor. This venous tumor sits directly beneath the ME and can invade the tympanum (Lustig and Jackler, 1997). If such invasion does occur, the pathology can result in pulsatile tinnitus, conductive hearing loss, and abnormal tympanograms (usually flat). Of special interest here is that in some of these cases, immittance recordings made over a time period of several seconds at atmospheric pressure may reveal periodic oscillations consistent with the pulsations of sounds (pulsatile tinnitus) that are often noted by the patient with this condition (Jerger and Jerger, 1981). This can be a valuable, objective documentation of pulsatile tinnitus, and as such can herald the consideration of a vascular disorder in the ME such as the glomus jugulare tumor.

Hemorrhage into the ME space is another vascular disorder that can affect the auditory periphery (Schuknecht, 1974). This condition is usually secondary to a longitudinal or transverse fracture of the temporal bone, but it can also occur with other types of head injury that do not result in temporal bone fractures (e.g., concussions, contusions, etc.). Bleeding into the ME can also result from trauma to the tympanic membrane, surgical intervention, and idiopathic causes. If blood collects in the ME space, the patient typically presents with a conductive hearing loss and a flat tympanogram for the involved ear. This latter vascular condition is one that typically improves over time.

Vascular Abnormities Affecting the Cochlea and the Eighth Nerve The inner ear can also be affected by vascular abnormalities, such as vessel occlusion, spasm, hemorrhage, vasculitis, and hypercoagulation (Goodhill, 1979). Occlusions that affect the peripheral system can occur anywhere along the vascular anatomy of the brainstem, IAM, and cochlea. One of the most studied occlusions is that of the IAA or labyrinthine artery. Occlusion of the IAA often results in permanent sensorineural hearing loss (usually of a severe to profound degree) and vestibular dysfunction (usually vertigo). Although the vestibular system may compensate over time, the hearing loss usually remains. Occlusion of the cochleo-vestibular branch of the IAA most often results

in high-frequency hearing loss because this branch primarily supplies the basal aspect of the cochlea (Baloh, 1995). It would also stand to reason that if the spiral modiolar artery was occluded, a low-frequency hearing loss might result, as this artery supplies the apical segment of the cochlea (recall the earlier discussion of these arteries). Occlusions of major vessels to the cochlea initially result in necrosis of the membranous tissue in the cochlea and the vestibular apparatus. Over time, however, the cochlea ossifies and the membranes become fixed (Baloh, 1995).

Ischemia of blood vessels can also reduce blood flow to important auditory and vestibular structures. Vertebrobasilar ischemia can result in various degrees of peripheral hearing loss and vestibular impairments that are highly dependent on the severity and the extent of the involvement. This condition can also affect the central auditory system, but this will be discussed in the next section of this chapter. Ischemia-like occlusions can occur anywhere along the vascular course of the AN and cochlea, with the locus of involvement dictating the nature of the symptoms. Ischemia may affect some areas of the cochlea more than others. Reduced blood supply to the stria vascularis, because of its high vascular demands, could result in compromise of the metabolic function of the organ of Corti (Martini and Prosser, 2003). The increased demand for blood supply at the basal end of the cochlea perhaps makes it more susceptible to damage from blood volume reductions than other portions of the cochlea.

Inner ear hemorrhage is often secondary to temporal bone fractures, head trauma without temporal bone involvement (cochlear contusions), and systemic diseases that affect the vascular system such as leukemia. In these conditions not only may the tissues and cells be deprived of blood supply, but the reduction in blood supply may cause chemical and mechanical compromises of cochlear function. Subarachnoid hemorrhage can result in blood in the IAM, Rosenthal's canal, and the cochlea via the cochlear aqueduct (see Schuknecht, 1974). Inner ear hemorrhage often results in sensorineural hearing loss.

Vascular loops are a vascular disorder that has been identified more recently (Jannetta, 1975). This condition exists when a vessel in the cerebellopontine angle (CPA) loops into the area of the opening of the IAM. This can result in contact of the blood vessel with the auditory, facial, and/or vestibular nerves in the IAM.

(continued)

It is sometimes difficult to determine which vessel is usually involved, but the AICA is a likely possibility. This contact can create abnormal neural activity and perhaps injury to the nerve itself (Moller, Moller, Jannetta, and Jho, 1993). Facial nerve dysfunction (**hemifacial spasm**), **tinnitus**, **hyperacusis**, vestibular abnormalities, and hearing loss can occur from vascular compression related to vascular loops. Vascular loops are diagnosed with MRI and auditory brainstem response (ABR) studies. Audiological findings in cases with vascular compressions are similar to those noted in patients with acoustic tumors; however, it is not uncommon for the findings to be a bit more subtle in these patients. The ABR is typically abnormal, with the I–III interwave interval being extended, and there are often, but not always, pure-tone deficits and reduced speech recognition scores associated with vascular loops (Moller and Moller, 1985). Interestingly, surgical decompression often results in improved hearing function in these patients (Moller and Moller, 1985). ●

VASCULAR ANATOMY OF THE CENTRAL AUDITORY SYSTEM

Two main vascular systems supply the CANS. One is the vertebral-basilar system, which is primarily responsible for the auditory structures in the brainstem. The other is the internal carotid system that supplies the auditory structures in the cerebrum. The vertebral-basilar system begins with the vertebral arteries, which branch from the subclavian artery (Barr, 1972; Waddington, 1974). The vertebral arteries ascend on each side of the upper six vertebrae through a small foramen. At the level of the foramen magnum the vertebral arteries course anteriorly (ventrally) and medially to run along the lateral aspect of the medulla. Usually about a few millimeters inferior to the ponto-medullary junction, the vertebral arteries join to form the main artery of the brainstem: the basilar artery.

CLINICAL CORRELATE

Some evidence shows that at or near the point where one artery splits into two arteries is an area of weakness in the vessel that might give rise to such abnormalities as aneurysms. This is thought to happen because at the locus of the bifurcation there is a thinning of the muscle layer in the vessel (Wilkinson, 1988). An aneurysm is a ballooning of a vessel, usually related to a weakness in the arterial wall.

An aneurysm at the bifurcation of the vertebral to basilar arteries may sometimes present with symptoms similar to those of a CPA tumor, especially if the lesion is large. The position of an aneurysm at the vertebral-basilar junction would be anterior to the CPA, but if the aneurysm were large, it could easily extend posteriorly into the CPA recess, placing pressure on the auditory, vestibular, and facial nerves. Musiek, Geurkink, and Spiegel (1987) provided a report for a patient where a large aneurysm encompassed the CPA and invaded most of the brainstem. In this case the aneurysm arose from a weakened area in the artery wall just a few millimeters from the bifurcation between the vertebral and basilar arteries. Initially this lesion was presumed to be a large CPA tumor, but computerized tomography showed it to be vascular in origin (see Figure 14.7). The patient's symptoms were similar to those typically noted in cases with large CPA lesions. The patient in this study reported decreased facial sensation and hearing loss on the involved side, as well as dizziness, headaches, and diplopia (on gaze to the involved side). However, unlike what is commonly observed in patients with CPA tumors, this patient demonstrated a low frequency sensorineural hearing loss on the involved side. The ABR showed the early waves to be present and the later waves to be absent or severely distorted for both ears (Figure 14.7). This ABR profile would be unusual for a CPA tumor, where typically abnormal ABR findings are noted only for the ear on the involved side and where the most prominent ABR abnormality is an extension of the I–III interwave interval (i.e., it is unlikely that the later waves would be absent or severely distorted). ●

● **Figure 14.7**

(a) Auditory brainstem response (ABR) showing replicable waves I, II, and III for the left ear (LE) at the slower repetition rate and only waves I and II for the right ear (RE) for a patient with a basilar artery aneurysm (see text). (b) Computerized tomography scan showing a large basilar artery aneurysm (arrows).

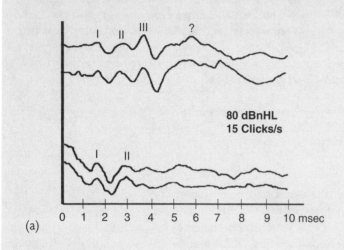

80 dBnHL
15 Clicks/s

(a)

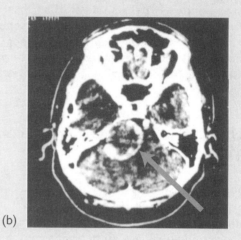

(b)

The basilar artery is located on the ventral (anterior) side of the pons and ascends most of the pons at midline. This artery has some major and minor branches. One of the key branches, located at the caudal portion of the pons, is the AICA (Figure 14.8). The AICA courses to the cerebellum but also sends circumferential branches posteriorly to supply the cochlear nucleus (CN).

In about 50% of the specimens studied by Portmann et al. (1975), the AICA gave rise to a branch that coursed to the IAM, known as the IAA, or labyrinthine artery (see discussion in earlier section of this chapter). In the other 50% of the specimens, the IAA branched directly from the basilar artery, with the IAA being rostral to the AICA (Waddington, 1974; Portmann et al., 1975).

Along most of the length of the basilar artery, small arteries penetrate the pons (pontine paramedian arteries) to supply structures deep in the pons, such as the superior olivary complex (SOC) and the cochlear stria. At the most rostral aspect of the pons, the basilar artery gives rise to the superior cerebellar artery, which supplies the cerebellum but also circumferentially supplies the inferior colliculus (IC) and lateral lemniscus (LL) (Barr, 1972; Waddington, 1974). The basilar artery also gives rise to the posterior cerebral artery, which supplies the splenium of the corpus callosum (CC) and forms the posterior segment of the **circle of Willis**. The circle of Willis is composed of the posterior cerebral artery segment, the posterior communicating artery, the internal carotid segment, the anterior cerebral artery, and the anterior communicating artery (Figure 14.9).

The circle of Willis provides an indirect connection between the vertebral-basilar system and the **internal carotid** system. Barr (1972) provides a detailed account of the arteries that course away from the circle of Willis. Four main groups of arteries come off the circle of Willis, including the anteromedial group, the anterolateral

● **Figure 14.8**

The basilar artery. 1 = vertebral artery, 2 = posterior inferior cerebellar artery (PICA), 3 = anterior inferior cerebellar artery (AICA), 4 = internal auditory, or labyrinthine artery, 5 = basilar artery, 6 = pontine penetrating arteries, 7 = superior cerebellar artery, 8 = posterior cerebral artery.

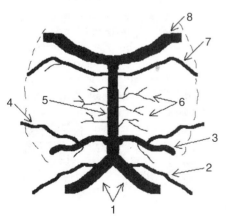

Figure 14.9

The arteries contributing to and forming the circle of Willis (from Waddington, 1974, with permission).

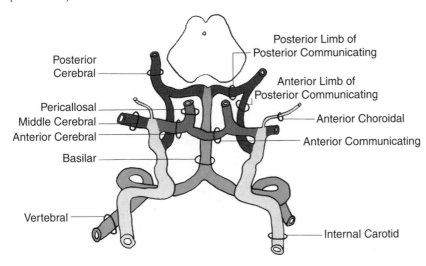

group, the posteromedial group, and the posterolateral group. The anterolateral and posteromedial group are of import in regard to auditory structures. The anteroganglionic arteries, which are part of the anterolateral group, send vessels to the internal capsule, the external capsule, and the claustrum. The posteroganglionic artery sends branches to the thalamus (anterior [ventral] and medial portions).

The other main vascular supply to the CANS comes from the internal carotid artery (ICA). The ICA divides into the **anterior cerebral artery** (ACA) and **middle cerebral artery** (MCA) branches (Kulenovic et al., 2003). The MCA is of special importance to the cerebral auditory system, and this is reflected by the "early branches" of the MCA. The early branches are the vessels that are proximal to the major bifurcation or trifurcation of the MCA (Tanriover, Kawashima, Rhoton, Ulm, and Mericle, 2003). A high percentage of these early branches lead to the temporal lobe and some lead to the frontal lobe. The **lenticulostriate arteries,** which supply the caudate, putamen, and globus pallidus, more commonly arise from frontal branches than from the temporal branches of the early branches (Waddington, 1974; Tanriover et al., 2003). The MCA can be followed for either a short distance before it branches extensively or it may course along most of the Sylvian fissure before it disappears into diffuse branching (Waddington, 1974). The MCA running from an anterior to posterior direction sends off a number of important vessels to the auditory substrate in the Sylvian and perisylvian areas (Figures 14.10 and 14.11).

Figure 14.10

The main branches of the middle cerebral artery. 1a = fronto-orbital (anterior) and 1b = (superior) branches, 2 = fronto-opercular, 3 = central sulcus, 4a = posterior parietal (superior), 4b =(inferior) branches, 5 = angular, 6 = (a) anterior temporal, (b) middle temporal, (c) posterior temporal arteries (from Waddington, 1974, with permission).

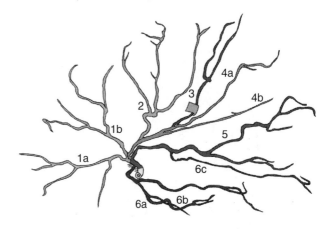

● **Figure 14.11**

(a) Photo of the human brain showing the branches of the middle cerebral artery running over the insula and temporal lobe. (b) Drawing of the brain depicted in (a) with the vessels labeled corresponding to Figure 14.10. 1 = not shown, 2 = fronto-opercular, 3 = central sulcus, 4 = posterior parietal, 5 = angular (running over the posterior parietal), 6a,b,c = temporal arteries (from Waddington, 1974, with permission).

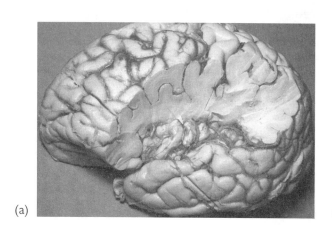

(a)

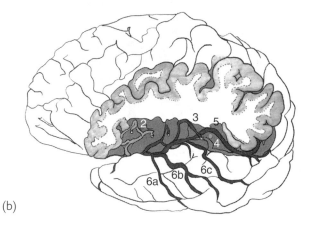

(b)

One of the first major branches of the MCA is the **fronto-opercular artery,** which courses superiorly and posteriorly, supplying the anterior section of the insula. The middle and posterior portions of insula are supplied by smaller branches of the MCA that arise further posteriorly along the MCA as well as by the central sulcus artery. The arteries that lie directly on the insula are termed insular arteries, which are believed to arise from either the fronto-opercular artery or from the smaller insular branches from the MCA.

The **central sulcus branch** of the MCA also courses superiorly (rostrally) and supplies the posterior frontal lobe and the pre-and post-central gyri. This branch and its secondary branches provide the blood supply to auditory areas in the inferior parietal and posterior inferior frontal lobes as has been previously discussed. The MCA in many specimens sends three **temporal branches**, the anterior, mid, and posterior segments, to supply the temporal lobe. Usually toward the posterior aspect of the MCA an angular branch evolves to carry blood to the supramarginal and angular gyri. At times the **angular artery** may look as if it is a continuation of the MCA proper. Also, some specimens have only two temporal branches, not three. The angular, mid, and posterior branches supply most of the primary auditory cortex (Figures 14.12 and 14.13).

The CC receives its blood supply from two main sources: the pericallosal artery and the posterior cerebral artery. The **pericallosal artery** arises from the ACA, one of the branches of the ICA (Figure 14.15). The pericallosal artery courses from near the anterior commissure around the genu and then on the superior surface of CC. It turns superiorly away from the CC, usually just anterior to the splenium. Therefore, usually only the anterior four-fifths of the CC is supplied by the pericallosal artery. The posterior one-fifth of the CC is supplied by the posterior cerebral

● **Figure 14.12**

Regions of the cerebrum's blood supply correlated with cerebral arteries. 1 = fronto-orbital, 2 = fronto-opercular, 3 = central sulcus, 4 = posterior parietal, 5 = angular, 6 = anterior, middle, and posterior temporal region (from Waddington, 1974, with permission).

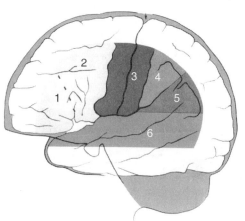

Figure 14.13

Carotid angiogram showing key branches of the middle cerebral artery. The black rectangle indicates vessels along the Sylvian fissure. Most prominent in this view are the angular, temporal, and posterior parietal branches (from Waddington, 1974, with permission).

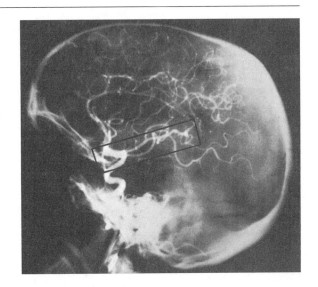

CLINICAL CORRELATE

Several types of cerebral vascular disorders can affect the auditory areas of the CANS. As was discussed in the case study presented above, aneurysms can affect auditory function. In addition, intracerebral hemorrhage, usually secondary to weakening of the artery wall by trauma, disease, or genetics, is a significant cause of auditory deficits. There is also occlusive disease that is secondary to obstruction of or reduced blood flow. Occlusive disease can result in ischemia (brief period of time without blood supply) or infarction (long periods without blood supply), which is when neural tissue begins to necrotize (Kaufman, 1990). Stroke is a cerebral (or brainstem) infarction that results in a fixed neurological deficit lasting more than several days (Reeves, 1989). Stroke can be viewed as an infarcted tissue in the area supplied by a major vessel (Reeves, 1989). Finally, there are arteriovenous malformations, which are abnormalities in the structural anatomy of the blood vessels, that result in entanglement and disruption of proper blood flow.

Figure 14.14

(a) Computerized tomography scan documenting the lesioned area of the brain that was secondary to a stroke in the temporal-parietal region for the patient described in the accompanying text. (b) The middle latency response for this patient showing a difference between the two ears and (c) the central auditory test results for three behavioral tests (dichotic digits, frequency pattern sequences, and dichotic rhymes) showing below-normal performance for the left ear (i.e., the ear contralateral to the lesion site). (Note: The calibration bar shown at the left top of panel (B) represents an amplitude of 0.3 μV.)

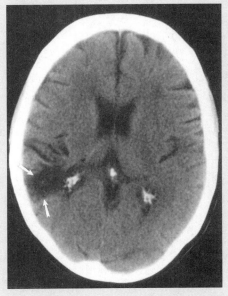

(a)

(continued)

● **Figure 14.14**

Continued

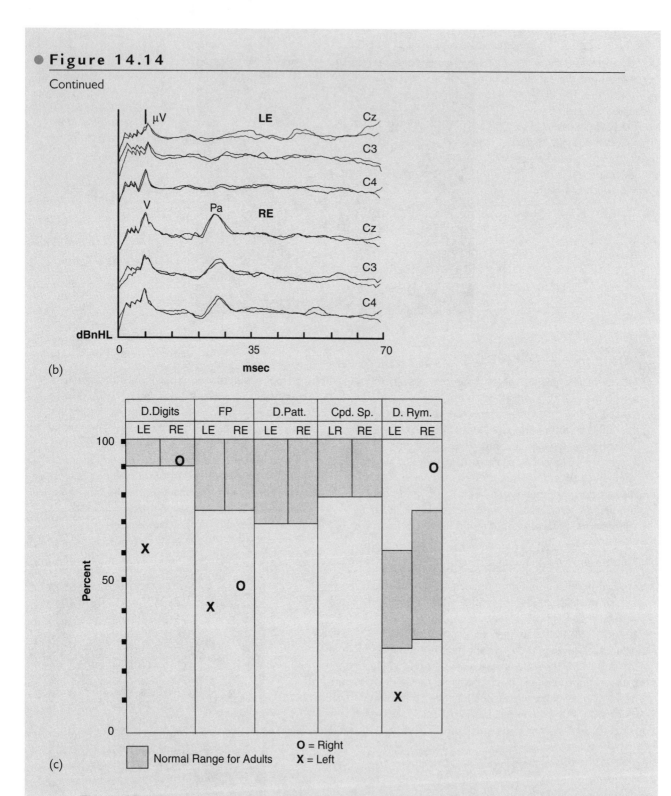

(b)

(c)

This case, by way of example, demonstrates the neuroaudiological correlates to one of these vascular disorders. This case is that of a middle-aged patient who was diagnosed with a temporal-parietal stroke secondary to occlusion of some of the branches of the right MCA. The patient reported that he had experienced confusion and a headache at the time of the stroke and that later he experienced intermittent

(continued)

episodes of vertigo and imbalance. Upon testing, the patient demonstrated essentially normal pure-tone thresholds and excellent speech recognition scores bilaterally. The computed tomography scan for this patient showed a lesion in the region of the temporal-parietal junction (Figure 14.14a). The middle latency response (MLR) showed no response following a normal ABR response for left ear stimulation using clicks for electrodes placed at C3, C4, and Cz. Right ear stimulation did show a Pa response and a normal ABR response (Figure 14.14b). Results for the frequency pattern test were abnormal bilaterally, and the dichotic digits and dichotic rhyme test results showed the "classic" contralateral left ear deficit (Figure 14.14c). These audiological results are typical for what is often observed in stroke cases involving the temporal lobe. ●

● Figure 14.15

Midsaggital view of a human corpus callosum showing the pericallosal artery running along the top (see arrows). Note that this artery only runs about four-fifths of the length of the corpus callosum. It courses away from the corpus callosum just anterior to the splenium. The splenium's blood supply comes from the posterior cerebral artery.

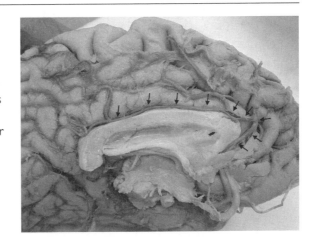

artery (Barr, 1972; Waddington, 1974; Carpenter and Sutin, 1983). There also can be an additional pericallosal artery that arises from the **anterior communicating** artery. This callosal artery is much smaller than the other pericallosal artery arising from the ACA (Kulenovic, Dilberovic, and Ovcina, 2003).

SUMMARY

The external ear (auricle and external auditory meatus) acquires its blood supply from the external carotid artery by two key artery branches: the STA and the PAA. The ME derives its blood supply from branches of the subclavian, internal carotid, and external carotid arteries, while the basis for the blood supply in the cochlea and the AN is the vertebro-basilar system. The basilar artery gives rise to the IAA (often termed the labyrinthine artery) in two possible ways. One way is that the IAA branches directly from the basilar artery, and the other is that the IAA arises from the AICA. The IAA courses through the IAM where branches supply the auditory, facial, and vestibular nerves. Key branches (cochleo-vestibular artery) then go on to the cochlea and vestibular apparatus. The cochleo-vestibular artery gives rise to radiating arterioles that supply the membranous structures of the cochlea. There is, of course, a venous system that is the counterpart of the arterial system in the periphery.

The central vascular system has two main origins, the basilar artery and the MCA, the latter a branch of the internal carotid artery. The basilar artery gives off branches such as the AICA, which indirectly supplies the CN; the penetrating arteries, which supply deep auditory structures like the SOC; and the superior cerebellar artery, which circumferentially supplies the LL and its nuclei and possibly the IC. The MCA also has branches that supply the structures along and around the Sylvian fissure. The fronto-opercular artery supplies the insula, and the temporal and angular branches supply the superior temporal gyrus and plane and retrosylvian auditory areas. The central sulcus artery supplies the auditory regions of the inferior frontal and parietal lobe, while the CC's vascular supply is from the pericallosal artery, which arises from the ACA and supplies the anterior four-fifths of the CC, and the posterior cerebral artery, which supplies the posterior one-fifth of the CC. Aneurysms, occlusive disease, hemorrhage, and vascular steal are vascular disorders that can affect hearing function if their loci are in or near the auditory system.

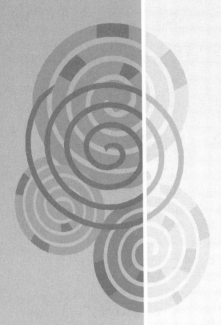

15

The Efferent System

Introduction

One of the mysteries of the auditory system is the function of the **efferent auditory system** or as it is sometimes termed, the "descending system." Although much progress has been made in elucidating many of the functions of this system and the role it plays in hearing, there are still many aspects of the system that have not been fully defined. The efferent auditory system is essentially the counterpart to the afferent system. Like the afferent pathway, the efferent system connects the brain to the cochlea, but in the reverse order of that which is seen in the afferent system. The efferent anatomy appears to be more loosely connected and less extensive than the afferent system. However, it is fair to say that the anatomy, especially that of the more rostral system, is not well defined and many questions still surround the morphology and function of this system.

Most of what will be covered in this chapter pertains to small animals and, in particular, the cat, as little is known about the human efferent system. However, some clinical measures will be discussed that may allow some insight into the structure and function of the human descending pathway. Advances in evoked potentials (EPs) and otoacoustic emissions (OAEs) have provided some clinical measures that look to be particularly useful for studying this system.

Even though comparatively little is known about the efferent pathway and its mechanisms, most researchers and clinicians who study this system would agree that it plays an important role in the functioning of the auditory system. It has been documented that the efferent system plays a role in modulating input from the periphery. It may also interact with the ascending system in some simple, as well as some extremely complex, ways. Early studies seemed to indicate that the descending system was primarily an inhibitory system. Certainly there is evidence of this, which will be discussed later in this chapter. However, evidence is also emerging that indicates that the efferent system is involved in excitatory processes. Perhaps it is not just the inhibitory or excitatory roles that the efferent system plays that are important, but rather the role that the system plays in the modulation and control of excitatory and inhibitory interactions within the auditory system. As mentioned in Chapter 1, there is growing interest in the idea that the auditory system has to have a balance of inhibitory and excitatory actions for it to work optimally. When there is an imbalance between the excitatory and inhibitory processes in the auditory system, hearing disorders may occur. It seems reasonable that the efferent system might play a role in maintaining this inhibitory–excitatory balance.

Whatever the ultimate role of the efferent system, the journey of discovery along the way will be an interesting one. It is anticipated that clinical studies may play a part in further discovery of the significance of this system, although at this point in time clinical correlates to the system are sparse. The discussion of the efferent system in this chapter will begin at the cortex and descend down the auditory system, as this approach appears to be a logical one. Wherever possible, clinical correlates will be introduced to help establish links between the research findings being discussed and their potential clinical applications. However, the number of these will be limited.

OVERVIEW OF THE EFFERENT SYSTEM

The efferent auditory pathway begins at the auditory cortex and association areas and courses from these areas down through the internal capsule to the medial geniculate body (MGB); from here the efferent pathway continues to course along a similar route as the ascending pathway (but in an opposite direction) until it finally terminates in the cochlea (Figure 15.1). The descending system has fewer fibers associated with it and it is not, at least at the present time, known to be as anatomically distinct as the ascending system. Finally, at certain points along the

● **Figure 15.1**

A general view of the efferent system based on the cat model and adapted to the human model. AC = auditory cortex, Int. Cap. = internal capsule, MGB = medial geniculate body, IC = inferior colliculus, LL = lateral lemniscus, CN = cochlear nucleus, SOC = superior olivary complex, (A. = contralateral medial olivocochlear bundle, B. = ipsilateral medial olivocochlear bundle, C. = lateral olivocochlear bundle), IAM = internal auditory meatus.

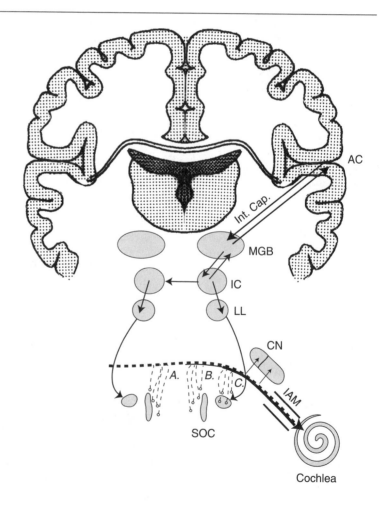

● **Figure 15.2**

Neural connections of the rostral efferent system based on the cat model. I = insula, AII = association area, AI = primary auditory cortex, P = pulvinar, RN = reticular nucleus, (D), (V) = dorsal and ventral segments of the medial geniculate body (MGB), Br. = brachium of the inferior colliculus, I.C. = inferior colliculus, S.C. = superior colliculus, SOC = superior olivary complex.

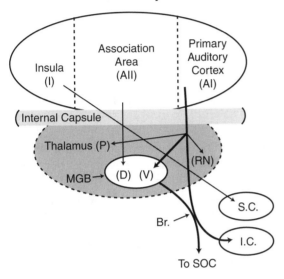

pathway from the cortex to the cochlea, the efferent system connects with distinct portions of the ascending system to form various **feedback loops**—making for a rather complex array of auditory neural connections.

Although it may be somewhat artificial, it may be best to view the descending auditory system in two segments. The more rostral segment is the part of the system rostral to the superior olivary complex (SOC) (Figure 15.2). The other segment is the **olivocochlear bundle** (OCB) and its caudal connections to the cochlea. The rostral segment is not as well studied as the OCB; hence, there is considerably less information available for the rostral portion of the efferent system than there is for the caudal segment (i.e., the OCB). The OCB segment arises primarily from around the SOC and has a lateral segment and a medial segment. The lateral segment is primarily an ipsilateral system, whereas the medial segment is a crossed system (e.g., left SOC region to right cochlea).

THE ROSTRAL EFFERENT SYSTEM

Anatomy of the Rostral Efferent System

The efferent system will be viewed first at the auditory cortex, using the cat as our primary model (see Spangler and Warr, 1991; Warr, 1992; Sahley, Nodar, and Musiek, 1997). The efferent system at this level includes the primary auditory area and secondary association areas. The efferent fibers leave the auditory areas (layers IV and V) of the cortex and proceed down through the internal capsule. These fibers then take an ipsilateral route to the pulvinar and the reticular nuclei of the

Figure 15.3

Reciprocal (loop) connections in the rostral efferent system from the auditory cortex (AC) and association areas to the medial geniculate body (MGB) and inferior colliculus (IC).

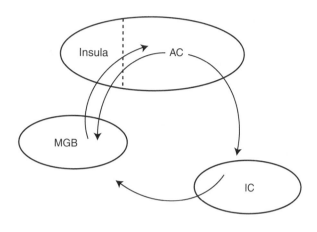

thalamus. The fibers then course, for the most part, to the ventral and medial MGB and proceed on to the brachium of the inferior colliculus (IC). Efferent fibers arising from the insula project to the superior colliculus. The efferent projections to the IC can course through the MGB, as just stated, or they can project directly from the cortex to the IC. Most efferent projections are to the ipsilateral dorsal cortex and central nucleus of the IC. However, some of the fibers from the auditory cortex course to the contralateral IC via the commissure of the IC (Andersen, Synder, and Merzenich, 1980; Aitkin, 1986). The efferent fibers projecting to the IC are tonotopically organized.

One of the most interesting aspects of the rostral efferent system is its multiple feedback loops (Andersen et al., 1980; Imig and Morel, 1985; Spangler and Warr, 1991). One such reciprocal connection is between the auditory cortex and the ventral division of the MGB. These cortical-geniculate fibers are tonotopically organized. Descending connections from the auditory cortex to the IC are also tonotopically organized. The efferent fibers (likely second-order fibers) projecting from the auditory cortex to the IC travel to the ventral and medial segments of the MGB. This last connection creates one of the key feedback loops (Figure 15.3). This loop includes auditory cortex projections to the MGB (ventral portion) and to the IC (dorsal and central regions). The MGB then projects back to the auditory cortex and receives projections from the IC.

Another feedback loop involves auditory cortex projections to the posterior thalamic nuclei and to the IC with connections between the IC and the posterior thalamus (Figure 15.4). The third feedback loop that will be mentioned here is the insular feedback circuit. This loop starts with projections from the insula to the superior colliculus, which in turn project to the suprageniculate nuclei of the MGB. The MGB then projects to the insular cortex to complete the loop (Figure 15.5). Other reciprocal loops also involve different areas of the MGB, the reticular thalamus, and the IC, but these will not be discussed here. The reader interested in more information on these feedback loops is referred to the articles referenced above.

Physiology of the Rostral Efferent System

Little is known about the function of the rostral efferent system. Hypothetically, based on the anatomy just discussed, it would seem that this system has a role in controlling the afferent system—at least to some degree. It is also important to mention that the descending rostral system directly and indirectly projects to the auditory nuclei within the caudal brainstem and to the cochlea. Therefore, it is possible that there could be a cortical influence on the functions of the cochlea, the auditory nerve (AN), and the lower brainstem nuclei.

Figure 15.4

Reciprocal (loop) connections in the rostral efferent system from auditory cortex and association areas to the posterior thalamic group (PTG) and inferior colliculus (IC).

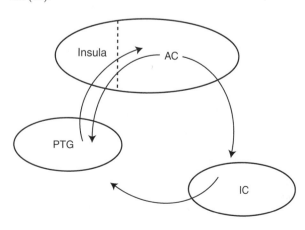

● Figure 15.5

Reciprocal (loop) connections in the rostral efferent system from the insula to the superior colliculus (SC) and the suprageniculate nucleus (SGN) of the medial geniculate body (MGB), AC = auditory cortex.

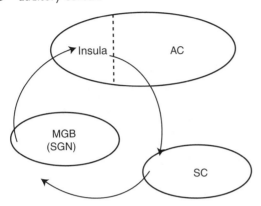

Studies of stimulation of the auditory cortex have shown inhibition and excitation at the MGB (Ryugo and Weinberger, 1976; Watanabe, Yanagisawa, Kanzaki, and Katsuki, 1966). Similarly, auditory cortex stimulation has resulted in both excitation and inhibition at the level of the IC (Mitani, Shimokouchi, and Nomura, 1983).

CLINICAL CORRELATE

Obviously, with little known about the physiology of the rostral efferent system, it is difficult to find information pertaining to clinical aspects of this system. However, there is one published article with clinical relevance to this topic (Efron, Crandall, Koss, Divenyi, and Yund, 1983). Efron and his colleagues, based on some early work with monkeys, theorized that there is an efferent auditory tract in the anterior temporal lobe. They then went on to theorize that the function of this efferent auditory tract is to enhance the ability of monkeys to hear nonspeech acoustic stimuli in the contralateral auditory space—especially in noise. These researchers supported this theory by demonstrating that when the anterior temporal lobe was damaged, the ability to hear targeted sounds in noise in the contralateral acoustic space was compromised in their experimental animals. Even though this effect could be explained by other mechanisms, Efron and colleagues support their idea well, arguing that inhibitory phenomena related to the efferent cortical tract may enhance hearing in noise. Although this research was done with monkeys, it is logical to assume that similar mechanisms are likely to exist in the human model, which would enhance one's ability to hear in noise. ●

THE CAUDAL EFFERENT SYSTEM

Anatomy of the Caudal Efferent System

The key player in the efferent system is clearly the OCB (medial and lateral components), which involves the auditory structures at the SOC and below. However, before the OCB is discussed, it is important to address the descending fiber tracts from the IC that contribute to the OCB and its related nuclei.

● Figure 15.6

Transverse hemisection through the mammalian caudal brainstem showing the superior olivary complex. The dotted line indicates the regions of the medial (left) and lateral (right) olivocochlear systems. DMPO = dorso-medial periolivary nucleus, MNTB = medial nucleus of the trapezoid body, VMPO = ventro-medial periolivary nucleus, VNTB = ventral nucleus of the trapezoid body, MSO = medial superior olivary nucleus, DPO = dorsal periolivary nucleus, DLPO = dorso-lateral periolivary nucleus, LSO = lateral superior olivary nucleus, LNTB = lateral nucleus of the trapezoid body (from Sahley et al., 1997 and the Cleveland Clinic Foundation, with permission).

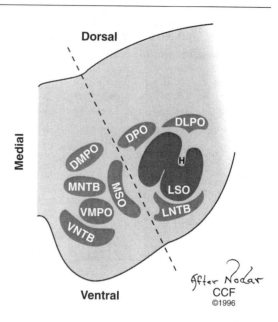

It appears that the central nucleus, the dorso-medial nucleus, and the commissure region of the IC are the main sources of the fibers that descend to the SOC area (Hashikawa and Kawamura, 1983). However, the superior colliculus, the ventral nucleus of the lateral lemniscus (LL), and the brachium of the IC may also be origins for some of the descending fibers (see Spangler and Warr, 1991). The course that these efferent fibers take is along the LL. This tract is in essence a descending correlate to the ascending LL pathway. Once the tract descends ipsilaterally to the area of the periolivary nuclei in the vicinity of the SOC, it terminates. Descending inputs are carried to the ventral nucleus of the trapezoid body (VNTB) and from there to the lateral nucleus of the trapezoid body (LNTB) and the dorso-medial periolivary nuclei (DMPO). These descending inputs to the VNTB, LNTB, and DMPO are primarily to the multipolar cells of these nuclei (Harrison and Howe, 1974). There are also contralateral descending projections from the IC to a variety of cells in and around the SOC (Lugo and Cooper, 1982) (see Figures 15.1 and 15.2).

● The Olivocochlear Bundle (OCB) System

In general, the OCB system is the neuron complex of descending fibers that originates in periolivary regions of the SOC. From the SOC the fibers travel to the cochlear nucleus (CN) and then through the internal auditory meatus (IAM) to end up as direct connections to the outer hair cells (OHCs) (medial or crossed system) or to the afferent fibers beneath the inner hair cells (IHCs) (lateral system). The OCB system can perhaps be best discussed by dividing it into lateral and medial components (see Figures 15.6 and 15.7).

LATERAL OLIVOCOCHLEAR BUNDLE (LOC)   The LOC fibers are essentially unmyelinated fibers that are smaller in diameter than their medial counterparts. There are approximately 800 fibers in the LOC. In the cat the fibers of the LOC range in diameter from 0.3 to 0.7 µm, while the fibers in the MOC range from 0.5 to 2.8 µm

● Figure 15.7

Transverse view of the olivocochlear bundle showing fiber connections in the right half of the caudal brainstem. DCN = dorsal cochlear nucleus, VCN = ventral cochlear nucleus (see Figure 15.6 for additional abbreviations) (from Sahley et al., 1997 and the Cleveland Clinic Foundation, with permission).

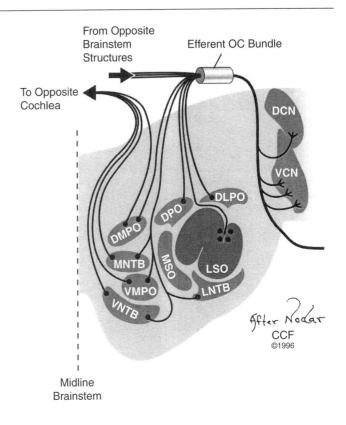

in their diameters (Warr, 1980; Guinan, Warr, and Norris, 1983; Sahley, Nodar, and Musiek, 1997). The origin of these fibers is in the LSO and surrounding area. The LOC pathway to the cochlea is ipsilateral for the most part, but this is species dependent. Some animals have strictly an ipsilateral route, while others have a small portion of contralateral fibers that contribute to the LOC. In the cat, about 90% of the lateral fibers are ipsilateral, whereas only 26 to 28% of the MOC fibers are ipsilateral (Warr, 1980; Guinan et al., 1983; Sahley et al., 1997) (Figure 15.8). The pathway of the LOC, including its origins and terminations, has been delineated and discussed by a number of investigators (Kane, 1976; Warr, 1980; Adams, 1983; Spangler, Cant, Henkel, Farley, and Warr, 1987; Sahley et al., 1997). There is fairly good agreement among these investigators that neurons from the **dorso-lateral periolivary nuclei** travel via the intermediate stria to the posterior ventral cochlear nucleus (PVCN). The **dorsal periolivary nuclei** and LSO send fibers to the PVCN, the anterior ventral cochlear nucleus (AVCN), and the dorsal cochlear nucleus (DCN). The LNTB sends fibers bilaterally to the DCN through the dorsal acoustic stria and sends ipsilateral fibers through the ventral acoustic stria to the AVCN and PVCN. Although less well defined, the medial periolivary nuclei, the MNTB, and the VNTB also project to the CN and into the cochlea.

The LOC bundle pathway has various descriptions, but the account here will synthesize descriptions by Galambos (1956), Warr, (1980, 1992) and Sahley et al. (1997). The LOC fibers, as they leave the periolivary areas, form a bundle, or tract, as they

● Figure 15.8

The percentage of ipsilateral and contralateral fibers in the lateral (LOCB) and medial olivo-cochlear bundle (MOCB) in the cat (based on data from Sahley et al., 1997).

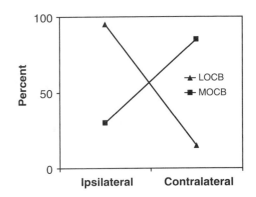

● **Figure 15.9**

Transverse section through the caudal brainstem showing the olivocochlear bundle (OCB) and its pathway components running to the cochlea, IV = fourth ventricle, DCN = dorsal cochlear nucleus, VCN = ventral cochlear nucleus, MSO = medial superior olive, LSO = lateral superior olive.

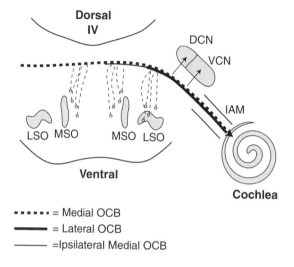

course dorsally along the floor of the fourth ventricle. The efferent fibers proceed laterally (near but caudal to the dorsal acoustic stria) around the vestibular nerve root and then run with the vestibular fibers as they enter the IAM (Figures 15.7 and 15.9). As these efferent fibers course through the IAM, they exit via the habenula perforata and then enter the cochlea between its first (basal) and second turns. These fibers form an **inner spiral bundle** that courses apically and basally to terminate on type I fibers as they leave the IHCs on their afferent path.

THE MEDIAL OLIVOCOCHLEAR BUNDLE (MOC)   The following discussion will focus on the work of Galambos (1956), Kane (1976), Warr (1980), Adams (1983), Spangler et al. (1987), and Sahley et al. (1997). The MOC bundle has mostly myelinated fibers that are larger in diameter than the lateral efferent fibers. In the cat, there are about 500 fibers in the MOC bundle. In most species, 65 to 75% of medial fibers are crossed, while the remaining 25 to 35% of the fibers are uncrossed (Figure 15.10). The medial fibers arise from the MNTB, the VNTB, the DMPO, and the VMPO in the vicinity of the MSO and contribute collaterals to the AVCN and the DCN bilaterally but with greater input to the contralateral nuclei. The VNTB also projects to the contralateral PVCN. The MOC fibers follow a similar route as the LOC bundle in the brainstem. The crossed MOC fibers that course across the midline combine with the fibers in the LOC bundle (forming the OCB proper) and then course to the cochlea, where they terminate.

Once in the cochlea, the medial efferents cross the tunnel of Corti above the afferent type II fibers. (Note: In most drawings of the tunnel of Corti, the fibers usually depicted are lateral efferents, as the afferent fibers are often found more toward the base of the tunnel and are more difficult to observe.) The medial efferents course through the space of Neul and bypass the medial aspect of the Deiters' cells to connect to the lower part of the OHCs (Figures 15.10, 15.11, 15.12 and 15.13).

● **Figure 15.10**

Lateral and medial olivocochlear connections to the inner and outer hair cells (from Sahley et al., 1997 and the Cleveland Clinic Foundation, with permission).

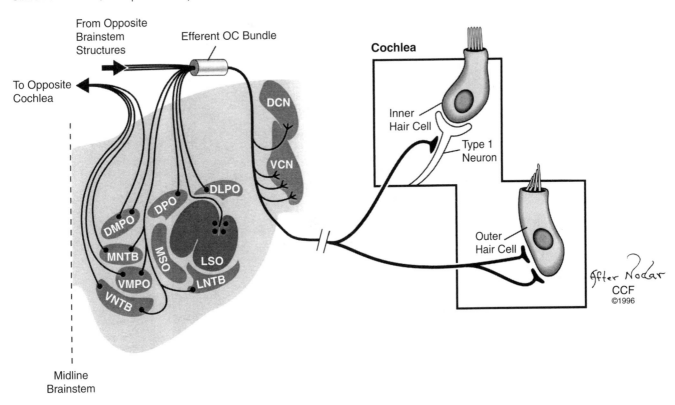

● **Figure 15.11**

The olivocochlear fibers in the organ of Corti. TR = tunnel crossing radial efferent fibers (from Sahley et al., 1997 and the Cleveland Clinic Foundation, with permission).

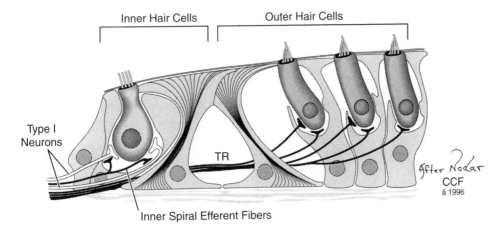

● **Figure 15.12**

The tonotopic fibers of the lateral olivocochlear system and their arrangement in the organ of Corti for connection to the inner hair cells. OC = olivocochlear, BM = basilar membrane, DPO = dorsal periolivary nucleus, LSO = lateral superiorolive (from Sahley et al., 1997 and the Cleveland Clinic Foundation, with permission; based in part on data from Warr et al., 1986).

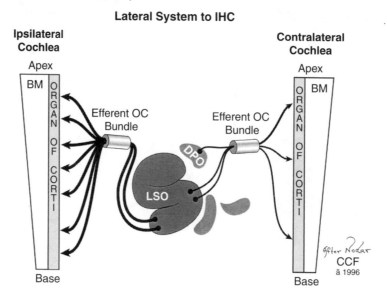

● **Figure 15.13**

The tonotopic fibers of the medial olivocochlear system and their arrangement in the organ of Corti for connection to the outer hair cells. OC = olivocochlear, BM = basilar membrane, MNTB = medial nucleus of the trapezoid body, MSO = medial superiorolive (from Sahley et al., 1997 and the Cleveland Clinic Foundation, with permission; in part based on data from Warr et al., 1986).

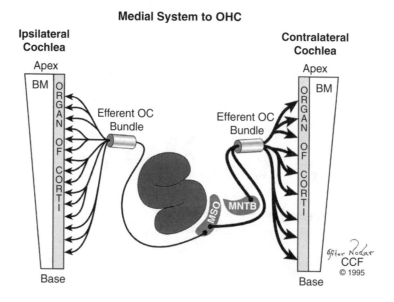

● *Tonotopicity*

The OCB neurons are tonotopically organized. Although it is believed that both the LOC and MOC fibers have a tonotopic organization, most of the information that is available only addresses the frequency representation within the MOC bundle. This is most likely because these fibers are myelinated and larger than the LOC fibers (as well as because they are probably easier to locate and record from). The available evidence suggests that higher frequencies are located on a medial plane and lower frequencies on a lateral plane within the OCB (Goldberg and Brown, 1968).

Physiology of the Caudal Efferent System

The discussion of the physiology of the OCB will center on the MOC bundle. Fibers of the MOC, as stated earlier, are myelinated and their response properties are much easier to measure. Therefore, there is much more data available for this system compared to that for the LOC system. In addition, there is some clinical precedent for measuring the MOC system. The suppression effect on OAEs is a clinical measure that is becoming widely used in diagnostic audiology.

● *Poststimulus Time Histograms*

Tsuchitani's (1977) early work and discussions by Sahley et al. (1997) indicate that there are three main poststimulus time histograms (PSTHs) for the OCB. These include a wide, or W-chopper, response; a sustained, or S-chopper, response; and an off type response. Comparison of the W and S types of chopper responses reveal that the S response has higher spike rates, shorter interspike intervals, and quicker onset times than the W chopper type response.

● *Other Response Properties*

The response thresholds of the MOC fibers vary considerably. Some of the fibers have thresholds as low as 10 to 15 dB SPL, while others may have thresholds as high as 80 dB SPL. This is a greater range of threshold sensitivity than that noted for the afferent fibers from the same cochlea (Liberman, 1988). The dynamic intensity range of most MOC fibers is about 40 to 60 dB (see Liberman, 1988 and Sahley et al., 1997 for reviews).

The onset latencies of the neural discharges of the MOC fibers to brief tonal stimuli at the fibers' characteristic frequencies (CFs) has been reported to range from 5 to 60 msec (Robertson and Gummer, 1985; Brown, de Venecia, and Guinan, 2003). The shorter latencies represented by the lower end of this response range may protect the auditory system from potentially damaging effects that might otherwise be associated with over-stimulation of the fibers (Brown et al., 2003). However, most of the MOC fibers have latencies to tonal stimuli that are greater than 10 msec—even at high intensities. It appears that in rodents, there are shorter latencies for contralateral versus ipsilaterally presented stimuli (Robertson and Gummer, 1985). These latencies are far more variable and longer than those obtained from the ascending fibers. The greater latencies noted for these fibers may suggest the presence of certain inhibitory phenomena and complex circuitry in this efferent region.

The spontaneous firing rate of the MOC neurons is of interest in that it is quite different from that seen in the afferent system. It has been reported that approximately 80% of MOC neurons demonstrate little or no spontaneous activity. The fibers that do exhibit spontaneous activity show relatively low firing rates, ranging from 1 to 10 spikes per second (see Fex, 1962; Liberman and Brown, 1986; and Sahley et al., 1997 for reviews). It is interesting that MOC fibers have essentially little or no spontaneous activity but that at least some of these fibers are highly sensitive to acoustic stimulation (low thresholds).

The tuning curves (TCs) of MOC fibers, as measured in rodents, are sharp—indicating good frequency selectivity. These TCs are very similar to those seen for the type I fibers of the AN (Robertson and Gummer, 1985).

The MOC system can respond equally well to either monaural or binaural stimuli, depending on the condition. Also, these fibers respond similarly to either ipsilateral or contralateral acoustic stimuli. Binaurally sensitive fibers seem to respond more to lower frequencies (<2 kHz in the cat) (Liberman and Brown, 1986; Sahley et al., 1997). It is difficult to determine what role these binaural fibers may play in sound localization or other binaural hearing processes. Perhaps they may help prevent the upward spread of masking that is often caused by low-frequency environmental noise.

Medial Olivocochlear Bundle Effects on Cochlear Nucleus Activity

The MOC fiber tract projects several collaterals to the CN on its way to the cochlea. Therefore, it would seem as though this system would have the capacity to exert considerable influence on the modulation of physiological activity within the afferent auditory system (e.g., the alteration of spontaneous firing rates of the CN). However, it is interesting to note that electrical stimulation of the MOC bundle has no measurable effect on more than half the fibers of the CN. In about one-third of the CN units there is a decrease in spontaneous activity, while in only a small number of fibers is there an increase in spontaneous activity (Starr and Wernick, 1968).

There is a wide, varied, and complex set of interactions between the MOC bundle and the CN when acoustic stimuli are presented to the ear. The stimulation of the MOC bundle (usually electrical) does in some cases influence how the CN responds to acoustic stimulation. Some fibers are unaffected, others are inhibited, and still others are excited. The details of how these responses are mediated is beyond the scope of this discussion. Moreover, not all studies are in agreement as to the manner in which these responses are mediated, and much of the interpretation is dependent on which part of the CN is being measured and which procedures are involved. The reader interested in this topic is directed to Sahley et al. (1997) for an additional review of this topic.

Medial and Lateral Olivocochlear Bundle Effects on the Auditory Nerve

The discussion of the OCB influences on the AN provides the first example in which there is a central-to-peripheral interaction. This is important in several aspects. One is that there is some control or modulation of the auditory periphery by central auditory structures. Another is that OCB–peripheral interactions demonstrate how the peripheral and central auditory systems must work together. Finally, the OCB–peripheral relationship shows the multidimensionality of the auditory system. New and different types of auditory functions may evolve from this central to peripheral interaction, not only from signals ascending but also from signals descending the auditory pathway. All of this points to the fact that it is shortsighted for either the researcher or the clinician to look only at the periphery or at the central mechanisms to explain the many facets of hearing and hearing disorders.

Perhaps the most cited study on the OCB involves the direct modulation of the AN. Galambos (1956) applied low-level electrical current to the MOC bundle of cats while recording the action potential (AP) from the AN. When current was applied to the MOC region of the floor of the fourth ventricle, the AP that was being recorded decreased in amplitude. This effect was most obvious when the click stimulus used to trigger the AP was presented at low-intensity levels, usually 25 dB sensation level (SL) or less. When the intensity of the acoustic stimulus became moderately intense, there was little or no influence from the activated MOC bundle. This study has been replicated many times with similar results. This classic study was the first one that suggested that the OCB was likely to have an inhibitory action on the AN and, in turn, the afferent auditory pathway. This explanation of the role of the OCB on modulating hearing was popular in the 1950s and 1960s and still remains valid today.

Although many studies subsequent to Galambos' investigation were performed with similar results, one particular study revealed an important twist to this research. In 1987, Folsom and Owsley conducted a study aimed at measuring OCB influences on the AP of the AN in humans. These investigators capitalized on an important principle of OCB stimulation brought forth earlier by Fex (1962, 1963) and Buno (1978). This principle was that the OCB could be stimulated not only by direct electrical current applied to the neural bundle but also by presenting noise (or other acoustic stimulation) to the contralateral ear. This method would allow the use of human subjects for OCB research. Folsum and Owsley (1987), using essentially typical ABR recordings and an ear canal electrode to enhance wave I, showed a decrease in the AP of the AN when noise was applied to the contralateral ear. This study showed similar findings as had been found with electrical stimulation of the OCB in animals (Figure 15.14).

CLINICAL CORRELATE

The work of early investigators such as Fex, Buno, and Folsom on the measurements of the OCB effects on the AN's AP has profound clinical implications. The idea of being able to trigger OCB (mostly MOC) activity by using contralateral acoustic stimulation has provided a new and highly applicable way of testing MOC function. Moreover, the procedure (a modification of the traditional ABR procedure by introducing noise to the contralateral ear) was totally noninvasive and therefore could be used with human subjects and patients. The results of the Folsum and Owsley study (1987) indicated that the procedure works and that its application is similar to classic methods of electrical stimulation to activate the MOC bundle. This study has also paved the way for the development of a clinical procedure to measure OCB (MOC) bundle function.

It is surprising that this procedure or modifications of it have not been further developed. Certainly the same technique using otoacoustic emissions (OAEs) has started to be clinically utilized (see discussion later). A major question is whether or not wave I suppression measurements (in the ABR protocol) are useful clinically. Little data is available in this regard. Could this measurement be as useful as or more useful than OAEs obtained with contralateral masking? Again additional research is needed to answer this question. Perhaps using both OAEs and ABRs to measure OCB influences on the peripheral system may have diagnostic merit. ●

It is anatomically difficult to separate the roles played by the MOC and the LOC systems in the auditory efferent system. Therefore, interpretations of what constitutes LOC versus MOC effects have to be considered with caution. In answering the question of whether or not the LOC can influence the AP of the AN, a review of the work of Gifford and Guinan (1987) may provide some insights. These investigators electrically stimulated the LOC region in the brainstem and showed no effect on the AP. However, Le Prell, Shore, Hughes, and Bledsoe (2003) demonstrated that by disrupting the LOC, the AP amplitude of the AN was

● Figure 15.14

Mean amplitude of the human action potential (AP) of the auditory nerve (wave I of the ABR) with and without contralateral tone stimulation. This AP was obtained for click stimuli at 30 and 40 dB sensation levels (based on data from Folsum and Owsley, 1987).

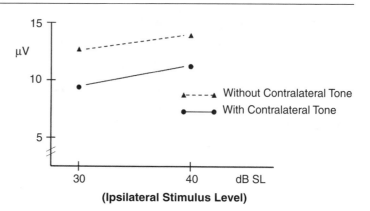

reduced with no effect on its latency. As will be discussed later, the LOC has a pharmacological influence on the AP. Hence, it appears that the LOC may exert an influence on the AP of the AN, but that the effects are likely to be smaller and less robust than those exerted by the MOC.

Returning to a discussion of the MOC bundle, Fex (1962) was one of the first to show the effect of MOC stimulation on the discharge rate of AN fibers. Fex observed that the discharge rate of type I AN fibers to tonal stimuli was most reduced when the tonal stimuli were presented at low levels (5 to 10 dB SL). At slightly higher levels (15 to 25 dB SL) some suppression effects were observed, but the effects were smaller than those noted at the lower levels of tonal stimulation. Interestingly, the latency of the suppressive effect in Fex's study was on the order of 75 to 100 msec following electrical stimulation of the MOC. In general the amount of reduction in firing rate was highly variable, but the results did show a definite influence of level of intensity of acoustic stimulation (Figure 15.15). Other studies have shown similar results, along with considerable variability in firing rate patterns (see Sahley et al., 1997 for review).

Stimulation of the MOC bundle also has an influence on AN frequency tuning (see Guinan and Gifford, 1988a,b,c for detailed coverage). The TCs of the AN afferent fibers are less sharp during MOC stimulation, with reductions in TCs measured via Q10s ranging from less than 10% to around 30%. Although there is considerable variability depending on the species studied, the greatest effects on frequency selectivity are generally in the mid-frequency range, with less influence noted at very low and high frequencies.

● Figure 15.15

The authors' interpretation of the effect of acoustic level on the amount of decrease (in percent) in the firing rate of auditory nerve fibers during electrical stimulation of the medial olivocochlear bundle (see text). At mid or higher intensities, MOC stimulation has essentially no effect on auditory nerve firing rate.

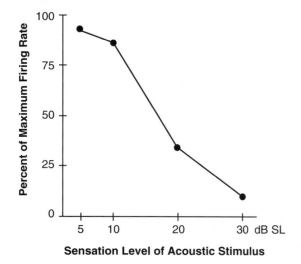

● Medial Olivocochlear Bundle Functions in Noise

In the discussion above, it is clear that either electrical stimulation or noise presented to the contralateral ear will result in a suppression of AN activity via the MOC system. This has been shown both in animals and humans. What follows is a discussion that extends the possible influences of MOC in a most intriguing manner. This discussion will highlight the idea that the MOC bundle can result in an

● **Figure 15.16**

Resultant action potential amplitudes from (a) a signal presented to one ear in quiet, (b) a signal embedded in noise in the same ear, and (c) a signal and noise in the same ear and noise in the contralateral ear, AP = action potential (8th nerve).

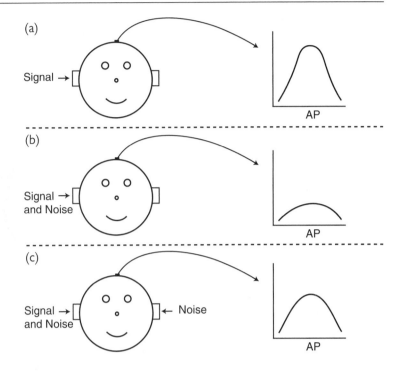

unmasking effect or a release from a masking effect when the stimulus presented to the test ear is imbedded in noise. The discussion that follows will focus on the unmasking of the AP (Desmedt, 1962; Dewson, 1967; Dolan and Nuttall, 1988; Winslow and Sachs, 1988; Kawase and Liberman, 1993). This phenomenon will be explained under three experimental conditions.

Condition one is a situation in which an AP is recorded from the AN in a quiet environment. This could be recorded as wave I of an ABR performed on humans or a near-field recording of the AP in animals. When this is done, the AP will be relatively large (Figure 15.16a). Condition two is similar to condition one, except that a noise is introduced at a given signal-to-noise ratio into the same ear as the response-eliciting stimulus while deriving the AP response. As expected, because of the addition of noise in this condition, the amplitude of the resultant AP will be reduced (Figure 15.16b). Finally, in condition three, an additional noise is delivered to the contralateral ear. The results of testing under this condition are rather startling. Introducing an additional noise to the contralateral ear results in the AP becoming larger than in condition two. This increase in AP amplitude represents a release from masking or an unmasking effect, which is presumed to be related to the fact that the MOC system has been activated by this contralateral noise (Figure 15.16c). In animals, condition three can also be achieved by stimulating the MOC system electrically at the brainstem. This unmasking phenomenon has been associated with the concept that the MOC bundle, when activated, helps hearing in noise. It has also been shown that this unmasking effect increases the dynamic range of the AN fibers from what it would have been in the ipsilateral noise condition (condition two) (Winslow and Sachs, 1987). Similar findings have been noted with pharmacological stimulation of the MOC system (see discussion later in this section).

● Figure 15.17

Dynamic range of an auditory nerve fiber (A) in quiet, (B) in noise, and (C) in noise with stimulation of the medial olivocochlear bundle (see text).

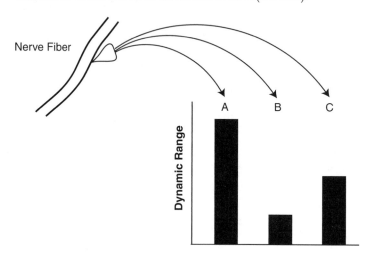

May, Budelis, and Niparko (2004) demonstrated that localization accuracy in noise was decreased when the OCB was sectioned in cats. This poorer localization was only manifested in a background noise situation. This study is another example of a type of unmasking created by function of the MOC bundle.

The unmasking effect by the MOC system in a noise condition works best when the signal-to-noise ratio in the test ear is good; as the signal-to-noise ratio becomes poorer, there is less release from masking (Fex, 1962; Dewson, 1967; Winslow and Sachs, 1987, 1988). Almost by inference, this also means that the acoustic signal in the test ear should be of a moderate intensity. It appears that MOC bundle activation also increases the dynamic range of the AN neurons. When a noise and a signal are presented to the ear, the AN fibers (as well as other fibers) allocate a portion of their dynamic range to the noise, leaving a restricted dynamic range to be devoted to the coding of the signal. Hence, this is not an optimal situation for hearing the signal. The MOC bundle, when activated, apparently increases the dynamic range of the AN so there is more capacity to code the intensity of the signal (see Sahley et al., 1997). To interpret this phenomenon further, the greater the dynamic range, the better the possibility of achieving a good signal-to-noise ratio (Figure 15.17). When individual or groups of fibers have improved signal-to-noise ratios caused by MOC bundle actions, it is likely that a number of hearing functions will improve.

CLINICAL CORRELATE

The concept just put forth in terms of the antimasking ability of the MOC has profound clinical implications. This is typified by a recent study showing that speech perception in noise in one ear was improved by adding noise to the contralateral ear. This enhancement, however, was only noted when the signal-to-noise ratios were +10 to +15 dB (Kumar and Vanaja, 2004). Unfortunately, one cannot make full use of this knowledge at this time because of a number of practical factors that limit the application of this

(continued)

information. Certainly the idea of developing ways to clinically measure whether the MOC bundle is functioning properly in people who have trouble hearing in noise is a key goal.

As will be discussed later, the use of OAEs to measure suppressive effects of the MOC system is a step in the right direction. However, the clinician needs additional measures of MOC system function. A test to measure the release from masking would be an advance. Having said this, one has to ponder the question: How is what we are seeing in this unmasking effect with OAEs different from the effects seen with masking-level differences (MLDs)—or could they both be part of the same mechanism? There are some differences in test administration procedures; e.g., MLDs are tested (clinically) at relatively high levels and at much poorer signal-to-noise ratios. However, MLDs are primarily mediated at the caudal brainstem (SOC) similar to unmasking effects of the MOC for OAEs. A release from masking can be obtained using an MLD paradigm that is essentially the same as that discussed in condition three mentioned above. That is, when a noise and a tone are presented to one ear alone, the perception of the tone is at a much higher level (≈ 10 dB) than when another noise is presented to the contralateral ear (Moore, 2003). Simply adding another noise to the opposite ear (in-phase with the noise and tone in the test ear) causes a release from masking. This procedural and resultant similarity argues for similar mechanisms underlying MOC activation in both the unmasking and MLD effects. So perhaps clinically one does have a procedure that may measure MOC activity. Certainly both the MLD and MOC unmasking effects need to be studied, from both an applied perspective and a basic science point of view. Clinically, it is necessary to determine what kinds of pathologies and what sites of involvement may lead to compromise of MOC unmasking. Would these be similar to abnormalities noted in MLDs and for OAE suppression studies? Would a lesion in the caudal brainstem result in the lack of MOC unmasking as well as an abnormal release from masking assessed with the MLD procedure and little or no suppression assessed with an OAE test? These are key questions that need answering.

Influences of Medial Olivocochlear System Stimulation on the Cochlea

The influences of the MOC bundle on the cochlea occur by way of the efferent terminals located at the lower portion of the OHCs. The endocochlear potential is reduced on the order of 6 to 7% when the MOC bundle is stimulated (Gifford and Guinan, 1987). Despite this decrease, it has been demonstrated repeatedly that MOC bundle stimulation results in an increase in the cochlear microphonic (CM). However, this enhancement seems to be confined to low and mid frequencies (Konishi and Slepian, 1971; see Sahley et al., 1997 for review). This is rather surprising given the extensive data that shows how the AP is suppressed with MOC bundle activity. Interestingly, the summating potential (SP) seems to be suppressed by MOC bundle activation—similar to what is seen at the AN (Fex, 1959).

Medial Olivocochlear Bundle and Otoacoustic Emissions

OAEs have been discussed a number of times in this book, but a discussion of them is again relevant here. This time the amplitude of the OAEs is the dependent measure following manipulation of the MOC system. By recording either transient or distortion product OAEs (TEOAEs or DPOAEs) and then applying noise to the opposite (nontest) ear, a suppression of the OAE amplitude can be measured (Collet, Kemp, Veuillet, Duclaux, Moulin, and Morgon, 1990). When a noise is presented to the contralateral ear, it is common to see a 1- to 4-dB decrease in the amplitude of either type of OAE (Collet et al., 1990; Moulin, Collet, and Duclaux, 1993). The change in amplitude of the OAEs with the presentation of contralateral noise is considered a measure of MOC system suppression (Collet et al., 1990; Berlin, Hood, Cecola, Jackson, and Szabo, 1993).

● Figure 15.18

The effect of varying contralateral noise levels on the amplitude of transient evoked otoacoustic emissions (TEOAEs) in one human subject.

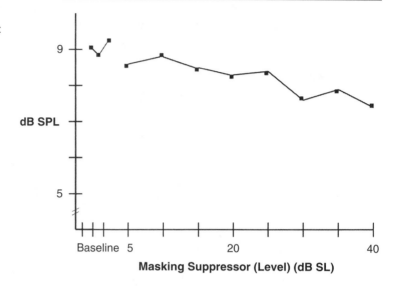

The **OAE suppression** can be best achieved by using broadband noise to activate the MOC system. It also appears that similar effects can be obtained by using narrowband masking at a wide variety of frequency bands. These findings have been interpreted to mean that the MOC system suppression, at least measured by TEOAEs, may not be frequency specific (Berlin et al., 1993). Distortion product OAEs seem to have slightly more frequency specificity in regard to measuring MOC suppression—especially if the narrowband masking noise used as the suppressor is close in frequency to the DPOAE test frequency. Otherwise, broadband contralateral noise used with DPOAEs provides the greatest suppression effect in the 1- to 3-kHz range (Berlin et al., 1993; Moulin, et al., 1993; see also Hood, 2002 for review). The amount of MOC system suppression on OAEs is a function of the intensity level of the noise in the contralateral ear. As the level of noise increases, so does the amount of suppression (Collet et al., 1990; Berlin et al., 1993) (Figure 15.18). The time period for which most suppression takes place is usually in the 8- to 18-msec range (poststimulation), at least for TEOAEs (Berlin et al., 1993).

The effect of intensity level for the OAE stimulus can also influence the amount of suppression. Consistent with the information previously presented in this chapter, suppression effects are greater if the OAE stimulus is less than 65 dB SPL. Higher intensities are more resistant to suppression effects of the MOC bundle (Hood, Hurley, Leonard, and Berlin, 1996).

CLINICAL CORRELATE

Measuring suppression of OAE amplitudes as an index of MOC system function has developed clinically. Various populations have been tested with OAE suppression techniques with similar results. Patients with cochlear hearing losses yield data that are difficult to interpret because most of these individuals, unless the hearing loss is very mild, do not have measurable OAEs. When suppressive effects are measured in subjects with mild hearing loss, the amount of suppression is typically reduced (see Hood, 2002). This finding may

(continued)

or may not be related to dysfunction of the MOC bundle. That is, the reduced suppression might be associated with the fact that the OAE amplitudes in individuals with mild hearing loss are reduced to begin with; hence, proportionately the amount of suppression may be reduced and thus it becomes more difficult to document the effects in these patients.

In patients with acoustic tumors, OAE suppression is often absent or reduced. However, as was the case with patients with cochlear hearing losses, many patients with acoustic tumors do not have measurable OAEs; thus, the suppression effect cannot be measured.

In cases of auditory neuropathy, OAE suppression is also typically absent or reduced. However, much depends on how auditory neuropathy is defined. In many cases of auditory neuropathy, the presence of the hearing loss disallows recording of the OAEs (Starr, Picton, Sininger, Hood, and Berlin, 1996; Hood, 2002). In cases where auditory neuropathy does not affect cochlear hearing sensitivity, OAEs can be utilized and can provide useful clinical information in regard to suppressive influences.

One of the more interesting clinical populations in which to measure OAE suppression includes patients who have undergone vestibular neurectomies. This population is interesting since the efferent fibers course along with the vestibular fibers in the IAM. Therefore, when the vestibular fibers are sectioned during the surgical procedure, the OCB fibers are also severed. Williams, Brooks, and Prasher (1994) studied this population and compared the amount of OAE suppression exhibited by these patients to the amounts shown by normal controls. The normals demonstrated mean suppression values of 27% (of OAE amplitude), while the neurectomy patients showed negligible amounts of suppression. This study is a powerful one in that the site-of-lesion is specific and the findings are consistent with what would be expected. Moreover, the Williams et al. study was performed on humans, making it clinically relevant.

In patients with brainstem lesions, OAE suppression is commonly reduced or absent. The available evidence in this area is based on studies of patients with lesions in the vicinity of the SOC (Prasher, Ryan, and Luxon, 1994).

Finally, children with auditory processing disorders (APDs) often complain of difficulty hearing in noise. In a recent study, children with APD demonstrated reduced OAE suppression effects. This finding raised the following question: In these children is the MOC system compromised, and is this why they have trouble hearing in noise (Muchnik, Ari-Even Roth, Othman-Jebara, Putter-Katz, Shabtai, and Hildesheimer, 2004)?

There are also a number of nonpathological factors that can influence the extent of the suppressive effects in certain populations. For example, it has been shown that age influences OAE suppression (see Hood, 2002 for review). Older adults appear to have less suppression than younger adults. Comparisons of preterm and term infants show mixed results, although the trend seems to be that term infants have greater suppression effects than preterm infants.

Since it appears that the MOC bundle likely plays a role in hearing in noise, it would seem appropriate to test individuals for OAE suppression who have distinct problems hearing in noise—especially if they have normal hearing sensitivity. This may provide clinical insight to the patients' complaints.

Measuring OAE suppression as an indicator of MOC integrity is an attractive procedure—especially to the clinician. However, some concerns surround the use of this measure clinically. It should be acknowledged that OAE suppression values are small. Therefore, even slight variability can disrupt accurate interpretation. Also, a number of normal subjects do not have measurable suppression effects, and some patients with lesions of the brainstem regions at or near the MOC bundle do have suppression effects. Moreover, little data on sensitivity and specificity of this measure is currently available. Therefore, although OAE suppression techniques are fairly well founded and relatively easy to perform, more clinical research is needed before they can be used routinely for clinical assessment of MOC function. ●

● *Neurotransmitters in the Olivocochlear System*

The **neurotransmitters** of the MOC and the LOC systems have become a rather popular area of research. However, there remain some inconsistencies in regard to the neurotransmitters presumed to be present in the MOC versus the LOC. Some of this variance has at its root differences in neurotransmitters among animal species. Other differences could be related to methodological approaches. The following discussion represents the best interpretation of the data as it now stands.

The MOC system has both **acetylcholine** (Ach) and **γ-aminobutyric acid** (GABA), as well as possibly **calcitonin gene-related peptide** (CGRP) (Sahley et al., 1997). The LOC system's neurotransmitters include acetylcholine, **opioids** (enkephalin and dynorphin,) GABA, CGRP, dopamine, and possibly urocortin (Fex and Altschuler, 1981; Sahley et al., 1997; Gil-Loyzaga, Bartolome, Vincent-Torres, and Carricondo, 2000).

Anticholinergic drugs have been shown to compromise MOC bundle function, and profusion in the cochlea with ACh has been shown to increase the CM amplitude (an MOC characteristic). Inhibitory actions have also been attributed to GABA in the MOC bundle (and essentially throughout the auditory system) (see Sahley et al., 1997 for review). It is difficult to state what hearing functions are related to each of the LOC system's neurotransmitters. However, some interesting experiments on the opioids of the LOC may provide some insight as to functions of this system as well as future clinical applications.

In pharmacological experiments conducted by Sahley and associates (1991, 1992, 1995, 1997) an opioid agonist, pentazocine, was used to determine if this neurotransmitter—exclusive to the LOC system—had any effect on the auditory function of the chinchilla (pentazocine maximizes the effects of opioid dynorphins found in the cochlea). After intravenous administration, a marked change in the amplitude of the AP was noted. Approximately a 100% change in the mean amplitude of the AP was observed, with essentially no change in the latency of the response. Interestingly, the increase in amplitude of the AP was graded. The largest effect was noted at threshold, with progressively smaller effects noted at suprathreshold levels. At intensity levels of greater than 20 dB SL, there was no effect of the drug (Figure 15.19). In addition, the amplitude effect was only on the neural response (AP) with no amplitude effect on the CM. Larger changes in amplitude were noted for a 16mg/kg compared to an 8 mg/kg drug administration. This increase in amplitude of the AP with **pentazocine** translated to an improvement of AP thresholds ranging from 6 to 8 dB across normal hearing animals.

In one of the early and important studies using pharmacological methods, Pickles and Comis (1973) applied atropine sulfate to the area immediately above the

● **Figure 15.19**

The change in the action potential amplitude of the auditory nerve as a result of intravenous administration of pentazocine (based on data from Sahley et al., 1991).

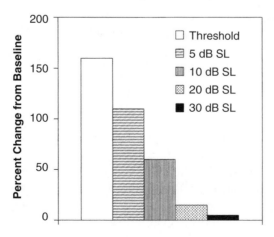

CN. The result was that cats performed poorer on hearing in noise measures following the administration of the pharmacological agent than before the agent was administered. This has been interpreted as evidence showing compromise of the OCB (probably the MOC) precipitated by the effects of the drug. This finding was similar to the release in noise functions mediated by the MOC discussed earlier.

CLINICAL CORRELATE

The pharmacological studies by Sahley and colleagues just mentioned have some strong clinical implications. Granted, this type of research is in its infancy and its clinical application is a bit premature, but these kinds of investigations impact our thinking about hearing and its disorders. One key concept regarding the aforementioned research is that by applying certain drugs to the auditory system of animals, hearing (at least its physiological response) is improved. Even in normal hearing animals, AP thresholds are improved. This is a rather amazing situation. Of course there is much that is currently not known about the effects of drugs on the auditory system and much additional research is needed before the application of drugs is used as a routine intervention strategy. Although pentazocine seems to enhance the evoked potentials (EPs) and improve thresholds, it may negatively affect other aspects of hearing. For example, it is possible that even though EPs are improved, perhaps auditory discrimination abilities may suffer. Therefore, extensive evaluations of pharmacological effects are necessary. In addition, the long- and short-term effects of drugs that may be used need to be investigated. Perhaps the drug may result in hearing improvement initially but may compromise hearing in the long term. All of these kinds of factors (and many others) need to be investigated before routine application of pharmacological agents is undertaken.

In the meantime, pharmacological studies of the hearing system have great potential for increasing our understanding of the function and dysfunction of the auditory system. They may provide a key to help unlock the mysteries of the efferent system and its clinical correlates.

● Olivocochlear Bundle and Protection from High-Intensity Sound

The OCB suppressive effects on the cochlea and AN might cause one to consider that the amount of acoustic energy that is reaching the auditory system is likely reduced when the OCB is activated. If this is the case, and certainly it seems to be, then one could hypothesize that OCB suppression could also be protective against the damaging effects of high-intensity sound. Experiments from Reiter and Liberman (1995) show this to be the case. In guinea pigs, electrical stimulation of the OCB during exposure to high-intensity tonal stimuli resulted in a reduced amount of **temporary threshold shift** (TTS) compared to control conditions. In this study there was a 10 to 15 dB less TTS when the OCB was electrically stimulated compared to when the OCB was not stimulated as well as when the OCB was stimulated but surgically severed. The protection effect noted from OCB stimulation was dependent on the frequency of the high-intensity "damaging" tone. The TTS from high-frequency tones (8 kHz and above) was more affected by OCB activity than the TTS from lower-frequency tones. This frequency dependency may have something to do with slow and fast OCB actions (see Liberman and Kujawa, 1999, for review). The concept of fast versus slow OCB action is important not only for this discussion of acoustic protection but in general. Fast–slow OCB action can be noted when measuring the amount of AP suppression in the AN. At the beginning of electrical stimulation of the OCB, there is a rapid decrease of the AP. After a few more seconds of electrical stimulation, there is a slow, additional decrement in the AP amplitude, which is followed by a leveling off of the AP amplitude until the electrical stimulation stops. At the offset of stimulation, there is a fast increment in the AP, followed by a slow offset that can last for close to 100 seconds after the electrical stimulation has stopped. The slow effects may be related to increased calcium concentrations in the OHCs that slowly increase the thresholds of these cells. These slow effect mechanisms of OCB action seem to manifest more at the higher frequencies, which is where most of the protection from acoustic trauma takes place.

There is also evidence that not only TTS but also **permanent threshold shift** (PTS) can be lessened by normal and stimulated activity of the OCB (see Liberman and Kujawa, 1999 for review). Animals that were exposed to high levels of noise with the OCB cut incurred more hearing loss than control animals (OCB intact) (Kujawa and Liberman, 1997).

A factor in the research on protection from acoustic trauma by the OCB is the acoustic reflex. The acoustic reflex is thought to also provide protection from high-intensity noise. However, in the previously mentioned studies on the protective effects of the OCB on hearing, the stapedius tendons of the experimental animals were cut to ensure that the acoustic reflex did not confound the experimental results. Obviously, there may be some interesting interactions between the OCB suppressive effects and the acoustic reflex as they relate to protection against acoustic trauma. These, however, will need to await further investigation.

SUMMARY

The efferent system has long been a mystery to those studying the structure and function of the auditory system. Although much is still unknown about this part of the auditory system, many significant strides have led to a clearer understanding of the role that the efferent system plays in normal and impaired hearing. In this chapter the efferent system was divided into the rostral and caudal systems. The rostral system involves the auditory cortex, the MGB, the IC, and the LL. It is further composed of a series of loop subsystems that feed back to the brain. Particular functions of the rostral system are not known, but perhaps some effects on inhibitory–excitatory balance in hearing processes are possible. The caudal olivocochlear system is in essence the OCB, which can be divided into medial and lateral systems. The MOC system is primarily a crossed system, while the LOC system is an uncrossed system. The MOC and LOC systems send efferents to the CN, the AN, the IHC afferents, and the OHCs on the contralateral and ipsilateral sides, respectively. The OCB from the brainstem courses with the vestibular nerves through the IAM.

The MOC bundle can be stimulated by electric current or by applying noise (or other acoustic stimuli) to the contralateral ear. When the MOC system is stimulated in quiet, it results in a reduction of the AN's AP and cochlear SP amplitudes. Conversely, MOC stimulation results in an increase in the CM amplitude but a decrease in the measured amplitudes of the OAEs. Of great interest is that in a noisy situation, MOC stimulation will result in an unmasking phenomenon that translates to better hearing in noise. Hence, the ability to measure MOC integrity becomes clinically important for the audiologist. Measuring suppressive effects of OAEs is a step in the right direction, but this procedure needs more research.

Little is known about functions of the LOC. Some indications are that it may also be inhibitory, but again more work needs to be done in this area.

The neurotransmission for the OCB is interesting and complex. The MOC system has both acetylcholine (Ach) and γ-aminobutyric acid (GABA) and probably calcitonin gene-related peptide (CGRP) (Sahley et al., 1997). The LOC system's neurotransmitters include acetylcholine, opioids (enkephalins and dynorphins), GABA, calcitonin gene-related peptide, dopamine, and possibly urocortin. Of interest are studies showing that opioids (of the LOC) may enhance the AP of the AN. These enhancements seem to be relegated to low-intensity levels.

A newly discovered role for the OCB may be tied into protection from high-intensity noise. Studies have shown that the amount of TTS and PTS is greater when the OCB is nonfunctioning. Investigations have also shown that when stimulated, the intact MOC reduces the amount of PTS and TTS to high-intensity sound.

The efferent system remains challenging and a mystery. However, it does appear that we are learning more about this system, and what we are learning is indeed intriguing. Such information may profoundly improve our knowledge of hearing and hearing disorders.

Glossary

Auditory Brainstem Response (ABR)   A series of averaged synchronous neural responses generated by the auditory nerve and brainstem auditory pathway, which usually occurs within the first 10 msec after stimulus onset.

Acetylcholine (Ach)   A neurotransmitter in the auditory system (and other neural systems) that may have differential excitatory/inhibitory effects.

Acoustic Impedance   The resistance to the flow of energy. It is determined by mass, stiffness, and friction of the system.

Acoustic patterns   Changes in frequency, duration, and intensity in a signal or group of signals that retain some overall relationship. In contemporary audiology, some common tests are frequency and duration pattern tests.

Acoustic reflex (AR)   The contraction of the middle ear muscles in response to the presentation of an intense sound.

Acoustic startle reflex (ASR)   A test for hearing sensitivity in which an intense sound will result in an abrupt movement (jump) on the part of the individual or animal. This type of response may be an indication that the structures of hearing underlying this response are functional.

Acoustic tumor or vestibular schwannoma   A tumor that most often arises from the vestibular nerve(s) in the internal auditory meatus and encroaches upon the auditory nerve. These types of tumors are typically benign but are serious in that they are typically located in close proximity to the brainstem.

Adaptation   The decrease in the amplitude of the auditory nerve action potential over the course of stimulus presentation without a coincident change in stimulus characteristics.

Admittance   The amount of sound energy that is admitted into the cochlea from the middle ear.

Agenesis of the corpus callosum   A congenital malformation of the midline structures of the cerebrum disallowing the development of the corpus callosum.

Amplitude-modulated (AM)   Signals in which the amplitude of the stimulus change over time (similar to a warble tone).

Amygdala   A set of subcortical nuclei located just beneath the surface of the front, medial part of the temporal lobe observed as a bulge in the surface called the uncus. It is a component of the limbic system responsible for emotional or affective behaviors and feelings.

Aneurysm   A bulge in an artery usually related to a vascular wall weakness.

Angular Gyrus   A gyrus located in the parietal lobe that is situated posterior and superior to the supramarginal gyrus (in the cortex).

Anterior Commissure   A middle structure located inferiorly to the anterior one-third of the corpus callosum. It connects fibers from the orbital frontal cortex and anterior superior and inferior temporal cortex on one side of the brain to the other.

Anterior inferior cerebellar artery (AICA)   A branch of the basilar artery.

Anterior sulcus of Heschl's gyrus (or temporal sulcus)   The sulcus immediately anterior to Heschl's gyrus in the temporal lobe.

Anterior ventral cochlear nucleus (AVCN)   One of the three major subdivisions of the cochlear nucleus. It is located on the lateral, caudal side of the pons in the human brainstem.

Aspartate   A main excitatory neurotransmitter in several of the nuclei of the auditory system (e.g., cochlear nucleus).

Atherosclerosis   A condition in which fatty material is deposited along the walls of arteries. This fatty material thickens, hardens, and may eventually block the arteries.

Auditory bottleneck   Areas in the central auditory system where most of the auditory information being transmitted from lower to higher areas in the auditory system must pass (e.g, the auditory nerve).

Auditory nerve (AN)   The nerve that connects the cochlea with the brainstem, relaying information about the intensity, frequency, and timing of a sound. It is part of the eighth cranial nerve.

Auditory neuropathy   A relatively newly defined disorder with an uncertain pathophysiology. It presents with a range of hearing symptoms related to dysfunction of the auditory nerve. Also termed auditory desynchrony.

Auditory processing disorder (APD)   A condition in which the affected individual generally has normal hearing but experiences difficulty in understanding and utilizing acoustic information. Also termed central auditory processing disorder (CAPD).

Auditory steady-state responses (ASSRs)   An evoked potential response of the brainstem and cortex to amplitude-modulated (AM) and or frequency-modulated (FM) signals.

Auricle   The cartilaginous portion of the external ear. Also termed the pinna.

Basilar membrane   A structure within the cochlea composed of membranous fibers that is connected to the spiral ligament on the outer wall of the bony cochlea and to the osseous spiral lamina to form the floor of the cochlear duct.

"Belt" or "core" regions   The core area refers to the primary auditory area, which is surrounded by a region (belt) of secondary auditory cortical tissue. The core is located on the superior temporal plane and gyrus.

Binaural interactions Neural processes that require interaction between the two ascending pathways and cortices for normal processing to occur, such as would be needed for normal localization.

Body or trunk The middle one-third of the corpus callosum, anterior to the sulcus, where the somatosensory and motor fibers from the parietal lobe cross the midline of the brain.

Bony labyrinth A bony structure that provides support and protection for the delicate anatomical structures of hearing and balance. Within the bony labyrinth are membranous structures that line the channels and canals of the temporal bone and form the inner ear.

Calcium channels Voltage-dependent cell membrane glycoproteins that are selectively permeable to calcium ions.

Central nucleus One of three main divisions of the inferior colliculus. It is a key auditory region and is an obligatory connection for fibers originating in the lower brainstem structures.

Characteristic frequency (CF) The frequency to which a hair cell (or neuron) best responds. It is generally determined by the hair cell's (or neuron's) lowest threshold or greatest magnitude of response to a tone.

Chloride (Cl-) Chloride ions.

Cisternae Smooth endoplasmic reticula on the lateral wall of the outer hair cells that supports expansion and contraction of the wall.

Cochlear amplifier A response mediated by outer hair cell (OHC) function. It sharpens frequency tuning and enhances basilar membrane movement—especially for low-intensity sounds. Briefly, this is accomplished by the OHCs contracting on upward movement of the basilar membrane and expanding on downward deflection of the membrane. The "cochlear amplifier" response is dependent on metabolic activity.

Cochlear aqueduct (CA) A structure (containing perilymph) that courses from the basal turn of the scala tympani only a few millimeters from the round window to the subarachnoid space near the jugular fossa. It runs parallel to the inferior margin of the internal auditory meatus. The CA allows transfer of cerebral spinal fluid.

Cochlear hearing loss One of the most common forms of hearing loss, which is attributed primarily to damage to the hair cells and membranes of the cochlea.

Cochlear microphonic (CM) An alternating current (AC) sound-evoked cochlear potential. The response of the CM mimics that of the stimulus.

Cochlear nucleus (CN) The initial neural complex in the central auditory nervous system.

Cocktail party effect The inability to hear well in background noise.

Commissure of Probst A neural connection between the two dorsal nuclei of the lateral lemniscus.

Commissure of the inferior colliculus A neural tract connecting the two inferior colliculi.

Commissurotomy The medical term for a surgical procedure in which a commissure is sectioned or severed (e.g., split-brain surgery).

Compound action potential (CAP) An electrical potential that is generated when an array of neurons depolarizes at about the same time, giving rise to a physiological response (e.g., wave I of the ABR, which is generated by the auditory nerve).

Concha The hollowed-out portion of the external ear.

Conduction velocity The speed at which an impulse travels down the axon of a nerve cell.

Corona radiata An area of nerve fibers in the subcortical white matter primarily seen in the parietal lobe that connects and crosses with the internal capsule at its most rostral region.

Corpus callosum (CC) A major part of the brain responsible for connecting the two hemispheres. It transfers information from one hemisphere to the other.

Cortex The gray matter (or nuclei of neurons) composed of six neuronal layers defined by the cell types and arrangement, located on the periphery of the brain.

Cytoarchitecture/cytoarchitectonics Cell pattern and structure of a particular anatomic region of the brain.

Depolarization A process in which an adequate stimulus changes the permeability of the cell membrane allowing for sodium to flow into the cell, changing the potential difference from a large negative value to a positive value.

Dichotic listening A listening condition that requires that two different words, numbers, consonant–vowels (CVs), etc., are presented to the ears simultaneously.

Deiters' cells Supporting cells for the outer hair cells, which rest on the "seats" of these cells.

Dorsal acoustic stria One of the three primary neural outputs from the cochlear nucleus. Output fibers from the dorsal cochlear nucleus run along the dorsal acoustic stria.

Dorsal cochlear nucleus (DCN) One of the three major subdivisions of the cochlear nucleus that can be seen on the posterior aspect of the caudal pons of the human brainstem.

Dorsal nucleus of the lateral lemniscus (DNLL) One of two groups of nuclei of the lateral lemniscus located in the upper pons of the brainstem.

Ductus reunions A small membranous channel that allows endolymph communication between the cochlea and vestibular system.

Ear effect An effect observed during electrophysiological testing in which one ear yields significantly smaller amplitude or latency responses across all electrode sites compared to the other ear for a potential such as the middle latency response (MLR) or the late potentials (N1, P2, P300).

Efferent system The portion of the auditory system that is also referred to as the descending system. It runs from the brain down to the cochlea following a similar pathway as the afferent system.

Electrode effect An effect observed during electrophysiological testing in which major differences in amplitude or latency measures are noted when comparing the responses derived from electrodes placed over analogous sides of the two hemispheres. These comparisons are usually made for the middle latency response (MLR) or late potentials (N1, P2, P300); any differences noted can be indicative of pathology in the hemisphere yielding the reduced amplitude.

Electromotility The longitudinal motion of outer hair cells in response to changes in transmembrane voltage.

Endocochlear potential A resting, electric polarization of the endolymph in the scala media. It is positively charged relative to perilymph in the scala vestibuli and scala tympani.

Endolymph A cochlear fluid (low sodium, high potassium) found in the cochlear duct.

Eustachian tube A tube connecting the middle ear to the nasopharynx that regulates and equalizes pressure in the middle ear space.

Evoked potentials (EP) Averaged electrical responses occurring over a given time period in response to an acoustic stimulus. These can be recorded from the auditory nervous system and, when recordings are made, they often reflect large numbers of fibers firing synchronously (i.e., a number of action potentials).

Excitatory response A neural response that shows increased activity in a neural network.

External auditory meatus The external ear canal.

Extra-axial lesions Lesions affecting the brainstem that arise from outside of a brainstem structure, such as from the cranial nerves.

Feedback loops Neural systems that are found mostly in the efferent system. They represent circuits that connect to another structure and then run back to the structure from which they originated.

Fourth ventricle A large, cerebral spinal fluid–filled recess that is located in the middle of the brainstem.

Free radical A destructive and unstable oxygen atom or a reactive molecule.

Fronto-opercular artery A branch of the middle cerebral artery that supplies the insula.

Fusion An integration of the information from the two ears for comparison, often happening at the superior olivary complex.

Gamma aminobutyric acid (GABA) An inhibitory neurotransmitter found in the auditory system.

Genu The anterior one-third of the corpus callosum and the locus of most of the frontal lobe fibers that cross the midline.

Glutamate An excitatory neurotransmitter found in the inner hair cells, the cochlear nucleus, and the dorsal nucleus of the lateral lemniscus.

Glycine An inhibitory neurotransmitter found in the cochlear nucleus and the ventral nucleus of the lateral lemniscus.

Gray matter Nuclei nerves that are most obvious in the auditory cortex (peripheral surface of the brain) and some subcortical regions of the brain.

Habenula perforata A bony structure of the osseous spiral lamina that has small openings through which auditory nerve fibers pass.

Helicotrema The area at the apex of the cochlea where the scala vestibuli and scala tympani communicate.

Hensen's stripe An eminence protruding downward from the underside of the tectorial membane immediately above the inner hair cells.

Heschl's gyrus A gryus located in the posterior one-fourth to one-third of the superior temporal plane. It is considered to be the primary auditory cortex.

Heterolateral fibers Fibers that connect to different sites in each hemisphere after running through the corpus callosum.

Homolateral fibers Fibers that connect one site in one hemisphere to essentially the same site in the opposite hemisphere via the corpus callosum.

Hyperacusis A condition in which an individual is highly sensitive to loud sounds.

Hyperbilirubinemia A condition that is the result of high bilirubin levels in the blood that can affect the health of the nuclei within the central auditory nervous system.

Incus One of the three ossicles of the middle ear. It is connected to the malleus at the malleo-incudal joint and the stapes at the incudo-stapedial joint.

Inferior colliculus (IC) One of the most recognized structures of the ascending auditory pathway. It is an obligatory synapse for most of the fibers arising from lower auditory nuclei in the brainstem.

Inhibitory response A response that shows suppressed activity in a neural network.

Inner hair cells (IHCs) Flask-shaped sensory cells of the cochlea.

Insula (Island of Reil) The cortex that lies deep in the Sylvian fissure and plays a role in auditory, visceral, motor, vestibular, and somatosensory actions.

Interaural intensity difference (IID) The sensitivity of neurons within the central system to interaural signal intensity differences arriving at the two ears; of the signal mechanisms that serve as the bases for localization and lateralization abilities.

Interaural time difference (ITD) The sensititivty of neurons within the central system to interaural time differences; related to auditory mechanisms that serve as the bases for localization and lateralization abilities.

Interhemispheric transfer time (IHTT) or transcallosal transfer time (TCTT) A measurement made to determine the latency of impulses that travel from one site on the cortex to its counterpart in the other cortex via the corpus callosum.

Intermediate acoustic stria One of the three primary neural outputs from the cochlear nucleus. The posterior ventral cochlear nucleus fibers exit via the intermediate acoustic stria.

Internal auditory artery (also labyrinthine artery) A branch of the basilar artery or anterior inferior cerebellar artery that supplies the inner ear and structures of the internal auditory meatus.

Internal auditory meatus (IAM) A small canal in the temporal bone where the auditory, facial, and vestibular nerves course from the cochlea to the brainstem.

Internal capsule A large white-matter pathway that runs from subcortical areas to the cortex.

Intra-axial lesions Lesions within the brainstem that arise intrinsically within the brainstem strucutres.

Ion channels Mechanically gated chemical channels. In hair cells they are believed to be located near the tips of the stereocilia.

Isthmus or sulcus A region of the corpus callosum located immediately anterior to the splenium where the auditory fibers cross the midline of the brain.

Jugular bulb A bulge in the jugular vein directly beneath the middle ear cavity.

Kernicterus A pathological condition that can evolve if hyperbilirubinemia is not properly managed. This condition often affects structures within the brainstem, resulting in auditory deficits.

Koniocortex A granular appearing cerebral cortex particularly characteristic of sensory areas.

Late potentials (Auditory) evoked potentials commonly termed N1 and P2 that are generated by the primary auditory cortex. These responses are larger than the middle latency response (MLR) and generally occur between 70 and 300 msec.

Lateral lemniscus (LL) A major lateral auditory pathway in the pons and midbrain, formed by fibers of the cochlear nucleus combining with fibers of the superior olivary complex (SOC). It contains both efferent and afferent fibers.

Lateral superior olive (LSO) An important nucleus of the superior olivary complex. Although in some animals it has a characteristic S-shape, in humans it is more circular in appearance.

Lateralization The determination by a subject of the apparent direction of a sound as being either left or right of the frontal-medial plane of the head.

Localization The determination by a subject of the apparent direction and/or distance of a sound source.

Malleus The largest of the middle ear ossicles. This bone attaches to the tympanic membrane at the umbo.

Masking-level difference (MLD) The difference in masked thresholds between binaurally presented signals that are presented in two conditions, an in-phase condition and an out-of-phase condition.

Medial geniculate body A major nucleus located in the postero-inferior thalamus that represents the last in a series of stations along the auditory pathway to the cerebral cortex.

Medial nucleus of the trapezoid body (MNTB) One of the main nuclei of the superior olivary complex located medial to the medial superior olive.

Medial superior olive (MSO) The largest and one of the most important of the superior olivary complex nuclei (in humans).

Membranous labyrinth A membranous, elastic structure that lines the bony labyrinth and houses a number of important auditory structures, including the cochlea or the end organ for hearing and five sensory structures that are part of the vestibular end organ (three semicircular canals, the utricle, and the saccule). The labyrinth is divided into three channels or ducts by the basilar membrane and Reissner's membrane.

Meningioma A slow-growing encapsulated tumor arising from the meninges that often causes damage by exerting pressure upon adjacent structures within the brain.

Middle cerebral artery (MCA) A key branch of the internal carotid artery that supplies auditory structures along the Sylvian fissure.

Middle latency response (MLR) An evoked potential that occurs with latencies ranging from roughly 12 to 75 msec and is generated by the primary auditory cortex, thalamo-cortical pathway, and reticular nuclei of the thalamus.

Mismatched negativity (MMN) An auditory evoked response that is obtained by having subjects listen to and discriminate standard and deviant sounds. The response when it is present occurs at a latency around 200 msec.

Mitochondria An organelle found in the cell body of a neuron that is important for cell metabolism and supplying energy to the cell.

Modiolus A central, cone-shaped, perforated bony core (of the bony cochlea) that encompasses nerve fibers from the hair cells, as well as blood vessels.

Monotonic fibers Neural fibers that respond in a linear fashion to increases in intensities.

Myelin maturation The increase in the amount of myelin within the central nervous system that occurs as the child develops. This increase in myelination occurs throughout the brain but is especially noticeable in the corpus callosum.

Neural arborization The branching of neurons.

Neurotransmitter A chemical substance (such as acetylcholine, glutamate, etc.) that provides for neural communication from one nerve fiber to another at a synaptic junction.

Nonmonotonic fibers Fibers that are characterized by varied dynamic ranges for intensity coding at different intensity levels. These fibers generally decrease their firing rates at high intensities.

Oligdendrocyte myelin A neuron covering similar to the type of myelin found in the brain; it is often referred to as central myelin.

Olivocochlear bundle A neuronal complex in the caudal brainstem that is part of the efferent system that runs from regions around the lateral and medial superior olives to the cochlea. This complex of neural fibers is also known as Rassmussen's bundle.

Opioids A class of neurotransmitters (e.g., enkephlin and dynorphin) that are found primarily in the lateral olivocochlear bundle.

Osseous spiral lamina A shelf-like structure that winds around the modiolus from the base to the apex of the cochlea.

Ossicular chain A series of three interconnected bones within the middle ear that connect the eardrum to the cochlear (oval window). These bones include the malleus, the incus, and the stapes.

Otoacoustic emissions suppression A phenomenon that occurs during otoacoustic emissions testing in which the introduction of noise to the contralateral ear results in the reduction of the amplitude of the measured emission via actions of the (medial) olivocochlear bundle.

Outer hair cells Sensory cells of the cochlea that have motile properties.

Oval window An opening into the cochlea that interacts with the stapes of the middle ear and opens into the scala vestibuli.

P300 or P3 An evoked potential that occurs at a latency of about 300 msec when the subject must listen for and make a cognitive response to infrequently occurring stimuli that are interspersed among a greater number of frequently occurring signals (odd-ball paradigm).

Parabelt region A region of the cortex that runs around the belt region and is located on the surface of the superior temporal gyrus; it has two divisions: the rostral and caudal parabelt regions.

Pars flaccida A region of the tympanic membrane that only has two of the three layers that typically form the tympanic membrane. This reduction in the number of layers in this region of the membrane causes it to be less tense than those parts of the membrane that have three layers (two epithelial layers and a fibrous center layer).

Pars tensa A region of the tympanic membrane that has three layers (two epithelial layers and a fibrous center layer). This region of the tympanic membrane provides a more effective vibratory surface than the pars flaccida.

Pericallosal artery A branch of the anterior cerebral artery that supplies the anterior four-fifths of the corpus callosum.

Perilymph A cochlear fluid (high sodium, low potassium) similar to cerebral spinal fluid found in the scalae tympani and vestibuli.

Phase-locking A clear and fixed relationship between some aspect of the neural response and the phase (or time) of some aspect of the stimulus.

Pinna The cartilaginous portion of the external ear.

Planum parietale A segment of the Sylvian fissure, the posterior ascending ramus, that runs superiorly (rostrally) to the parietal lobe.

Planum temporale A segment of the temporal lobe located on the superior temporal plane immediately posterior to Heschl's gyrus, which has been shown to be sensitive to a variety of types of acoustic stimuli.

Poststimulus time histogram (PSTH) The envelope of a nerve fiber's firing rate over the time period that it fires.

Posterior nucleus (PN) A nucleus in the thalamus that can be responsive to acoustic stimulation.

Posterior sulcus of Heschl's gyrus or Heschl's sulcus The sulcus immediately posterior to Heschl's gyrus.

Posterior ventral cochlear nucleus (PVCN) One of the three major subdivisions of the cochlear nucleus; it is located on the lateral side of the human brainstem.

Potassium (K+) Potassium ions.

Potassium channels Voltage-dependent cell membranes that are selectively permeable to potassium ions.

Precedence effect A phenomenon that occurs during sound localization tasks. It is assessed by presenting pairs of click stimuli through speakers on opposite sides of a sound room with one speaker leading the other in time, resulting in the perception of a sound image in a particular place in the sound field.

Prestin A motor protein found in outer hair cells.

Primary auditory area The main auditory area of the brain, typically considered to be Heschl's gyrus.

Promontory A protrusion of the bony cochlea into the middle ear space that is located between the oval and round windows.

Radiating arterioles Small arteries mostly found in a network on the lateral wall of the cochlea.

Refractory period The time during which an excitable neuron does not respond to a stimulus that would otherwise normally generate a response.

Reissner's membrane (RM) A thin, avascular membrane that forms the roof of the cochlear duct and the floor of the scala vestibuli.

Reticular lamina A structure within the cochlea that forms the ceiling of the sensory and supporting cells of the organ of Corti, through which the cilia of the hair cells protrude.

Reticular nucleus (RN) A nucleus in the thalamus that can be responsive to acoustic stimulation.

Roll-over   A reduction in the firing rate of nerve fibers that may be seen with increases in intensity once the fiber has reached or exceeded its maximal firing rate.

Root entry zone   The area in the low brainstem where the auditory nerve fibers project relatively deeply into the cochlear nucleus.

Rosenthal's canal   A slightly enlarged area where the ganglion cells of the auditory nerve converge.

Rostrum   The segment of the corpus callosum that is located inferior to the genu and that carries fibers of the medial prefrontal cortex as well as fibers that have olfactory functions across the midline.

Round window   An opening into the cochlea that is inferior to the oval window. This window opens into the scala tympani and is covered by a membrane.

Scala media   The duct or scala in the middle of the organ of Corti, which houses the sensory structures for hearing. It is often called the cochlear duct.

Scala tympani   The most inferior of the three ducts in the cochlea.

Scala vestibuli   One of three ducts within the cochlea, this one is located superiorly to the other ducts.

Septum pellucidum   A thin tissue, inferior to the corpus callosum, that divides the lateral ventricles.

Sodium (Na+)   Sodium ions.

Spiral ligament (SL)   A ligment situated between the otic capsule wall and the stria vascularis. It covers the entire lateral wall of the scala media and extends inferiorly into the upper part of the scala tympani, providing support to the organ of Corti.

Splenium   The posterior segment of the corpus callosum where the occipital fibers cross from one visual cortex to the other.

Split-brain   A condition in which the corpus callosum has been surgically sectioned.

Spontaneous firing rate   The neural discharge activity (from a sensory or nerve cell) that is present even in the absence of acoustic stimulation.

Stapedial reflex   The contraction of the stapedius muscle in response to intense sounds.

Stapedius muscle   The muscle (tendon) that connects the posterior wall of the middle ear to the neck of the stapes. It contracts in response to intense sounds.

Stapes   The smallest of the three ossicles of the middle ear. The footplate of the stapes articulates with the oval window, sending mechanical energy into the vestibule of the cochlea.

Stereocilia or cilia   Hair-like projections on the top of hair cells.

Stria vascularis   A highly vascular structure on the lateral wall of the cochlear duct that probably produces endolymph.

Summating potential (SP)   A sound-evoked cochlear potential. The response generally follows the envelope of the stimulus.

Superior colliculus   A nuclei that occupies, along with the inferior colliculus, most of the dorsal aspect of the midbrain. The superior colliculus is primarily a visual nucleus.

Superior olivary complex (SOC)   The next major group of nuclei in the ascending auditory pathway after the cochlear nucleus. It is located within the brainstem and it is the first place in the auditory system where binaural representation (left and right SOCs) from monaural input is noted.

Supramarginal gyrus   The gyrus that surrounds the ascending terminal ramus of the Sylvian fissure and is activated by acoustic stimulation.

Sylvian or lateral fissure   An anatomical demarcation that is the separation between the superior temporal gyrus and the inferior aspect of the frontal and parietal lobes.

Temporal bone   An osseous structure that is part of the cranium and houses a portion of the external ear, as well as the middle ear, the inner ear including the cochlea and the vestibular apparatus, and the seventh and eighth cranial nerves. There are four main parts of the temporal bone, including the squamous, mastoid, petrous, and tympanic portions.

Temporal processing   The encoding of an acoustic stimulus (waveform and/or envelope) over time and an essential component of auditory processing capability. The subprocesses are (1) temporal masking, (2) temporal ordering or sequencing, (3) temporal integration or summation, and (4) temporal resolution or discrimination.

Tensor tympani muscle   The muscle (tendon) connected to the manubrium of the malleus. It contracts in response to intense sounds in animals.

Terminal buttons   Small regions of the auditory nerve fiber where the fibers contact the hair cells.

Thalamo-cortical pathway   The pathway from the medial geniculate body to the cortex.

Tip-links   Small filaments found among the cilia of the hair cells that have several orientations in their connections to other cilia and hair cells. These filaments connect the cilia in such a manner that when the more prominent cilia (i.e., the tallest) are deflected, the other cilia are deflected in a similar direction.

Tonotopic   The sensory or neural-spatial representation of frequency in the cochlea as well as the central auditory structures.

Tragus   A cartilagenous projection of the external ear in front of the external auditory meatus.

Transcallosal auditory pathway (TCAP)   Auditory fibers of the corpus callosum that radiate outward to connect the various auditory areas of the brain.

Transcallosal pathway   A pathway of callosal fibers that connect the two hemispheres.

Transtympanic electrocochleography   Recording of cochlear and auditory nerve potentials using a needle electrode is passed through the tympanic membrane to the promontory or near the round window. This allows enhanced recordings of the action potential (AP) of the auditory nerve but also permits the recording of the cochlear microphonic (CM) and summating potential (SP).

Traveling wave (TW) The movement of the cochlear partition in response to a sound stimulus. This movement of the cochlear partition (and in turn the basilar membrane) is caused by fluid displacement (that travels down the cochlea). The TW is initiated by the in and out movement of the stapes of the oval window.

Tuning curves (TCs) A plot of the intensity needed to make a hair cell (or neurons) fire (above spontaneous rate) across a range of frequencies.

Two-tone inhibition or two-tone suppression The interaction between two tones presented at the same time, such that, a response from an auditory nerve fiber to one tone can be inhibited by the presentation of a second tone if the second tone is within a certain frequency range of the first tone.

Tympanic membrane A thin membrane separating the middle ear from the outer ear. It transmits incoming acoustic energy to mechanical energy in the middle ear. It is also referred to as the eardrum.

Tympanum An air-filled cavity in the temporal bone behind the tympanic membrane (middle ear space).

Vascular loop An artery that loops around nerves in the cerebellopontine angle resulting in symptoms of hearing and balance difficulty and perhaps hemi-facial spasm.

Vein of Labbe A large superficial vein running near the anterior auditory areas of the temporal lobe.

Ventral acoustic stria One of the three primary neural outputs from the cochlear nucleus. The anterior ventral cochlear nucleus fibers leave along the ventral acoustic stria.

Ventral nucleus of the lateral lemniscus (VNLL) One of two groups of nuclei of the lateral lemniscus.

Vertebral-basilar system Vertebral arteries that form the basilar artery that branches and supplies the inner ear, the auditory nerve, and several auditory structures in the brainstem.

Vestibular aqueduct The bony channel that encompasses the endolymphatic duct (ED) and contains endolymph. The ED runs from the postero-lateral wall of the vestibule to the endolymphatic sac, which is located on the posterior surface of the petrous pyramid of the temporal bone.

Volley principle The principle that states that multiple nerve fibers will be recruited to respond to some frequencies (usually high) because a single nerve fiber cannot fire fast enough to code a particular frequency. This recruitment of additional fibers increases the ability of the auditory nerve to code to high frequencies.

Wernicke's area The receptive auditory–language associational cortex that *may* include part of the planum temporale and the postero-superior temporal gyrus.

We acknowledge the use of the following books in helping us with the terms in the Glossary:

Stach's Comprehensive Dictionary of Audiology Illustrated 2nd edition (2003).

Gelfand's Hearing: An Introduction to Psychological and Physiological Acoustics (1998).

References

Aboitiz, F., Ide, A., & Olivares, R. (2003). Corpus callosum morphology in relation to cerebral asymmetries in the postmortem human. In: E. Zaidel & M. Iacoboni (Eds.), *The Parallel Brain: The Cognitive Neuroscience of the Corpus Callosum* (pp. 33–49). Cambridge, MA: MIT Press.

Aboitiz, F., Rodriguez, E., Olivares, R., & Zaidel, E. (1996). Age-related changes in fibre composition of the human corpus callosum: Sex differences. *Neuroreport, 7,* 1761–1764.

Abou-Madi, L., Pontarotti, P., Tramu, G., Cupo, A., & Eybalin, M. (1987). Coexistence of putative neuroactive substances in lateral olivocochlear neurons of rat and guinea pig. *Hearing Research, 30,* 135–146.

Achor, L.J. & Starr, A. (1980). Auditory brain stem responses in the cat. I. Intracranial and extracranial recordings. *Electroencephalography and Clinical Neurophysiology, 48,* 154–173.

Adams, J.C. (1979). Ascending projections to the inferior colliculus. *Journal of Comparative Neurology, 183,* 519–538.

Adams, J.C. (1981). Cytology of the nuclei of the lateral lemniscus. *Anatomy Record, 199,* 6A.

Adams, J.C. (1983). Cytology of periolivary cells and the organization of their projections in the cat. *Journal of Comparative Neurology, 215,* 275–289.

Adams, J.C. & Wenthold, R.J. (1987). Immunostaining of ascending auditory pathways with glycine antiserum. *Abstract from the Association for Research of Otolaryngology, 10,* 63.

Aidan, D., Avan, P., & Bonfils, P. (1999). Auditory screening in neonates by means of transient evoked otoacoustic emissions: A report of 2,842 recordings. *Annals of Otology, Rhinology, and Laryngology, 108,* 525–531.

Aitkin, L.M. (1986). *The Auditory Midbrain: Structure and Function in the Central Auditory Pathway.* Clifton, NJ: Humana Press.

Aitkin, L.M. (1988). Properties of central auditory neurons of cats responding to free-field acoustic stimuli. In: J. Syka & R.B. Masterton (Eds.), *Auditory Pathway Structure and Function* (pp. 335–347). New York: Plenum Press.

Aitkin, L.M. (1990). *The Auditory Cortex: Structure and Functional Bases of Auditory Perception.* London: Chapman and Hall.

Aitkin, L.M., Anderson, D.L., & Brugge, J.F. (1970). Tonotopical organization and discharge characteristics of single neurons in the nuclei of the lateral lemniscus of the cat. *Journal of Neurophysiology, 33,* 421–440.

Aitkin, L.M., Pettigrew, J.D., Calford, M.B., Phillips, S.C., & Wise, L.Z. (1985). Representation of stimulus azimuth by low-frequency neurons in inferior colliculus of the cat. *Journal of Neurophysiology, 53,* 43–59.

Aitkin, L.M. & Webster, W.R. (1971). Tonotopic organization in the medial geniculate body of the cat. *Brain Research, 26,* 402–405.

Aitkin, L.M. & Webster, W.R. (1972). Medial geniculate body in the cat: Organization and responses to tonal stimuli of neurons in ventral division. *Journal of Neurophysiology, 35,* 365–380.

Aitkin, L.M., Webster, W.R., Veale, J.L., & Crosby, D.C. (1975). Inferior colliculus. I. Comparison of response properties of neurons in central, pericentral, and external nuclei of the adult cat. *Journal of Neurophysiology, 38,* 1196–1207.

Alexander, M.P. & Warren R.L. (1988). Localization of callosal auditory pathways: A CT case study. *Neurology, 38,* 802–804.

Altman, J.A. & Kalmykova, I.V. (1986). Role of the dog's auditory cortex in discrimination of sound signals simulating sound source movement. *Hearing Research, 24,* 243–253.

Altschuler, R.A. & Fex, J. (1986). Efferent neurotransmitters. In: R.A. Altschuler, R.P. Bobbin, & D.W. Hoffman (Eds.), *Neurobiology of Hearing: The Cochlea* (pp. 383–396). New York: Raven Press.

Altschuler, R.A., Hoffman, D.W., & Wenthold, R.J. (1986). Neurotransmitters of the cochlea and cochlear nucleus: Immunocytochemical evidence. *American Journal of Otolaryngology, 7,* 100–106.

American National Standards Institute (ANSI). (1989). American national specifications for audiometers. ANSI S3.6-1989. New York: ANSI.

Andersen, R.A., Snyder, R.L., & Merzenich, M.M. (1980). The topographic organization of corticocollicular projections from physiologically identified loci in the AI, AII, and anterior auditory cortical fields of the cat. *Journal of Comparative Neurology, 191,* 479–494.

Anderson, S.D. & Kemp, D.T. (1979). The evoked cochlear mechanical response in laboratory primates. A preliminary report. *Archives of Otorhinolaryngology, 224,* 47–54.

Ando, M. & Takeuchi, S. (1999). Immunological identification of an inward rectifier K+ channel (Kir4.1) in the intermediate cell (melanocyte) of the cochlear stria vascularis of gerbils and rats. *Cell and Tissue Research, 298,* 179–183.

Anson, B.J. & Donaldson, J.A. (1967). *The Surgical Anatomy of the Temporal Bone and Ear.* Philadelphia: W.B. Saunders.

Arslan, E., Santarelli, R., Sparacino, G., & Sella, G. (2000). Compound action potential and cochlear microphonic extracted from electrocochleographic responses to condensation or rarefaction clicks. *Acta Otolaryngologica, 120,* 192–196.

Ashmore, J.F. (1987). A fast motile response in guinea-pig outer hair cells: The cellular basis of the cochlear amplifier. *Journal of Physiology, 388,* 323–347.

Ashmore, J.F. & Brownell, W.E. (1986). Kilohertz movements induced by electrical stimulation in outer hair cells isolated from the guinea-pig cochlea. *Journal of Physiology, 377,* 41.

Assad, J.A., Shepherd, G.M., & Corey, D.P. (1991). Tip-link integrity and mechanical transduction in vertebrate hair cells. *Neuron, 7,* 985–994.

Augustine, J.R. (1985). The insular lobe in primates including humans. *Neurological Research, 7,* 2–10.

Augustine, J.R. (1996). Circuitry and functional aspects of the insular lobe in primates including humans. *Brain Research Reviews, 22,* 229–244.

Axelsson, A. & Ryan, A.F. (2001). Circulation of the inner ear. I. Comparative study of the vascular anatomy in the mammalian cochlea. In: A.F. Jahn & J. Santos-Sacchi (Eds.), *Physiology of the Ear* (2nd ed.) (pp. 301–320). San Diego: Singular Publishing Group.

Baloh, R.W. (1995). Vertebrobasilar insufficiency and stroke. *Otolaryngology-Head and Neck Surgery, 112,* 114–117.

Bamiou, D.E., Musiek, F.E., & Luxon, L.M. (2003). The insula (Island of Reil) and its role in auditory processing: Literature review. *Brain Research Reviews, 42,* 143–154.

Bamiou, D.E., Musiek, F.E., Sisodiya, S.M., Free, S.L., Davies, R.A., Moore, A., van Heyningen, V., & Luxon, L.M. (2004). Deficient auditory interhemispheric transfer in patients with PAX6 mutations. *Annals of Neurology, 56,* 503–509.

Baran, J.A., Musiek, F.E., & Reeves, A.G. (1986). Central auditory function following anterior sectioning of the corpus callosum. *Ear and Hearing, 7,* 359–362.

Barr, M.L. (1972). *The Human Nervous System: An Anatomical Viewpoint.* New York: Harper and Row.

Barsz, K., Benson, P.K., & Walton, J.P. (1998). Gap encoding by inferior collicular neurons is altered by minimal changes in signal envelope. *Hearing Research, 115,* 13–26.

Batra, R. & Fitzpatrick, D.C. (2002). Monaural and binaural processing in the ventral nucleus of the lateral lemniscus: A major source of inhibition to the inferior colliculus. *Hearing Research, 168,* 90–97.

Beitel, R.E. & Kaas, J.H. (1993). Effects of bilateral and unilateral ablation of auditory cortex in cats on the unconditioned head orienting response to acoustic stimuli. *Journal of Neurophysiology, 70,* 351–369.

Bellis, T.J. & Wilber, L.A. (2001). Effects of aging and gender on interhemispheric function. *Journal of Speech, Language and Hearing Research, 44,* 246–263.

Benson, T.E. & Brown, M.C. (2004). Postsynaptic targets of type II auditory nerve fibers in the cochlear nucleus. *Journal of the Association for Research in Otolaryngology, 5,* 111–125.

Berlin, C.I. & Cullen, J.K. (1975). The physical bases of impedance measurements. In: J. Jerger (Ed.), *Handbook of Clinical Impedance Audiometry* (pp. 1–20). Dobbs Ferry, NY: American Electromedics Corporation.

Berlin, C.I., Cullen, J.K., Berlin, H., Tobey, E., & Mouney, D. (1975). Dichotic listening in a patient with presumed lesion of the medial geniculate bodies. Paper presented at the meeting of the Acoustical Society of America, San Francisco.

Berlin, C.I., Hood, L.J., Cecola, R.P., Jackson, D.F., & Szabo, P. (1993). Does type I afferent neuron dysfunction reveal itself through lack of efferent suppression? *Hearing Research, 65,* 40–50.

Berlucchi, G. (1983). Two hemispheres but one brain. *Behavioral Brain Science, 6,* 171–172.

Berlucchi, G. (2003). From the physiology of callosal connections to the understanding of the mind: Still a long way to go. In: E. Zaidel & M. Iacoboni, (Eds.), *The Parallel Brain: The Cognitive Neuroscience of the Corpus Callosum* (pp. 166–169). Cambridge, MA: MIT Press.

Berry, I., Demonet, J.F., Warach, S., Viallard, G., Boulanouar, K., Franconi, J.M., Marc-Vergnes, J.P., Edelman, R., & Manelfe, C. (1995). Activation of association auditory cortex demonstrated with function MRI. *Neuroimage, 2,* 215–219.

Bilecen, D., Seifritz, D., Scheffler, K., Henning, J., & Schulte, A.C. (2002). Amplitopicity of the human auditory cortex: An fMRI study. *Neuroimage, 17,* 710–718.

Binder, J.R., Frost, J.A., Hammeke, T.A., Rao, S.M., & Cox, R.W. (1996). Function of the left planum temporale in auditory and linguistic processing. *Brain, 119,* 1239–1247.

Blauert, J. (1983). *Spatial Hearing. The Psychophysics of Human Sound Localization.* Cambridge, MA: MIT Press.

Boehnke, S.E. & Phillips, D.P. (1999). Azimuthal tuning of human perceptual channels for sound location. *Journal of the Acoustical Society of America, 106,* 1948–1955.

Bohne, B.A. & Harding, G.W. (2000). Degeneration in the cochlea after noise damage: Primary versus secondary events. *American Journal of Otology, 21,* 505–509.

Bookstein, F.L. (2003). Morphometrics for callosal shape studies. In: E. Zaidel & M. Iacoboni, (Eds.), *The Parallel Brain: The Cognitive Neuroscience of the Corpus Callosum* (pp. 75–91). Cambridge, MA: MIT Press.

Borg, E. (1973). On the neuronal organization of the acoustic middle ear reflex: A physiological and anatomical study. *Brain Research, 49,* 101–123.

Boudreau, J.C. & Tsuchitani, C. (1968). Binaural interaction in the cat superior olive S segment. *Journal of Neurophysiology, 31,* 442–454.

Boudreau, J.C. & Tsuchitani, C. (1970). Cat superior olive S-segment cell discharge to tonal stimulation. *Contributions to Sensory Physiology, 4,* 143–213.

Bourk, T.R. (1976). *Electrical responses of neural units in the anteroventral cochlear nucleus of the cat.* Ph.D. dissertation, Cambridge, MA: MIT Press.

Bourk, T.R., Mielcarz, J.P., & Norris, B.E. (1981). Tonotopic organization of the anteroventral cochlear nucleus of the cat. *Hearing Research, 4,* 215–241.

Brask, T. (1978). Extratympanic manometry in man: Clinical and experimental investigations of the acoustic stapedius and tensor tympani contractions in normal subjects and in patients. *Scandinavian Audiology, 7(Suppl.),* 1–199.

Bray, P. & Kemp, D. (1987). An advanced cochlear echo technique suitable for infant screening. *British Journal of Audiology, 21,* 191–204.

Bremer, F., Brihaye, J., & Andre-Balisaux, G. (1956). Physiologie et pathologie du corps calleux. *Arch Suisses de Neurol et de Psychiat, 78,* 31–32.

Brown, A.M., McDowell, B., & Forge, A. (1989). Acoustic distortion products can be used to monitor the effects of chronic gentamicin treatment. *Hearing Research, 42,* 143–156.

Brown, M.C., Berglund, A.M., Kiang, N.Y.S., & Ryugo, D.K. (1988). Central trajectories of type II spiral ganglion neurons. *Journal of Comparative Neurology, 278,* 581–590.

Brown, M.C., de Venecia, R.K., & Guinan, J.J. (2003). Responses of medial olivocochlear neurons. Specifying the central pathways of the medial olivocochlear reflex. *Experimental Brain Research, 153,* 491–498.

Brown, M.C. & Nuttall, A.L. (1984). Efferent control of cochlear inner hair cell responses in the guinea-pig. *Journal of Physiology, 354,* 625–646.

Brown, M.C., Nuttall, A.L., & Masta, R.I. (1983). Intracellular recordings from cochlear inner hair cells: Effects of stimulation of the crossed olivocochlear efferents. *Science, 222,* 69–72.

Brownell, W.E., Bader, C.R., Bertrand, D., & de Ribaupierre, Y. (1985). Evoked mechanical responses of isolated cochlear outer hair cells. *Science, 227,* 194–196.

Brugge, J.F., Anderson D.J., & Aitkin, L.M. (1970). Responses of neurons in the dorsal nucleus of the lateral lemniscus of cat to binaural tonal stimulation. *Journal of Neurophysiology, 33,* 441–458.

Brugge, J.F. & Geisler, C.D. (1978). Auditory mechanisms of the lower brainstem. *Annual Review of Neuroscience, 1,* 363–394.

Brunso-Bechtold, J.K., Thompson, G.C., & Masterton, R.B. (1981). HRP study of the organization of auditory afferents ascending to central nucleus of inferior colliculus in cat. *Journal of Comparative Neurology, 197,* 705–722.

Buno, W. (1978). Auditory nerve fiber activity influenced by contralateral ear sound stimulation. *Experimental Neurology, 59,* 62–74.

Burton, H. & Jones, E.G. (1976). The posterior thalamic region and its cortical projection in New World and Old World monkeys. *Journal of Comparative Neurology, 168,* 249–301.

Buser, P. & Imbert, M. (1992). *Audition.* Cambridge, MA: MIT Press.

Butler, R.A. & Musicant, A.D. (1993). Binaural sound localization: Influence of stimulus frequency and the linkage to convert peak areas. *Hearing Research, 67,* 220–229.

Cable, J., Barkway, C., & Steel, K.P. (1992). Characteristics of stria vascularis melanocytes of viable dominant spotting (Wv/Wv) mouse mutants. *Hearing Research, 64,* 6–20.

Cable, J., Huszar, D., Jaenisch, R., & Steel, K.P. (1994). Effects of mutations at the W locus (c-kit) on inner ear pigmentation and function in the mouse. *Pigment Cell Research, 7,* 17–32.

Caird, D. (1991). Processing in the colliculi. In: R.A. Altschuler, R.P. Bobbin, B.M. Clopton, & D.W. Hoffman (Eds), *Neurobiology of Hearing: The Central Auditory System* (pp. 253–292). New York: Raven Press.

Calford, M.B. (1983). The parcellation of the medial geniculate body of the cat defined by the auditory response properties of single units. *Journal of Neuroscience, 3,* 2350–2364.

Calford, M.B. & Aitkin, L.M. (1983). Ascending projections of the medial geniculate body of the cat: Evidence for multiple parallel auditory pathways through the thalamus. *Journal of Neuroscience, 3,* 2365–2380.

Calford, M.B., Webster, W.R., & Semple, M.M. (1983). Measurement of frequency selectivity of single neurons in the central auditory pathway. *Hearing Research, 11,* 395–401.

Campain, R. & Minckler, J. (1976). A note on the gross configurations of the human auditory cortex. *Brain and Language, 3,* 318–323.

Campbell, A. (1905). *Physiological Studies on Localization of Cerebral Function.* Cambridge: Cambridge University Press.

Campbell, K.C., Larsen, D.L., Meech, R.P., Rybak, L.P., & Hughes, L.F. (2003). Glutathione ester but not glutathione protects against cisplatin-induced ototoxicity in a rat model. *Journal of the American Academy of Audiology, 14,* 124–133.

Campbell, K.C., Meech, R.P., Rybak, L.P., & Hughes, L.F. (2003). The effect of D-methionine on cochlear oxidative state with and without cisplatin administration: Mechanism of otoprotection. *Journal of the American Academy of Audiology, 14,* 144–156.

Cant, N.B. (1992). The cochlear nucleus: Neuronal types and their synaptic organization. In: D.B. Webster, A.N. Popper, & R.R. Fay (Eds.), *The Mammalian Auditory Pathway: Neuroanatomy* (pp. 66–116). New York: Springer-Verlag.

Carhart, R. (1950). The clinical application of bone conduction audiometry. *Archives of Otolaryngology, 51,* 798–808.

Carhart, R. (1957). Clinical determination of abnormal auditory adaptation. *Archives of Otolaryngology, 65,* 32–39.

Carlisle, L., Steel, K., & Forge, A. (1990). Endocochlear potential generation is associated with intercellular communication in the stria vascularis: Structural analysis in the viable dominant spotting mouse mutant. *Cell and Tissue Research, 262,* 329–337.

Carpenter, M.B. & Sutin, J. (1983). *Human Neuroanatomy.* Baltimore: Williams and Wilkins.

Casimiro, M.C., Knollmann, B.C., Ebert, S.N., Vary, J.C., Greene, A.E., Franz, M.R., Grinberg, A., Huang, S.P., & Pfeifer, K. (2001). Targeted disruption of the Kcnq1 gene produces a mouse model of Jervell and Lange-Nielsen syndrome. *Proceedings of the National Academy of Sciences of the United States of America, 98,* 2526–2531.

Caspary, D.M., Havey, D.C., & Faingold, C.L. (1983). Effect of acetylcholine on cochlear nucleus neurons. *Experimental Neurology, 82,* 491–498.

Celesia, G.G. (1976). Organization of auditory cortical areas in man. *Brain, 99,* 403–414.

Cetas, J.S., Price, R.O., Velenovsky, D.S., Crowe, J.J., Sinex, D.G., & McMullen, N.T. (2002). Cell types and response properties of neurons in the ventral division of the medial geniculate body of the rabbit. *Journal of Comparative Neurology, 445,* 78–96.

Chandrasekhar, S.S., Brackmann, D.E., & Devgan, K.K. (1995). Utility of auditory brainstem response audiometry in diagnosis of acoustic neuromas. *American Journal of Otology, 16,* 63–67.

Chang, H.T. (1953). Cortical response to activity of callosal neurons. *Journal of Neurophysiology, 16,* 117–131.

Chermak, G.D. & Musiek, F.E. (1997). *Central Auditory Processing Disorders: New Perspectives.* San Diego: Singular Publishing Group.

Chiappa, K. (1983). *Evoked Potentials in Medicine.* New York: Raven Press.

Clarke, S. (2003). Complexity of human interhemispheric connections. In: E. Zaidel & M. Iacoboni (Eds.), *The Parallel Brain: The Cognitive Neuroscience of the Corpus Callosum* (pp. 47–49). Cambridge, MA: MIT Press.

Clemis, J.D. & Sarno, C.N. (1980). The acoustic reflex latency test: Clinical application. *Laryngoscope, 90,* 601–611.

Code, R.A. & Winer, J.A. (1985). Commissural neurons in layer III of cat primary auditory cortex (AI): Pyramidal and non-pyramidal cell input. *Journal of Comparative Neurology, 242,* 45–510.

Cody, A.R. & Russell, I.J. (1987). The response of hair cells in the basal turn of the guinea-pig cochlea to tones. *Journal of Physiology, 383,* 551–569.

Cody, A.R. & Russell, I.J. (1992). Effects of intense acoustic stimulation on the nonlinear properties of mammalian hair cells. In: A.L. Dancer, D. Henderson, R.J. Salvi, & R.P. Hamernik (Eds.), *Noise-Induced Hearing Loss* (pp. 11–27). St. Louis: Mosby Year Book.

Colavita, F.B., Szeligo, F.V., & Zimmer, S.D. (1974). Temporal discrimination in cats with insular-temporal lesions. *Brain Research, 79,* 153–156.

Collet, L., Kemp, D.T., Veuillet, E., Duclaux, R., Moulin, A., & Morgon, A. (1990). Effect of contralateral auditory stimuli on active cochlear micro-mechanical properties in human subjects. *Hearing Research, 43,* 251–261.

Corey, D.P. & Hudspeth, A.J. (1979). Ionic basis of the receptor potential in a vertebrate hair cell. *Nature, 281,* 675–677.

Corey, D.P. & Hudspeth, A.J. (1983). Kinetics of the receptor current in bullfrog saccular hair cells. *Journal of Neuroscience, 3,* 962–976.

Corina, D.P., Richards, T.L., Serafini, S., Richards, A.L., Steury, K., Abbott, R.D., Echelard, D.R., Maravilla, K.R., & Berninger, V.W. (2001). fMRI auditory language differences between dyslexic and able reading children. *Neuroreport, 12,* 1195–1201.

Covey, E. & Casseday, J.H. (1986). Connectional basis for frequency representation in the nuclei of the lateral lemniscus of the bat Eptesicus fuscus. *Journal of Neuroscience, 6,* 2926–2940.

Cowell, P. & Hugdahl, K. (2000). Individual differences in neurobehavioral measures of laterality and interhemispheric function as measured by dichotic listening. *Developmental Neuropsychology, 18,* 95–112.

Cowell, P.E., Denenberg, V., Boehm, G., Kertesz, A., & Nasrallah, H. (2003). Using the corpus callosum as an effective anatomical probe in the study of schizophrenia. In: E. Zaidel & M. Iacoboni (Eds.), *The Parallel Brain: The Cognitive Neuroscience of the Corpus Callosum* (pp. 433–444). Cambridge, MA: MIT Press.

Cranford, J.L. (1979a). Auditory cortex lesions and interaural intensity and phase-angle discrimination in cats. *Journal of Neurophysiology, 42*, 1518–1526.

Cranford, J.L. (1979b). Detection versus discrimination of brief tones by cats with auditory cortex lesions. *Journal of the Acoustical Society of America, 65*, 1573–1575.

Cranford, J.L., Igarashi, M., & Stramler, J.H. (1976). Effect of auditory neocortex ablation on pitch perception in the cat. *Journal of Neurophysiology, 39*, 143–152.

Cranford, J.L., Stream, R.W., Rye, C.V., & Slade, T.L. (1982). Detection v discrimination of brief-duration tones. Findings in patients with temporal bone damage. *Archives of Otolaryngology, 108*, 350–356.

Crawford, A.C., Evans, M.G., & Fettiplace, R. (1989). Activation and adaptation of transducer currents in turtle hair cells. *Journal of Physiology, 419*, 405–434.

Crouch, J.J. & Schulte, B.A. (1995). Expression of plasma membrane Ca-ATPase in the adult and developing gerbil cochlea. *Hearing Research, 92*, 112–119.

Dallos, P. (1973). *The Auditory Periphery: Biophysics and Physiology.* New York: Academic Press.

Dallos, P. (1975). Cochlear potentials. In: D.D. Towers (Ed.), *The Nervous System.* Vol. 3. *Communication and Its Disorders* (pp. 69–80). New York: Raven Press.

Dallos, P. (1986). Neurobiology of cochlear inner and outer hair cells: Intracellular recordings. *Hearing Research, 22*, 185–198.

Dallos, P. (1992). The active cochlea. *Journal of Neuroscience, 12*, 4575–4585.

Dallos, P. (1996). Overview: Cochlea neurobiology. In: P. Dallos, A.N. Popper, & R.R. Fay (Eds.), *The Cochlea* (pp. 1–42). New York: Springer-Verlag.

Dallos, P., Billone, M.C., Durrant, J.D., Wang, C., & Raynor, S. (1972). Cochlear inner and outer hair cells: Functional differences. *Science, 177*, 356–358.

Dallos, P. & Cheatham, M.A. (1976). Production of cochlear potentials by inner and outer hair cells. *Journal of the Acoustical Society of America, 60*, 510–512.

Dallos, P. & Evans, B.N. (1995). High-frequency motility of outer hair cells and the cochlear amplifier. *Science, 267*, 2006–2009.

Dallos, P. & Fakler, B. (2002). Prestin, a new type of motor protein. *Nature Reviews. Molecular Cell Biology, 3*, 104–111.

Dallos, P. & Harris, D. (1978). Properties of auditory nerve responses in absence of outer hair cells. *Journal of Neurophysiology, 41*, 365–383.

Damasio, H. & Damasio, A. (1979). "Paradoxic" ear extinction in dichotic listening: Possible anatomic significance. *Neurology, 29*, 644–653.

Dankbaar, W.A. (1970). The pattern of stapedial vibration. *Journal of the Acoustical Society of America, 48*, 1021–1022.

Davis, H. (1962). A functional classification of auditory defects. *Annals of Otology, Rhinology, and Laryngology, 71*, 693–704.

Davis, H. (1965). A model for transducer action in the cochlea. *Cold Spring Harbor Symposia on Quantitative Biology, 30*, 181–190.

Davis, J. (1987). Anatomy of the ear. In: R. Stark (Ed.), *Plastic Surgery of the Head and Neck* (pp. 445–462). New York: Churchill Livingstone.

Davis, K.A. (2002). Evidence of a functionally segregated pathway from dorsal cochlear nucleus to inferior colliculus. *Journal of Neurophysiology, 87*, 1824–1835.

DeArmond, S., Fusco, M., & Dewey, M. (1989). *Structure and Function of the Human Brain* (3rd ed.). New York: Oxford University Press.

Deatherage, B.H. & Hirsh, I.J. (1959). Auditory localization of clicks. *Journal of the Acoustical Society of America, 31*, 486–492.

De Boer, E. (1983). No sharpening? A challenge for cochlear mechanics. *Journal of the Acoustical Society of America, 73*, 567–573.

Demeter, S., Rosene, D., & Van Hoesen, G.W. (1990). Fields of origin and pathways of the interhemispheric commissures in the temporal lobe of macaques. *Journal of Comparative Neurology, 302*, 29–53.

de No, R.L. (1937). The sensory endings of the cochlea. *Laryngoscope, 47*, 373–377.

de No, R.L. (1976). Some unresolved problems concerning the cochlear nerve. *Annals of Otology, Rhinology, and Laryngology, 6*(Suppl. 34), 1–28.

de Ribaupierre, F. (1997). Acoustical information processing in the auditory thalamus and cerebral cortex. In: G. Ehret & R. Romand (Eds.), *The Central Auditory System* (pp. 317–398). New York: Oxford University Press.

Derlacki, E.L. (1996). Otoslerosis. In: J.L. Northern (Ed.), *Hearing Disorders* (3rd ed.) (pp. 139–148). Boston: Allyn & Bacon.

Desmedt, J.E. (1962). Auditory-evoked potentials from cochlea to cortex as influenced by activation of the efferent olivocochlear bundle. *Journal of the Acoustical Society of America, 34*, 1478–1496.

Dewson, J.H. (1967). Efferent olivocochlear bundle: Some relationships to noise masking and to stimulus attenuation. *Journal of Neurophysiology, 30*, 817–832.

Diamond, I.T. & Neff, W.D. (1957). Ablation of temporal cortex and discrimination of auditory patterns. *Journal of Neurophysiology, 20*, 300–315.

Dolan, D.F. & Nuttall, A.L. (1988). Masked cochlear whole-nerve response intensity functions altered by electrical stimulation of the crossed olivocochlear bundle. *Journal of the Acoustical Society of America, 83*, 1081–1086.

Don, M., Masuda, A., Nelson, R., & Brackmann, D. (1997). Successful detection of small acoustic tumors using the stacked derived-band auditory brain stem response amplitude. *American Journal of Otology, 18*, 608–621.

Donnelly, K. (1992). *The auditory brainstem response and hydrocephalus.* Ph.D. dissertation. University of Texas, Dallas.

Dublin, W.B. (1974). Cytoarchitecture of the cochlear nuclei: Report of an illustrative case of erythroblastosis. *Archives of Otolaryngology, 100*, 355–359.

Dublin, W.B. (1976). The combined correlated audiohistogram. Incorporation of the superior ventral cochlear nucleus. *Annals of Otology, Rhinology, and Laryngology, 85*, 813–819.

Dublin, W.B. (1986). Central auditory pathology. *Otolaryngology-Head and Neck Surgery, 95*, 363–424.

Dunlop, C.W., Itzkowic, D.J., & Aitkin, L.M. (1969). Tone-burst response patterns of single units in the cat medial geniculate body. *Brain Research, 16*, 149–164.

Durrant, J.D. & Ferraro, J.A. (1999). Short latency auditory evoked potentials: Electrocochleography and auditory brainstem response. In: F.E. Musiek & W.F. Rintelmann (Eds.), *Contemporary Perspectives in Hearing Assessment* (pp. 197–242). Boston: Allyn & Bacon.

Durrant, J.D., Wang, J., Ding, D.L., & Salvi, R.J. (1998). Are inner or outer hair cells the source of summating potentials recorded from the round window? *Journal of the Acoustical Society of America, 104*, 370–377.

Duvall, A.J. & Rhodes, V.T. (1967). Reissner's membrane. An ultrastructural study. *Archives of Otolaryngology, 86*, 143–151.

Edeline, J.M. (2003). The thalamo-cortical auditory receptive fields: Regulation by the states of vigilance, learning and the neuromodulatory systems. *Experimental Brain Research, 153*, 554–572.

Efron, R., Crandall, P.H., Koss, B., Divenyi, P.L., & Yund, E.W. (1983). Central auditory processing. III. The "cocktail party" effect and anterior temporal lobectomy. *Brain Language, 19*, 254–263.

Efron, R., Yund, E.W., Nichols, D., & Crandall, P.H. (1985). An ear asymmetry for gap detection following anterior temporal lobectomy. *Neuropsychologia, 23*, 43–50.

Eggermont, J.J. (1993). Wiener and Volterra analyses applied to the auditory system. *Hearing Research, 66*, 177–201.

Eggermont, J.J. & Odenthal, D.W. (1974). Electrophysiological investigation of the human cochlea. Recruitment, masking and adaptation. *Audiology, 13*, 1–22.

Ehret, G. (1997). The auditory midbrain, a "shunting-yard" of acoustical information processing. In: G. Ehret & R. Romand (Eds.), *The Central Auditory System* (pp. 259–316). New York: Oxford University Press.

Ehret, G. & Merzenich, M.M. (1988). Neuronal discharge rate is unsuitable for encoding sound intensity at the inferior-colliculus level. *Hearing Research, 35*, 1–7.

Ehret, G. & Romand, R. (Eds.), (1997). *The Central Auditory System*. New York: Oxford University Press.

El-Badry, M. (2003). *Physiological and anatomical changes following demyelination of the auditory nerve in chinchillas*. Ph.D. dissertation. University of Buffalo, Buffalo, NY.

Elliot, L. (1994). Functional brain imaging and hearing. *Journal of the Acoustical Society of America, 96*, 1397–1408.

Engstrom, H. (1960). The cortolymph, the third lymph of the inner ear. *Acta Morphologica Neerlands Scandinavica, 3*, 195–204.

Erulkar, S.D. (1959). The responses of single units of the inferior colliculus of the cat to acoustic stimulation. *Proceedings of the Royal Society of London Series B Biological Sciences, 150*, 336–355.

Eslinger, P. & Darnasio, H. (1988). Anatomical correlates of paradoxic ear extinction. In: K. Hugdahl (Ed.), *Handbook of Dichotic Listening: Theories, Methods, and Research* (pp. 139–160). New York: John Wiley & Sons.

Estrem, S.A., Babin, R.W., Ryu, J.H., & Moore, K.C. (1981). Cisdiamminedichloroplatinum (II) ototoxicity in the guinea pig. *Otolaryngology-Head and Neck Surgery, 89*, 638–745.

Evans, E.F. (1972). The frequency response and other properties of single fibers in the guinea-pig cochlear nerve. *Journal of Physiology, 226*, 263–287.

Evans, E.F. (1974). Neural processes for the detection of acoustic patterns and for sound localization. In: F. Schmitt & F. Worden (Eds.), *Neurosciences. Third Study Program* (pp. 134–145). Cambridge, MA: MIT Press.

Evans, E.F. (1978). Place and time coding of frequency in the peripheral auditory system: Some physiological pros and cons. *Audiology, 17*, 369–420.

Eybalin, M. (1993). Neurotransmitters and neuromodulators of the mammalian cochlea. *Physiological Reviews, 73*, 309–373.

Eybalin, M., Charachon, G., & Renard, N. (1993). Dopaminergic lateral efferent innervation of the guinea-pig cochlea: Immunoelectron microscopy of catecholamine-synthesizing enzymes and effect of 6-hydroxydopamine. *Neuroscience, 54*, 133–142.

Fatterpekar, G.M., Mukherji, S.K., Alley, J., Lin, Y., & Castillo, M. (2000). Hypoplasia of the bony canal for the cochlear nerve in patients with congenital sensorineural hearing loss: Initial observations. *Radiology, 215*, 243–246.

Faure, P.A., Fremouw, T., Casseday, J.H., & Covey, E. (2003). Temporal masking reveals properties of sound-evoked inhibition in duration-tuned neurons of the inferior colliculus. *Journal of Neuroscience, 23*, 3052–3065.

Fausti, S.A., Henry, J.A., Schaffer, H.I., Olson, D.J., Frey, R.H., & Bagby, G.C. (1993). High-frequency monitoring for early detection of cisplatin ototoxicity. *Archives of Otolaryngology-Head and Neck Surgery, 119*, 661–666.

Fawcett, D.W. (1994). *A Textbook of Histology* (12th ed.). New York: Chapman & Hall.

Fechner, F.P., Nadol, J.B., Burgess, B.J., & Brown, M.C. (2001). Innervation of supporting cells in the apical turns of the guinea pig cochlea is from type II afferent fibers. *Journal of Comparative Neurology, 429*, 289–298.

Ferraro, J.A., Arenberg, I.K., & Hassanein, R.S. (1985). Electrocochleography and symptoms of inner ear dysfunction. *Archives of Otolaryngology, 111*, 71–74.

Ferraro, J.A., Blackwell, W.L., Mediavilla, S.J., & Thedinger, B.S. (1994a). Normal summating potential to tone bursts recorded from the tympanic membrane in humans. *Journal of the American Academy of Audiology, 5*, 17–23.

Ferraro, J.A., Thedinger, B.S., Mediavilla, S.J., & Blackwell, W.L. (1994b). Human summating potential to tone bursts: Observations on tympanic membrane versus promontory recordings in the same patients. *Journal of the American Academy of Audiology, 5*, 24–29.

Fettiplace, R., Ricci, A.J., & Hackney, C.M. (2001). Clues to the cochlear amplifier to the turtle ear. *Trends in Neurosciences, 24*, 169–175.

Fex, J. (1959). Augmentation of cochlear microphonic by stimulation of efferent fibres to the cochlea: Preliminary report. *Acta Otolaryngologica, 50*(Suppl. 189), 540–541.

Fex, J. (1962). Auditory activity in centrifugal and centripetal cochlear fibres in cat. A study of a feedback system. *Acta Physiologica Scandinavica, 55*, 1–68.

Fex, J. (1963). Crossed cochlear efferents activated by sound through both ears. *Acta Physiologica Scandinavica, 59*, 41.

Fex, J. & Altschuler, R.A. (1981). Enkephalin-like immunoreactivity of olivocochlear nerve fibers in cochlea of guinea pig and cat. *Proceedings of the National Academy of Sciences of the United States of America, 78*, 1255–1259.

Fex, J. & Altschuler, R.A. (1986). Neurotransmitter-related immunocytochemistry of the organ of Corti. *Hearing Research, 22*, 249–263.

Fifer, R.C. (1993). Insular stroke causing unilateral auditory processing disorder: Case report. *Journal of the American Academy of Audiology, 4*, 364–369.

Fisch, U. (1974). Facial paralysis and fractures of the petrous bone. *Laryngoscope, 84,* 2141–2154.

Fischer, C., Bognar, L., Turjman, F., & Lapras, C. (1995). Auditory evoked potentials in a patient with a unilateral lesion of the inferior colliculus and medial geniculate body. *Electroencephalography and Clinical Neurophysiology, 96,* 261–267.

Fitzgerald, R. (2002). Inhibition in the brain plays a key role in sound localization. *Physics Today, Oct.,* 13–14.

Flock, A., Bretscher, A., & Weber, K. (1982). Immunohistochemical localization of several cytoskeletal proteins in inner ear sensory and supporting cells. *Hearing Research, 7,* 75–89.

Flock, A. & Flock, B. (2003). Micro-lesions in Reissner's membrane evoked by acute hydrops. *Audiology and Neuro-otology, 8,* 59–69.

Folsum, R.C. & Owsley, R.M. (1987). N1 action potentials in humans. Influence of simultaneous contralateral stimulation. *Acta Otolaryngologica, 103,* 262–265.

Forbes, B.F. & Moskowitz, N. (1977). Cortico-cortical connections of the superior temporal gyrus in the squirrel monkey. *Brain Research, 136,* 547–552.

Forge, A. (1991). Structural features of the lateral walls in mammalian cochlear outer hair cells. *Cell and Tissue Research, 265,* 473–483.

Forge, A., Zajic, G., Li, L., Nevill, G., & Schacht, J. (1993). Structural variability of the subsurface cisternae in intact, isolated outer hair cells shown by florescent labelling of intracellular membranes and freeze-fracture. *Hearing Research, 64,* 175–183.

Frank, G., Hemmert, W., & Gummer, A.W. (1999). Limiting dynamics of high-frequency electromechanical transduction of outer hair cells. *Proceedings of the National Academy of Sciences of the United States of America, 96,* 4420–4425.

Fuchs, P.A. & Mann, A.C. (1985). Voltage oscillations and ionic currents in hair cells isolated from the apex of the chick's cochlea. *Journal of Physiology (London), 371,* 31.

Furst, M., Aharonson, V., Levine, R.A., Fullerton, B.C., Tadmor, R., Pratt, H., Polyakov, A., & Korczyn, A. (2000). Sound lateralization and interaural discrimination. Effects of brainstem infarcts and multiple sclerosis lesions. *Hearing Research, 143,* 29–42.

Furuta, S., Ogura, M., Higano, S., Takahashi, S., & Kawase, T. (2000). Reduced size of the cochlear branch of the vestibulocochlear nerve in a child with sensorineural hearing loss. *American Journal of Neuroradiology, 21,* 328–330.

Gadea, M., Marti-Bonmati, L., Arana, E., Espert, R., Casanova, V., & Pascual, A. (2002). Dichotic listening and corpus callosum magnetic resonance imaging in relapsing-remitting multiple sclerosis with emphasis on sex differences. *Neuropsychology, 16,* 275–281.

Galaburda, A.M. & Eidelberg, D. (1982). Symmetry and asymmetry in the human posterior thalamus, II. Thalamic lesions in a case of developmental dyslexia. *Archives of Neurology, 39,* 333–336.

Galaburda, A.M., Sherman, G.F., Rosen, G.D., Aboitiz, F., & Geschwind, N. (1985). Developmental dyslexia: Four consecutive patients with cortical anomalies. *Journal of Neurology, 18,* 222–233.

Galambos, R. (1956). Suppression of auditory nerve activity by stimulation of efferent fibers to the cochlea. *Journal of Neurophysiology, 19,* 424–437.

Galambos, R., Schwartzkopff, J., & Rupert, A. (1959). Microelectrode study of superior olivary nuclei. *American Journal of Physiology, 197,* 527–536.

Gazzaniga, M.S., Bogen, J.E., & Sperry R.W. (1962). Some functional effects of sectioning the cerebral commissures in man. *Proceedings of the National Academy of Sciences of the United States of America, 48,* 1765–1769.

Gazzaniga, M.S. & Hillyard, S.A. (1973). Attention mechanisms following brain bisection. In: S. Kornblum (Ed.), *Attention and Performance* (Vol. IV) (pp. 221–238). New York: Academic Press.

Geisler, C.D. (1998). *From Sound to Synapse: Physiology of the Mammalian Ear.* New York: Oxford University Press.

Gelfand, S.A. (1997). *Essentials of Audiology.* New York: Thieme Medical Publishers.

Gelfand, S.A. (1998). *Hearing: An Introduction to Psychological and Physiological Acoustics* (3rd ed.). New York: Marcel Dekker.

Gelfand, S.A. (2001). *Essentials of Audiology* (2nd ed.). New York: Thieme Medical Publishers.

Geniec, P. & Morest, D.K. (1971). The neuronal architecture of the human posterior collicullus. A study with the Golgi method. *Acta Otolaryngologica, 295(Suppl.),* 1–33.

Geschwind, N. & Levitsky, W. (1968). Human brain: Left-right asymmetries in temporal speech regions. *Science, 161,* 186–187.

Giebink, G.S. (1988). Epidemiology of otitis media with effusion. In: F.H. Bess (Ed.), *Hearing Impairment in Children* (pp. 75–90). Parkton, MD: York Press.

Giedd, J.N., Blumenthal, J., Jeffries, N.O., Castellanos, F.X., Liu, H., Zijdenbos, A., Paus, T., Evans, A.C., & Rapoport J.L. (1999). Brain development during childhood and adolescence: A longitudinal MRI study. *Nature Neuroscience, 2,* 861–863.

Giedd, J.N., Rumsey, J.M., Castellanos, F.X., Rajapakse, J.C., Kaysen, D., Vaituzis, A.C., Vauss, Y.C., Hamburger, S.D., & Rapoport J.L. (1996). A quantitative MRI study of the corpus callosum in children and adolescents. *Developmental Brain Research, 91,* 274–280.

Gifford, M.L. & Guinan, J.J. (1987). Effects of electrical stimulation of medial olivocochlear neurons on ipsilateral and contralateral cochlear responses. *Hearing Research, 29,* 179–194.

Gillespie, P.G. (1995). Molecular machinery of auditory and vestibular transduction. *Current Opinions in Neurobiology, 5,* 449–455.

Gil-Loyzaga, P., Bartolome, V., Vicente-Torres, A., & Carricondo, F. (2000). Serotonergic innervation of the organ of Corti. *Acta Otolaryngologica, 120,* 128–132.

Giraud, A.L. & Price, C.J. (2001). The constraints functional neuroimaging places on classic models of auditory word processing. *Journal of Cognitive Neuroscience, 13,* 754–765.

Glasscock, M.E., Haynes, D.S., Storper, I.S., & Bohrer, P.S. (1997). Surgery for chronic ear disease. In: G.B. Hughes & M.L. Pensak (Eds.), *Clinical Otology* (2nd ed.) (pp. 215–232). New York: Thieme Medical Publishers.

Glassman, R.B., Forgus, M.W., Goodman, J.E., & Glassman, H.N. (1975). Somesthetic effects of damage to cats' ventrobasal complex, medial lemniscus or posterior group. *Experimental Neurology, 48,* 460–492.

Glendenning, K.K., Baker, B.N., Hutson, K.A., & Masterton, R.B. (1992). Acoustic chiasm. V. Inhibition and excitation in the ipsilateral and contralateral projections of LSO. *Journal of Comparative Neurology, 319,* 100–122.

Glendenning, K.K., Brunso-Bechtold, J.K., Thompson, G.C., & Masterton, R.B. (1981). Ascending auditory afferents to the nuclei of the lateral lemniscus. *Journal of Comparative Neurology, 197,* 673–703.

Glendenning, K.K., Hutson, K.A., Nudo, R.J., & Masterton, R.B. (1985). Acoustic chiasm. II. Anatomical basis of binaurality in lateral superior olive of cat. *Journal of Comparative Neurology, 232,* 261–285.

Glendenning, K.K. & Masterton, R.B. (1983). Acoustic chiasm: Efferent projections of the lateral superior olive. *Journal of Neuroscience, 3,* 1521–1537.

Godfrey, D., Beranek, K., Carlson, L., Parli, J., Dunn, J., & Ross, C. (1990). Contribution of centrifugal innervation to choline acetyltransferase activity in the cat cochlear nucleus. *Hearing Research, 49,* 259–280.

Gold, T. (1948). Hearing. II. The physical basis of the action of the cochlea. *Proceedings of the Royal Society of London Series B Biological Sciences, 135,* 492–498.

Goldberg, J.M. & Brown, P.B. (1968). Functional organization of the dog superior olivary complex: An anatomical and electrophysiological study. *Journal of Neurophysiology, 31,* 639–656.

Goldberg, J.M. & Brown, P.B. (1969). Response of binaural neurons of dog superior olivary complex to dichotic tonal stimuli: Some physiological mechanisms of sound localization. *Journal of Neurophysiology, 32,* 613–636.

Goldstein, M. & Kiang, N.Y.S. (1958). Synchrony of neural activity in electric responses evoked by transient acoustic stimuli. *Journal of the Acoustical Society of America, 30,* 107–114.

Gollegly, K.M. & Musiek, F.E. (1993). Auditory dysfunction in patient with subcortical and insular involvement. *Seminars in Hearing, 14,* 245–253.

Gonchar, Y.A., Johnson, P.B., & Weinberg, R.J. (1995). GABA-immunopositive neurons in rat neocortex with contralateral projections to S-I. *Brain Research, 697,* 27–34.

Goodhill, V. (1979). *Ear Diseases, Deafness, and Dizziness.* New York: Harper and Row.

Gorga, M.P., Neely, S.T., Bergman, B., Beauchaine, K.L., Kaminski, J.R., Peters, J., & Jesteadt, W. (1993). Otoacoustic emissions from normal-hearing and hearing-impaired subjects: Distortion product responses. *Journal of the Acoustical Society of America, 93,* 2050–2060.

Gorga, M.P., Stover, L., Neely, S.T., & Montoya, D. (1996). The use of cumulative distributions to determine critical values and levels of confidence for clinical distortion product otoacoustic emission measurements. *Journal of the Acoustical Society of America, 100,* 968–1977.

Grafstein, B. (1963). Postnatal development of the transcallosal evoked response in cerebral cortex of the cat. *Journal of Neurophysiology, 26,* 79–99.

Green, D. (1985). Temporal factors in psychoacoustics. In: A. Michelsen (Ed.), *Time Resolution in Auditory Systems* (pp. 304–318). New York: Springer-Verlag.

Griffiths, T.D., Bates, D., Rees, A., Witton, C., Gholkar, A., & Green, G.G. (1997). Sound movement detection deficit due to a brainstem lesion. *Journal of Neurology, Neurosurgery and Psychiatry, 62,* 522–526.

Groff, J.A. & Liberman, M.C. (2003). Modulation of cochlear afferent response by the lateral olivocochlear system: Activation via electrical stimulation of the inferior colliculus. *Journal of Neurophysiology, 90,* 3178–3200.

Guinan, J.J. & Gifford, M.L. (1988a). Effects of electrical stimulation of efferent olivocochlear neurons on cat auditory-nerve fibers. I. Rate-level functions. *Hearing Research, 33,* 97–113.

Guinan, J.J. & Gifford, M.L. (1988b). Effects of electrical stimulation of efferent olivocochlear neurons on cat auditory-nerve fibers. II. Spontaneous rate. *Hearing Research, 33,* 115–127.

Guinan, J.J. & Gifford, M.L. (1988c). Effects of electrical stimulation of efferent olivocochlear neurons on cat auditory-nerve fibers. III. Tuning curves and thresholds at CF. *Hearing Research, 37,* 29–45.

Guinan, J.J., Guinan, S., & Norris, B. (1972). Single auditory units in the superior olivary complex. I. Responses of sounds and classifications based on physiological properties. *International Journal of Neuroscience, 4,* 101–120.

Guinan, J.J. & Peake, W.T. (1967). Middle-ear characteristics of anesthetized cats. *Journal of the Acoustical Society of America, 41,* 1237–1261.

Guinan, J.J., Warr, W.B., & Norris, B.E. (1983). Differential olivocochlear projections from lateral versus medial zones of the superior olivary complex. *Journal of Comparative Neurology, 221,* 358–370.

Gulya, A.J. (1997). Anatomy and embryology of the ear. In: G.B. Hughes & M.L. Pensak (Eds.), *Clinical Otology* (2nd ed.) (pp. 3–34). New York: Thieme Medical Publishers.

Gunnarson, A.D. & Finitzo, T. (1991). Conductive hearing loss during infancy: Effects on later auditory brainstem electrophysiology. *Journal of Speech and Hearing Research, 34,* 1207–1215.

Habib, M., Daquin, G., Milandre, L., Royere, M.L., Rey, M., Lanteri, A., Salamon, G., & Khalil, R. (1995). Mutism and auditory agnosia due to bilateral insular damage: Role of the insula in human communication. *Neuropsychologia, 3,* 327–339.

Hackett, T.A., Preuss, T.M., & Kaas, J.H. (2001). Architectonic identification of the core region in auditory cortex of macaques, chimpanzees, and humans. *Journal of Comparative Neurology, 441,* 197–222.

Hackett, T.A., Stepniewska, I., & Kaas, J.H. (1998). Thalamocortical connections of the parabelt auditory cortex in Macaque monkeys. *Journal of Comparative Neurology, 400,* 271–286.

Hall, J.W. (1985). The acoustic reflex in central auditory dysfunction. In: M.L. Pinheiro, & F.E. Musiek (Eds.), *Assessment of Central Auditory Dysfunction: Foundations and Clinical Correlates* (pp. 103–130). Baltimore: Williams and Wilkins.

Hall, J.W. (1992). *Handbook of Auditory Evoked Responses.* Boston: Allyn & Bacon.

Halipike, C.S. & Rawdon-Smith, A.E. (1937). The Wever-Bray phenomenon: Origin of the cochlear effect. *Annals of Otology, 46,* 976–990.

Hanekom, J.J. & Kruger, J.J. (2001). A model of frequency discrimination with optimal processing of auditory nerve spike intervals. *Hearing Research, 151,* 188–204.

Harada, J., Aoyagi, M., Suzuki, T., Kiren, T., & Koike, Y. (1994). A study on the phase spectral analysis of middle latency responses and 40-Hz event-related potential in central nervous system disorders. *Acta Otolarynologica, 511(Suppl.),* 34–39.

Harford, E.R. (1975). Tympanometry. In: J. Jerger (Ed.), *Handbook of Clinical Impedance Audiometry* (pp. 47–70). Dobbs Ferry, NY: American Electromedics Corporation.

Harris, F.P. (1990). Distortion-product otoacoustic emissions in humans with high frequency sensorineural hearing loss. *Journal of Speech and Hearing Research, 33,* 594–600.

Harris, F.P. & Probst, R. (1997). Otoacoustic emissions and audiometric outcomes. In: M.S. Robinette & T.J. Glattke (Eds.), *Otoacoustic Emissions: Clinical Applications* (pp. 151–180). New York: Thieme Medical Publishers.

Harrison, J., Buchwald, J., & Kaga, K. (1986). Cat P300 present after primary auditory cortex ablation. *Electroencephalography and Clinical Neurophysiology, 63,* 180–187.

Harrison, J.M. & Howe, M.E. (1974). Anatomy of the descending auditory system (mammalian). In: W.D. Keidel & W.D. Neff (Eds.), *Handbook of Sensory Physiology* (Vol. 5) (pp. 363–388). New York: Springer-Verlag.

Harrison, R.V. (1981). Rate-versus-intensity functions in related AP responses in normal and pathological guinea pig and human cochleas. *Journal of the Acoustical Society of America, 70*, 1036–1044.

Harrison, R.V. (2001). The physiology of the cochlear nerve. In: A.F. Jahn & J. Santos-Sacchi (Eds.), *Physiology of the Ear* (2nd ed.) (pp. 549–573). San Diego: Singular Publishing Group.

Harrison, R.V. & Mount, R.J. (2001). The sensory epithelium of the normal and pathological cochlea. In: A.F. Jahn & J. Santos-Sacchi (Eds.), *Physiology of the Ear* (2nd ed.) (pp. 285–300). San Diego: Singular Publishing Group.

Hashikawa, T. & Kawamura, K. (1983). Retrograde labeling of ascending and descending neurons in the inferior colliculus. A fluorescent double labelling study in the cat. *Experimental Brain Research, 49*, 457–561.

Hawkins, J.E. (1976). Drug ototoxicity: In: W.D. Keidel & W.D. Neff (Eds.), *Handbook of Sensory Physiology* (pp. 707–748). New York: Springer-Verlag.

Hawkins, J.E., Beger, V., & Aran, J.M. (1967). Antibiotic insults to Corti's organ. In: A.B. Graham (Ed.), *Sensorineural Hearing Processes and Disorders.* (pp. 411–425). Boston: Little, Brown and Company.

He, D.Z., Beisel, K.W., Chen, L., Ding, D.L., Jia, S., Fritzsch, B., & Salvi, R. (2003). Chick hair cells do not exhibit voltage-dependent somatic motility. *Journal of Physiology, 546*, 511–520.

He, D.Z. & Dallos, P. (2000). Properties of voltage-dependent somatic stiffness of cochlear outer hair cells. *Journal of the Association for Research in Otolaryngology, 1*, 64–81.

He, J. (2001). On and off pathways segregated at the auditory thalamus of the guinea pig. *Journal of Neuroscience, 21*, 8672–8679.

Heffner, H.E. (1997). The role of macaque auditory cortex in sound location. *Acta Otolaryngologica, 532*(Suppl.), 22–27.

Heffner, H.E. & Heffner, R.S. (1986). Effect of unilateral and bilateral auditory cortex lesions on the discrimination of vocalizations by Japanese macaques. *Journal of Neurophysiology, 56*, 683–701.

Heffner, H.E. & Heffner, R.S. (1989). Effect of restricted cortical lesions on absolute thresholds and aphasia-like deficits in Japanese macaques. *Behavioral Neuroscience, 103*, 158–169.

Heffner, H.E. & Heffner, R.S. (1990). Effect of bilateral auditory cortex lesions on absolute thresholds in Japanese macaques. *Journal of Neurophysiology, 64*, 191–205.

Heffner, R.S. & Heffner, H.E. (1984). Hearing loss in dogs after lesions of the brachium of the inferior colliculus and medial geniculate. *Journal of Comparative Neurology, 230*, 207–217.

Helfert, R.H. & Aschoff, A. (1997). Superior olivary complex and nuclei of the lateral lemniscus. In: G. Ehret & R. Romand (Eds.), *The Central Auditory System* (pp. 193–258). New York: Oxford University Press.

Helfert, R.H., Sneed, C.R., & Altschuler, R.A. (1991). The ascending auditory pathways. In: R.A. Altschuler, R.P. Bobbin, B.M. Clopton, & D.W. Hoffman (Eds.), *Neurobiology of Hearing: The Central Auditory System* (pp. 1–26). New York: Raven Press.

Henderson, D., McFadden, S., Liu, C., Hight, N., & Zheng, X. (1999). The role of antioxidants in protection from impulse noise. *Annals of the New York Academy of Sciences, 884*, 368–380.

Henson, M.M. & Henson, O.W. (1988). Tension fibroblasts and the connective tissue matrix of the spiral ligament. *Hearing Research, 35*, 237–258.

Henson, M.M., Henson O.W., & Jenkins, D.B. (1984). The attachment of the spiral ligament to the cochlear wall: Anchoring cells and the creation of tension. *Hearing Research, 16*, 231–242.

Hind, J.E. (1972). Physiological correlates of auditory stimulus periodicity. *Audiology, 11*, 42–57.

Hirsch, B.E., Durrant, J.D., Yetiser, S., Kamerer, D.B., & Martin, W.H. (1996). Localizing retrocochlear hearing loss. *American Journal of Otolaryngology, 17*, 537–546.

Hirsh, I. (1948). The influence of interaural phase on interaural summation and inhibition. *Journal of the Acoustical Society of America, 20*, 761–776.

Hofman, P. & van Opstal, J. (2003). Binaural weighting of pinna cues in human sound localization. *Experimental Brain Research, 148*, 458–470.

Hofstetter, P., Ding, D., Powers, N., & Salvi, R.J. (1997). Quantitative relationship of carboplatin dose to magnitude of inner and outer hair cell loss and the reduction in distortion product otoacoustic emission amplitude in chinchillas. *Hearing Research, 112*, 199–215.

Hogmoen, K. & Gundersen, T. (1977). Holographic investigation of stapes footplate movements. *Acustica, 37*, 198–202.

Holley, M.C. & Ashmore, J.F. (1988). A cytoskeletal spring in cochlear outer hair cells. *Nature, 335*, 635–637.

Holley, M.C., Kalinec, F., & Kachar, B. (1992). Structure of the cortical cytoskeleton in mammalian outer hair cells. *Journal of Cell Science, 102*, 569–580.

Hood, L.J. (2002). Suppression of otoacoustic emission in normal individuals and patients with auditory disorders. In: M.S. Robinette & T.J. Glattke (Eds.), *Otoacoustic Emissions: Clinical Applications* (pp. 325–347). New York: Thieme Medical Publishers.

Hood, L.J., Hurley, A., Leonard, L., & Berlin, C.I. (1996). Frequency characteristics of suppression of click-evoked otoacoustic emissions differ with binaural noise. *Abstract from the Association for Research in Otolaryngology, 19*, 23.

Horner, K.C. (1995). Auditory and vestibular function in experimental hydrops. *Otolaryngology-Head and Neck Surgery, 112*, 84–89.

House, W. & Luetje, C. (1979). *Acoustic Tumors* (Vol. 1). Baltimore: University Park Press.

House, W., Luetje, C., & Doyle, K. (1997). *Acoustic Tumors: Diagnosis and Management* (2nd ed.). San Diego: Singular Publishing Group.

Howard, J. & Hudspeth, A.J. (1988). Compliance of the hair bundle associated with gating of mechanolectrical transduction channels in the bullfrog's saccular hair cell. *Neuron, 1*, 189–199.

Howard, J., Roberts, W.M., & Hudspeth, A.J. (1988). Mechano-electrical transduction by hair cells. *Annual Review of Biophysics and Biophysical Chemistry, 17*, 99–124.

Huang, M.Y. & Lambert, P.R. (1997). Temporal bone trauma. In: G.B. Hughes & M.L. Pensack (Eds.), *Clinical Otology* (2nd ed.) (pp. 251–267). New York: Thieme Medical Publishers.

Hudspeth, A.J. (1982). Extracellular current flow and the site of transduction by vertebrate hair cells. *Journal of Neuroscience, 2*, 1–10.

Hudspeth, A.J. (1985). Models for mechanoelectrical transduction by hair cells. *Progress in Clinical and Biological Research, 176*, 193–205.

Hudspeth, A.J. (1986). The ionic channels of a vertebrate hair cell. *Hearing Research, 22*, 21–27.

Hudspeth, A.J. (1989a). How the ear works. *Nature, 341*, 397–404.

Hudspeth, A.J. (1989b). Mechanoelectrical transduction by hair cells of the bullfrog's sacculus. *Progress in Brain Research, 80*, 129–135.

Hudspeth, A.J. (2000a). Hearing. In: E.R. Kandel, J.H. Schwartz, & T.M. Jessell (Eds.), *Principles of Neural Science* (4th ed.) (pp. 591–612). New York: McGraw Hill.

Hudspeth, A.J. (2000b). Sensory transduction in the ear. In: E.R. Kandel, J.H. Schwartz, & T.M. Jessell (Eds.), *Principles of Neural Science* (4th ed.) (pp. 591–612). New York: McGraw Hill.

Hudspeth, A.J., Choe, Y., Mehta, A.D., & Martin, P. (2000). Putting ion channels to work: Mechanoelectrical transduction, adaptation, and amplification by hair cells. *Proceedings of the National Academy of Sciences of the United States of America, 97*, 11765–11772.

Hudspeth, A.J. & Corey, D.P. (1977). Sensitivity, polarity, and conductance change in the response of vertebrate hair cells to controlled mechanical stimuli. *Proceedings of the National Academy of Sciences of the United States of America, 74*, 2407–2411.

Hudspeth, A.J. & Jacobs, R. (1979). Stereocilia mediate transduction in vertebrate hair cells (auditory system/cilium/vestibular system). *Proceedings of the National Academy of Sciences of the United States of America, 76*, 1506–1509.

Hugdahl, K. (Ed.). (1988). *Handbook of Dichotic Listening: Theory, Methods, and Research*. New York: John Wiley & Sons.

Hugdahl, K., Bronnick, K., Kyllingsback, S., Law, I., Gade, A., & Paulson, O.B. (1999). Brain activation during dichotic presentations of consonant-vowel in musical instrument stimuli: A 15O-Pet study. *Neuropsychologia, 37*, 431–440.

Hugdahl, K., Wester, K., & Asbjornsen, A. (1991). Auditory neglect after right frontal lobe and right pulvinar thalamic lesions. *Brain and Language, 41*, 465–473.

Hurd, L.B., Hutson, K.A., & Morest, D.K. (1999). Cochlear nerve projections to the small cell shell of the cochlear nucleus: The neuroanatomy of extremely thin sensory axons. *Synapse, 33*, 83–117.

Huss, M. & Moore, B.C. (2003). Tone decay for hearing-impaired listeners with and without dead regions in the cochlea. *Journal of the Acoustical Society of America, 114*, 3283–3294.

Hyde, G.E. & Rubel, E.W. (1995). Mitochondrial role in hair cell survival after injury. *Otolaryngology-Head and Neck Surgery, 113*, 530–540.

Hyman, B.T. & Tranel, D. (1989). Hemianesthesia and aphasia. An anatomical and behavioral study. *Archives of Neurology, 46*, 816–819.

Hynd, G.W., Semrud-Clikeman, M., Lorys, A.R., Novey, E.S., & Eliopulos, D. (1990). Brain morphology in developmental dyslexia and attention deficit disorder/hyperactivity. *Archives of Neurology, 47*, 919–926.

Imig, T.J. & Morel, A. (1985). Tonotopic organization in lateral part of posterior group of thalamic nuclei in the cat. *Journal of Neurophysiology, 53*, 836–851.

Innocenti, G.M. & Bressoud, R. (2003). Callosal axons and their development. In: E. Zaidel & M. Iacoboni (Eds.), *The Parallel Brain: The Cognitive Neuroscience of the Corpus Callosum* (pp. 11–26). Cambridge, MA: MIT Press.

Irvine, D. (1986). The auditory brainstem. In: D. Ottoson (Ed.), *Progress in Sensory Physiology* (pp. 1–179, 208–279). New York: Springer-Verlag.

Irvine, D. (1992). Physiology of the auditory brainstem. In: A.N. Popper & R.R. Fay (Eds.), *The Mammalian Auditory Pathway: Neurophysiology* (pp. 170–175). New York: Springer-Verlag.

Ivarsson, C., de Ribaupierre, Y., & de Ribaupierre, F. (1988). Influence of auditory localization cues on neuronal activity in the auditory thalamus of the cat. *Journal of Neurophysiology, 59*, 586–606.

Jackler, R.K. & Hwang, P.H. (1993). Enlargement of the cochlear aqueduct: Fact or fiction? *Otolaryngology-Head and Neck Surgery, 109*, 14–25.

Jancke, L. & Steinmetz, H. (2003). Brain size: A possible source of interindividual variability in corpus callosum morphology. In; E. Zaidel & M. Iacoboni (Eds.), *The Parallel Brain: The Cognitive Neuroscience of the Corpus Callosum* (pp. 51–63). Cambridge, MA: MIT Press.

Jannetta, P.J. (1975). Neurovascular cross-compression in patients with hyperactive dysfunction symptoms of the eighth cranial nerve. *Surgical Forum, 26*, 467–469.

Jeeves, M. (1969). A comparison of interhemispheric transmission times in acallosals and normals. *Psychonomic Science, 16*, 245–246.

Jeeves, M.A. (1994). Callosal agenesis: A natural split-brain: Overview. In: M. Lassonde & M. Jeeves (Eds.), *Callosal Agenesis: A Natural Split Brain* (pp. 285–300). New York: Plenum Press.

Jeeves, M.A. & Moes, P. (1996). Interhemispheric transfer time differences related to aging and gender. *Neuropsychologia, 34*, 627–636.

Jenkins, W.M. & Masterton, R.B. (1982). Sound localization: Effects of unilateral lesions in the central auditory system. *Journal of Neurophysiology, 47*, 987–1016.

Jenkins, W.M. & Merzenich, M.M. (1984). Role of cat primary auditory cortex for sound-localization behavior. *Journal of Neurophysiology, 52*, 819–847.

Jerger, J., Alford, B., Lew, H., Rivera V., & Chmiel, R. (1995). Dichotic listening, event-related potentials, and interhemispheric transfer in the elderly. *Ear and Hearing, 16*, 482–498.

Jerger, J., Anthony, L., Jerger, S., & Mauldin, L. (1974). Studies in impedance audiometry. III. Middle ear disorders. *Archives of Otolaryngology, 99*, 165–171.

Jerger, J. & Hayes, D. (1983). Latency of the acoustic reflex in eighth-nerve tumors. *Archives of Otolaryngology, 109*, 1–5.

Jerger, J. & Jerger, S. (1974). Auditory findings in brain stem disorders. *Archives of Otolaryngology, 99*, 342–350.

Jerger, J., Jerger, S., & Mauldin, L. (1972). Studies in impedance audiometry. I. Normal and sensorineural ears. *Archives of Otolaryngology, 96*, 513–523.

Jerger, J., Neely, J.G., & Jerger, S. (1980). Speech, impedance, and auditory brainstem response audiometry in brainstem tumors: Importance of a multiple-test strategy. *Archives of Otolaryngology, 106*, 218–223.

Jerger, S. & Jerger, J. (1981). *Auditory Disorders: A Manual for Clinical Evaluation*. Boston: Little, Brown and Company.

Jirsa, R. & Clontz, K. (1990). Long latency auditory event related potentials from children with auditory processing disorders. *Ear and Hearing, 11,* 222–232.

John, M.S., Dimitrijevic, A., van Roon, P., & Picton, T.W. (2001). Multiple auditory steady-state responses to AM and FM stimuli. *Audiology and Neuro-otology, 6,* 12–27.

Johnson, D.H. (1978). The relationship of post-stimulus time in interval histograms to the timing characteristics of spike trains. *Biophysical Journal, 22,* 413–430.

Johnson, E.W. (1977). Auditory test results in 500 cases of acoustic neuromas. *Archives of Otolaryngology, 103,* 152–158.

Johnsson, L.G. (1972). Cochlear blood vessel pattern in the human fetus and postnatal vascular involution. *Annals of Otology, Rhinology, and Laryngology, 81,* 22–40.

Johnsrude, I.S., Giraud, A.L., & Frackowiak, R.S. (2002). Functional imaging of the auditory system: The use of positron emission tomography. *Audiology and Neuro-otology, 7,* 251–276.

Johnstone, B.M. & Boyle, A.J. (1967). Basilar membrane vibration examined with the Mossbauer technique. *Science, 158,* 389–390.

Jones, E.G. & Powell, T.P. (1970). An anatomical study of converging sensory pathways within the cerebral cortex of the monkey. *Brain, 93,* 793–820.

Joris, P.X., Schreiner, C.E., & Rees, A. (2004). Neural processing of amplitude-modulated sounds. *Physiological Reviews, 84,* 541–577.

Joris, P.X. & Yin T.C. (1995). Envelope coding in the lateral superior olive. I. Sensitivity to interaural time differences. *Journal of Neurophysiology, 73,* 1043–1062.

Kaas, J.H. & Hackett, T.A. (1998). Subdivisions of auditory cortex and levels of processing in primates. *Audiology and Neuro-otology, 3,* 73–85.

Kaas, J.H., Hackett, T.A., & Tramo, M.J. (1999). Auditory processing in primate cerebral cortex. *Current Opinion in Neurobiology, 9,* 164–170.

Kaltenbach, J.A. & Afman, C.E. (2000). Hyperactivity in the dorsal cochlear nucleus after intense sound exposure and its resemblance to tone-evoked activity: A physiological model for tinnitus. *Hearing Research, 140,* 165–172.

Kane, E.S. (1976). Descending projections to specific regions of cat cochlear nucleus: A light microscopic study. *Experimental Neurology, 52,* 372–388.

Kane, E.S. & Barone, L.M. (1980). The dorsal nucleus of the lateral lemniscus in the cat: Neuronal types and their distributions. *Journal of Comparative Neurology, 192,* 797–826.

Kaufman, D. (1990). *Clinical Neurology for Psychiatrists* (3rd ed.). Philadelphia: W.B. Saunders.

Kavanagh, G.L. & Kelly, J.B. (1988). Hearing in the ferret (Mustela putorius): Effects of primary auditory cortical lesions on thresholds for pure tone detection. *Journal of Neurophysiology, 60,* 879–888.

Kawase, T. & Liberman, M.C. (1993). Antimasking effects of the olivocochlear reflex. I. Enhancement of compound action potentials to masked tones. *Journal of Neurophysiology, 70,* 2519–2532.

Keidel, W.D., Kallert, S., & Korth, M. (1983). *The Physiological Bases of Hearing.* New York: Thieme-Stratton.

Keiler, S. & Richter, C.P. (2001). Cochlear dimensions obtained in hemicochleae of four different strains of mice: CBA/CaJ, 129/CD1, 129/SvEv and C57BL/6J. *Hearing Research, 162,* 91–104.

Kelly, J.B. & Kavanagh, G.L. (1986). Effects of auditory cortical lesions on pure-tone sound localization by the albino rat. *Behavioral Neuroscience, 100,* 569–575.

Kelly, J.B., Rooney, B.J., & Phillips, D.P. (1996). Effects of bilateral auditory cortical lesions on gap-detection thresholds in the ferret (Mustela putorius). *Behavioral Neuroscience, 110,* 542–550.

Kelly, J.P. & Wong, D. (1981). Laminar connections of the cat's auditory cortex. *Brain Research, 212,* 1–15.

Kemp, D.T. (1978). Stimulated acoustic emissions from within the human auditory system. *Journal of the Acoustical Society of America, 64,* 1386–1391.

Kemp, D.T. (1979). Evidence of mechanical nonlinearity and frequency selective wave amplification in the cochlea. *Archives of Otorhinolaryngology, 224,* 37–45.

Kiang, N.Y.S., (1975). Stimulus representation in the discharge patterns of auditory neurons. In: D.D. Towers (Ed.), *The Nervous System.* Vol. 3. *Communication and Its Disorders* (pp. 81–96). New York: Raven Press.

Kiang, N.Y.S., Watanabe, T., Thomas, E.C., & Clark, S.F. (1965). *Discharge Patterns of Single Fibers in the Cat's Auditory Nerve.* Cambridge, MA: MIT Press.

Kier, E.L. & Truwit, C.L. (1996). The normal and abnormal genu of the corpus callosum: An evolutionary, embryologic, anatomic, and MR analysis. *American Journal of Neuroradiology, 17,* 1631–1641.

Kikuchi, T., Adams, J.C., Miyabe, Y., So, E., & Kobayashi, T. (2000). Potassium ion recycling pathway via gap junction systems in the mammalian cochlea and its interruption in hereditary nonsyndromic deafness. *Medical Electron Microscopy, 33,* 51–56.

Kikuchi, T., Kimura, R.S., Paul, D.L., & Adams, J.C. (1995). Gap junctions in the rat cochlea: Immunohistochemical and ultrastructural analysis. *Anatomy and Embryology, 191,* 101–118.

Kileny, P., Paccioretti, D., & Wilson, A.F. (1987). Effects of cortical lesions on middle latency evoked responses (MLR). *Electroencephalography and Clinical Neurophysiology, 66,* 108–120.

Kim, D.O. & Parham, K. (1991). Auditory nerve spatial encoding of high frequency pure tones: Population response profiles derived from d′ measure associated with nearby places along the cochlea. *Hearing Research, 52,* 167–179.

Kim, D. & Parham, K. (1997). Physiology of the auditory nerve. In: M. Crocher (Ed.), *Encyclopedia of Acoustics* (pp. 1331–1378). New York: John Wiley & Sons.

Kimura, D. (1961). Some effects of temporal lobe damage on auditory perception. *Canadian Journal of Psychology, 15,* 156–165.

Klose, A.K. & Sollmann, W.P. (2000). Anatomical variations of landmarks for implantation at the cochlear nucleus. *Journal of Laryngology and Otology, 114* (Suppl.), 8–10.

Knight, R.T., Hillyard, S.A., Woods, D.L., & Neville, H.J. (1980). The effects of frontal and temporal-parietal lesions on the auditory evoked potential in man. *Electroencephalography and Clinical Neurophysiology, 50,* 112–124.

Knight, R.T., Scabini, D., Woods, D.L., & Clayworth, C.C. (1988). The effects of lesions of the superior temporal gyrus and inferior parietal lobe on temporal and vertex components of the human AEP. *Electroencephalography and Clinical Neurophysiology, 70,* 499–509.

Knight, R., Scabini, D., Woods, D., & Clayworth, C. (1989). Contributions of the temporal-parietal junction to human auditory P3. *Brain Research, 502,* 109–116.

Koch, M. (1999). The neurobiology of startle. *Progress in Neurobiology, 59*, 107–128.

Komune, S. & Snow, J.B. (1981). Potentiating effects of cisplatin and ethacrynic acid in ototoxicity. *Archives of Otolaryngology, 107*, 594–597.

Konishi, T. & Slepian, J.Z. (1971). Effects of the electrical stimulation of the crossed olivocochlear bundle on cochlear potentials recorded with intracochlear electrodes in guinea pigs. *Journal of the Acoustical Society of America, 49*, 1762–1769.

Krast, R. (1985). A new method for non-invasive measurement of short term cerebrospinal fluid pressure changes in humans. *Journal of Neurology, 232*, 260–261.

Kraus, N., Kileny, P., & McGee, T. (1994). Middle latency auditory evoked potentials. In: J. Katz (Ed.), *Handbook of Clinical Audiology* (4th ed.) (pp. 387–402). Baltimore: Williams & Wilkins.

Kraus, N. & McGee, T. (1994). Auditory event-related potentials. In: J. Katz (Ed.), *Handbook of Clinical Audiology* (4th ed.) (pp. 406–423). Baltimore: Williams & Wilkins.

Kraus, N. & McGee, T. (1995). The middle latency response generating system. *Electroencephalography and Clinical Neurophysiology, 44* (Suppl.), 93–101.

Kraus, N., McGee, T., & Comperatore, C. (1989). MLRs in children are consistently present during wakefulness, stage 1, and REM sleep. *Ear and Hearing, 10*, 339–345.

Kraus, N., McGee, T., Littman, T., & Nicol, T. (1992). Reticular formation influences on primary and non-primary auditory pathways as reflected by the middle latency response. *Brain Research, 587*, 186–194.

Kraus, N., Ozdamar, O., Heydemann, P.T., Stein, L., & Reed, N.L. (1984). Auditory brain stem responses in hydrocephalic patients. *Electroencephalography and Clinical Neurophysiology, 59*, 310–317.

Kryter, K.D. & Ades, H.W. (1943). Studies on the function of the higher acoustic centers in the cat. *American Journal of Psychology, 56*, 501–536.

Kujawa, S.G., Glattke, T.J., Fallon, M., & Bobbin, R.P. (1992). Intracochlear application of acetylcholine alters sound-induced mechanical events within the cochlear partition. *Hearing Research, 61*, 106–116.

Kujawa, S.G., Glattke, T.J., Fallon, M., & Bobbin, R.P. (1993). Contralateral sound suppresses distortion product otoacoustic emissions through cholinergic mechanisms. *Hearing Research, 68*, 97–106.

Kujawa, S.G. & Liberman, M.C. (1997). Conditioning-related protection from acoustic injury: Effects of chronic deefferentation and sham surgery. *Journal of Neurophysiology, 78*, 3095–3106.

Kulenovic, A., Dilberovic, F., & Ovcina, F. (2003). Variation in the flow and branching of the anterior and middle cerebral arteries. *Medical Archives, 57*, 3–5.

Kumar, U.A. & Vanaja, C.S. (2004). Functioning of olivocochlear bundle and speech perception in noise. *Ear and Hearing, 25*, 142–146.

Kutas, M., Hillyard, S., Volpe, B., & Gazzaniga, M. (1990). Late positive event-related potentials after commissural section in humans. *Journal of Cognitive Neuroscience, 2*, 258–271.

Kuwada, S., Yin, T.C., Syka, J., Buunen, T.J., & Wickesburg, R.E. (1984). Binaural interaction in low-frequency neurons in inferior colliculus of the cat. IV. Comparison of monaural and binaural response properties. *Journal of Neurophysiology, 51*, 1306–2325.

Lackner, J.R. & Teuber, H.L. (1973). Alterations in auditory fusion thresholds after cerebral injury in man. *Neuropsychologia, 11*, 409–415.

LaMantia, A.S. & Rakic, P. (1984). The number, size, myelination and regional variation of axons in the corpus callosum and anterior commissure of the developing Rhesus monkey. *Society of Neuroscience Abstracts, 10*, 1081.

Lang, J. (1981). Facial and vestibulocochlear nerve: Topographic anatomy and variations. In: M. Samii & P.J. Jannetta (Eds.), *The Cranial Nerves: Anatomy, Pathology, Pathophysiology, Diagnosis and Treatment* (pp. 363–277). New York: Springer-Verlag.

Lang, J. (1991). *Clinical Anatomy of the Posterior Cranial Fossa and its Foramina*. Stuttgart: Thieme-Verlag.

Langner, G. & Schreiner, C.E. (1988). Periodicity coding in the inferior colliculus of the cat. I. Neuronal mechanisms. *Journal of Neurophysiology, 60*, 1799–1822.

Lasota K.J., Ulmer J.L., Firszt, J.B., Biswal, B.B., Daniels, D.L., & Prost R.W. (2003). Intensity-dependent activation of the primary auditory cortex in functional magnetic resonance imaging. *Journal of Computer Assisted Tomography, 27*, 213–318.

Lassonde, M. (1986). The facilitory influence of the corpus callosum on interhemispheric processing. In: F. Lepore, M. Ptito, & H.H. Jasper (Eds.), *Two Hemispheres, One Brain: Functions of the Corpus Callosum* (pp. 385–401). New York: Allan R. Liss.

Lassonde, M.C., Sauerwein, H.C., & Lepore, F. (2003). Agenesis of the corpus callosum. In: E. Zaidel & M. Iacoboni (Eds.), *The Parallel Brain: The Cognitive Neuroscience of the Corpus Callosum* (pp. 357–369). Cambridge, MA: MIT Press.

Lauter, J.L., Herscovitch, P., Formby, C., & Raichle, M.E. (1985). Tonotopic organization in human auditory cortex revealed by positron emission tomography. *Hearing Research, 20*, 199–205.

Le, T.H., Patel, S., & Roberts, T.P. (2001). Functional MRI of human auditory cortex using block and event-related designs. *Magnetic Resonance in Medicine, 45*, 254–260.

LeDoux, J. (1986). The neurobiology of emotion. In: J. LeDoux & W. Hirst (Eds.), *Mind and Brain* (pp. 342–346). Cambridge. MA: Cambridge University Press.

Lee, M.P., Ravenel, J.D., Hu, R.J., Lustig, L.R., Tomaselli, G., Berger, R.D., Brandenburg, S.A., Litzi, T.J., Bunton, T.E., Limb, C., Francis, H., Gorelikow, M., Gu, H., Washington, K., Argani, P., Goldenring, J.R., Coffey, R.J., & Feinberg, A.P. (2000). Targeted disruption of the Kvlqt1 gene causes deafness and gastric hyperplasia in mice. *Journal of Clinical Investigation, 106*, 1447–1455.

Lennartz, R.C. & Weinberger, N.M. (1992). Frequency selectivity is related to temporal processing in parallel thalamocortical auditory pathways. *Brain Research, 583*, 81–92.

Leonard, C.M., Puranik, C., Kuldau, J.M., & Lombardino, L.J. (1998). Normal variation in the frequency and location of the human auditory cortex landmarks. Heschl's gyrus: Where is it? *Cerebral Cortex, 8*, 397–406.

Leonova, E.V. & Raphael, Y. (1997). Organization of cell junctions in cytoskeleton in the reticular lamina in normal and ototoxically damaged organ of corti. *Hearing Research, 113*, 14–28.

Le Prell, C.G., Shore, S.E., Hughes, L.F., & Bledsoe, S.C. (2003). Disruption of lateral efferent pathways: Functional changes in auditory evoked responses. *Journal of the Association for Research in Otolaryngology, 4*, 276–290.

Letts, V.A., Valenzuela, A., Dunbar, C., Zheng, Q.Y., Johnson, K.R., & Frankel, W.N. (2000). A new spontaneous mouse mutation in the Kcne1 gene. *Mammalian Genome, 11,* 831–835.

Levine, R.A., Gardner, J.C., Fullerton, B.C., Stufflebeam, S.M., Carlisle, E.W., Furst, M., Rosen, B.R., & Kiang, N.Y.S. (1993). Effects of multiple sclerosis brainstem lesions on sound lateralization and brainstem auditory evoked potentials. *Hearing Research, 68,* 73–88.

Levine, R.A., Gardner, J.C., Fullerton, B.C., Stufflebeam, S.M., Furst, M., & Rosen, B.R. (1994). Multiple sclerosis lesions of the auditory pons are not silent. *Brain, 117,* 1127–1141.

Lewis, R.S. & Hudspeth, A.J. (1983). Voltage- and ion-dependent conductances in solitary vertebrate hair cells. *Nature, 304,* 538–541.

Li, X.F., Phillips, R., & LeDoux, J.E. (1995). NMDA and non-NMDA receptors contribute to synaptic transmission between the medial geniculate body and the lateral nucleus of the amygdala. *Experimental Brain Research, 105,* 87–100.

Liberman, M.C. (1978). Auditory-nerve response from cats raised in a low-noise chamber. *Journal of the Acoustical Society of America, 63,* 442–455.

Liberman, M.C. (1982a). Single-neuron labeling in the cat auditory nerve. *Science, 216,* 1239–1241.

Liberman, M.C. (1982b). The cochlear frequency map for the cat: Labeling auditory-nerve fibers of known characteristic frequency. *Journal of the Acoustical Society of America, 72,* 1441–1449.

Liberman, M.C. (1988). Physiology of cochlear efferent and afferent neurons: Direct comparisons in the same animal. *Hearing Research, 34,* 179–191.

Liberman, M.C. & Brown, M.C. (1986). Physiology and anatomy of single olivocochlear neurons in the cat. *Hearing Research, 24,* 17–36.

Liberman, M.C., Gao, J., He, D.Z., Wu, X., Jia, S., & Zuo, J. (2002). Prestin is required for electromotility of the outer hair cell and for the cochlear amplifier. *Nature, 419,* 300–304.

Liberman, M.C. & Kujawa, S.G. (1999). The olivocochlear system and protection from acoustic injury: Acute and chronic effects. In: C.I. Berlin (Ed.), *The Efferent Auditory System: Basic Science and Clinical Applications* (pp. 1–29). San Diego: Singular Publishing Group.

Liberman, M.C. & Mulroy, M. (1982). Acute and chronic affects of acoustic trauma: Cochlear pathology and auditory nerve pathophysiology. In: R.P. Hamernik, D. Henderson, & R. Salvi (Eds.), *New Perspectives of Noise-Induced Hearing Loss* (pp. 105–135). New York: Raven Press.

Liegeois-Chauvel, C., Giraud, K., Badier, J.M., Marquis, P., & Chauvel, P. (2001). Intracerebral evoked potentials in pitch perception reveal a functional asymmetry of the human auditory cortex. *Annals of the New York Academy of Sciences, 930,* 117–132.

Lighthill, J. (1981). Energy flow in the cochlea. *Journal of Fluid Mechanics, 106,* 149–213.

Lim, D.J. (1972). Fine morphology of the tectorial membrane. Its relationship to the organ of Corti. *Archives of Otolaryngology, 96,* 199–215.

Litovsky, R.Y., Fligor, B.J., & Tramo, M.J. (2002). Functional role of the human inferior colliculus in binaural hearing. *Hearing Research, 165,* 177–188.

Long, G.R. & Tubis, A. (1988). Modification of spontaneous and evoked otoacoustic emissions and associated psychoacoustic microstructure by aspirin consumption. *Journal of the Acoustical Society of America, 84,* 1343–1353.

Lonsbury-Martin, B.L., Whitehead, M.L., & Martin, G.K. (1991). Clinical applications of otoacoustic emissions. *Journal of Speech and Hearing Research, 34,* 964–981.

Lugo, D.I. & Cooper, M.H. (1982). Descending efferent projections of the inferior colliculus: An autoradiographic study. Abstract from the *12th Annual Meeting of the Society for Neuroscience, 8,* 349.

Lustig, L.R. & Jackler, R.K. (1997). Benign tumors of the temporal bone. In: G.B. Hughes & M.L. Pensak (Eds.), *Clinical Otology* (2nd ed.) (pp. 313–334). New York: Thieme Medical Publishers.

Lynn, G.E., Gilroy, J., Taylor, P.C., & Leiser, R.P. (1981). Binaural masking-level differences in neurological disorders. *Archives of Otolaryngology, 107,* 357–362.

Maher, W.P. (1988). Microvascular networks in tympanic membrane, malleus periosteum, and annulus perichondrium of neonatal mongrel dog: A vasculoanatomic model for surgical considerations. *American Journal of Anatomy, 183,* 294–302.

Maison, S.F., Emeson, R.B., Adams, J.C., Luebke, A.E., & Liberman, M.C. (2003). Loss of alpha CGRP reduces sound-evoked activity in the cochlear nerve. *Journal of Neurophysiology, 90,* 2941–2949.

Maitland, C.G. (2001). Perilymphatic fistula. *Current Neurology and Neuroscience Reports, 1,* 486–491.

Mammano, F. & Ashmore, J.F. (1993). Reverse transduction measured in the isolated cochlea by laser Michelson interferometry. *Nature, 365,* 838–841.

Mammano, F., Kros, C.J., & Ashmore, J.F. (1995). Patch clamped responses from outer hair cells in the intact adult organ of Corti. *Pflugers Archive: European Journal of Physiology, 430,* 745–750.

Marchbanks, R. (2003). Measurement of inner ear fluid pressure and clinical applications. In: L. Luxon, J.M. Furman, A. Martini, & D. Stephens (Eds.), *Textbook of Audiological Medicine: Clinical Aspects of Hearing and Balance* (pp. 289–308). London: Martin Dunitz.

Marcus, D.C., Marcus, N.Y., & Thalmann, R. (1981). Changes in cation contents of stria vascularis with ouabain and potassium-free perfusion. *Hearing Research, 4,* 149–160.

Marcus, D.C., Sunose, H., Liu, J., Bennett, T., Shen, Z., Scofield, M.A., & Ryan, A.F. (1998). Protein kinase C mediates P2U purinergic receptor inhibition of K+ channel in apical membrane of strial marginal cells. *Hearing Research, 115,* 82–92.

Marcus, D.C., Wu, T., Wangemann, P., & Kofuji, P. (2002). KCNJ10 (Kir4.1) potassium channel knockout abolishes endocochlear potential. *American Journal of Physiology: Cell Physiology, 282,* C403–407.

Marshall, L. & Heller, L.M. (1996). Reliability of transient-evoked otoacoustic emissions. *Ear and Hearing, 17,* 237–254.

Marshall, L. & Heller, L.M. (1998). Transient-evoked otoacoustic emissions as a measure of noise-induced threshold shift. *Journal of Speech, Language and Hearing Research, 41,* 1319–1334.

Martini, A. & Prosser, S. (2003). Disorders of the inner ear in adults. In: L. Luxon, J.M. Furman, A. Martini, & D. Stephens (Eds.), *Textbook of Audiological Medicine: Clinical Aspects of*

Hearing and Balance (pp. 451–476). London: Martin Dunitz.

Mast, T.E. (1973). Dorsal cochlear nucleus of the chinchilla: Excitation by contralateral sound. *Brain Research, 62,* 61–70.

Masterton, R.B. & Granger, E.M. (1988). Role of acoustic stria in hearing: Contribution of dorsal and intermediate stria to the detection of noises and tones. *Journal of Neurophysiology, 60,* 1841–1860.

Masterton, R.B., Granger, E.M., & Glendenning, K.K. (1992). Psychoacoustical contribution of each lateral lemniscus. *Hearing Research, 63,* 57–70.

Masterton, R.B., Granger, E.M., & Glendenning, K.K. (1994). Role of acoustic stria in hearing: Mechanism for enhancement of sound detection in cats. *Hearing Research, 73,* 209–222.

Maxwell, A.P, Mason, S.M., & O'Donoghue, G.M. (1999). Cochlear nerve aplasia: Its importance in cochlear implantation. *American Journal of Otology, 20,* 335–337.

May, B.J. (2000). Role of the dorsal cochlear nucleus in sound localization behavior of cats. *Hearing Research, 148,* 74–87.

May, B.J., Budelis, J., & Niparko, J.K. (2004). Behavioral studies of the olivocochlear efferent system: Learning to listen in noise. *Archives of Otolaryngology-Head and Neck Surgery, 130,* 660–664.

McGee, T., Kraus, N., Littman, T., & Nicol, T. (1992). Contributions of medial geniculate body subdivisions to the middle latency response. *Hearing Research, 61,* 147–154.

McKeever, W., Sullivan, K., Ferguson, S., & Rayport, M. (1985). Hemispheric disconnection effects in patients with corpus callosum section. In: A.G. Reeves (Ed.), *Epilepsy and the Corpus Callosum* (pp. 451–466). New York: Plenum Press.

McPherson, D.L. (1996). *Late Potentials of the Auditory System.* San Diego: Singular Publishing Group.

McPherson, D.L. & Starr, A. (1995). Auditory time-intensity cues in the binaural interaction component of the auditory evoked potentials. *Hearing Research, 89,* 162–171.

Meloni, E.G. & Davis, M. (1998). The dorsal cochlear nucleus contributes to high intensity component of the acoustic startle reflex in rats. *Hearing Research, 119,* 69–80.

Merchan, M.A. & Berbel, P. (1996). Anatomy of the ventral nucleus of the lateral lemniscus in rats: A nucleus with a concentric laminar organization. *Journal of Comparative Neurology, 372,* 245–263.

Merzenich, M.M. & Brugge, J.F. (1973). Representation of the cochlear partition of the superior temporal plane of the macaque monkey. *Brain Research, 50,* 275–296.

Mesulam, M.M. & Mufson, E.J. (1985). The insular of Reil in man and monkey architectonics, connectivity, and function. In: E.G. Jones & A. Peters (Eds.), *Cerebral Cortex* (Vol. 4) (pp. 179–226). New York: Plenum Press.

Meyer, D.R. & Woolsey, C.N. (1952). Effects of localized cortical destruction on auditory discriminative conditioning in cat. *Journal of Neurophysiology, 15,* 149–162.

Middlebrooks, J.C., Dykes, R.W., & Merzenich, M.M. (1980). Binaural response to specific bands in primary auditory cortex (AI) of the cat: Topographical organization orthogonal to isofrequency contours. *Brain Research, 181,* 31–48.

Milner, A. & Rugg, M. (1989). Interhemispheric transmission times. In: J. Crawford & D. Parker (Eds.), *Developments in Clinical and Experimental Neuropsychology* (pp. 99–112). New York: Plenum Press.

Mitani, A., Shimokouchi, M., Itoh, K., Nomura, S., Kudo, M., & Mizuno, N. (1985). Morphology and laminar organization of electrophysiologically identified neurons in the primary auditory cortex of the cat. *Journal of Comparative Neurology, 235,* 430–437.

Mitani, A., Shimokouchi, M., & Nomura, S. (1983). Effects of stimulation of the primary auditory cortex upon colliculogeniculate neurons in the inferior colliculus of the cat. *Neuroscience Letters, 42,* 185–189.

Moller, A.R. (1962). The sensitivity of contraction of the tympanic muscles in man. *Annals of Otology, Rhinology, and Laryngology, 71,* 86–95.

Moller, A.R. (1972). Coding of amplitude and frequency modulated sounds in the cochlear nucleus of the rat. *Acta Physiologica Scandinavica, 86,* 223–238.

Moller, A.R. (1979). Coding of increments and decrements in stimuli intensity in single units in the cochlear nucleus of the rat. *Journal of Neuroscience Research, 4,* 1–8.

Moller, A.R. (1983). Frequency selectivity of phase-locking of complex sounds in the auditory nerve of the rat. *Hearing Research, 11,* 267–284.

Moller, A.R. (2000). *Hearing: Its Physiology and Pathophysiology.* New York: Academic Press.

Moller, A.R, Colletti, V., & Fiorino, F.G. (1994). Neural conduction velocity of the human auditory nerve: Bipolar recordings from exposed intracranial portion of the eighth nerve during vestibular nerve section. *Electroencephophalography and Clinical Neurophysiology, 92,* 316–320.

Moller, A.R. & Jannetta, P.J. (1982). Evoked potentials from the inferior colliculus in man. *Electroencephalography and Clinical Neurophysiology, 53,* 612–620.

Moller, A.R., Jannetta, P.J., & Jho, H.D. (1994). Click-evoked responses in cochlear nucleus: A study in human. *Electroencephalography and Clinical Neurophysiology, 92,* 215–224.

Moller, A.R., Jho, H.D., & Jannetta, P.J. (1994). Preservation of hearing and operations on acoustic tumors: An alternative to recording BAEP. *Neurosurgery, 34,* 688–693.

Moller, A.R., Jho, H.D., Yokota, M., & Jannetta, P.J. (1995). Contribution from crossed and uncrossed brainstem structures to the brainstem auditory evoked potentials: A study in humans. *Laryngoscope, 105,* 596–605.

Moller, M.B. & Moller, A.R. (1985). Auditory brainstem evoked responses (ABR) in diagnosis of eighth nerve and brainstem lesions. In: M.L. Pinheiro & F.M. Musiek (Eds.), *Assessment of Central Auditory Dysfunction: Foundations and Clinical Correlates* (pp. 43–66). Baltimore: Williams and Wilkins.

Moller, M.B., Moller, A.R., Jannetta, P.J., & Jho, H.D. (1993). Vascular decompression surgery for severe tinnitus: Selection criteria and results. *Laryngoscope, 103,* 421–427.

Monsell, E.M., Teixido, M.T., Wilson, M.D., & Hughes, G.B. (1997). Nonhereditary hearing loss. In: G.B. Hughes & M.L. Pensak (Eds.), *Clinical Otology* (2nd ed.) (pp. 295–301). New York: Thieme Medical Publishers.

Moore, B.C. (2003). *An Introduction to the Psychology of Hearing* (5th ed.). New York: Academic Press.

Moore, B.C., Alcantara, J.I., & Glasberg, B.R. (2002). Behavioural measurement of level-dependent shifts in the vibration pattern on the basilar membrane. *Hearing Research, 163,* 101–110.

Moore, C.A., Cranford, J.L., & Rahn, A.E. (1990). Tracking a "moving" fused auditory image under conditions that elicit the precedence effect. *Journal of Speech and Hearing Research, 33,* 141–148.

Moore, C.N., Cassedy, J.H., & Neff, W.D. (1974). Sound localization: The role of the commissural pathway of the auditory system in cat. *Brain Research, 82,* 13–26.

Moore, D.R., Sempel, M.N., & Addison, P.D. (1983). Some acoustic properties of neurones in the ferret inferior colliculus. *Brain Research, 269,* 69–82.

Moore, J.K. (1987). The human auditory brainstem: A comparative view. *Hearing Research, 29,* 1–32.

Moore, J.K. (2000). Organization of the human superior olivary complex. *Microscopy Research and Technique, 51,* 403–412.

Morel, A., Rouiller, E., de Ribaupierre, Y., & de Ribaupierre, F. (1987). Tonotopic organization in the medial geniculate body (MGB) of lightly anesthetized cats. *Experimental Brain Research, 69,* 24–42.

Morest, D.K. (1964). The neuronal architecture of the medial geniculate body of the cat. *Journal of Anatomy, 98,* 611–630.

Morest, D.K. (1965a). The laminar structure of the medial geniculate body of the cat. *Journal of Anatomy, 99,* 143–160.

Morest, D.K. (1965b). The lateral tegmental system of the midbrain and the medial geniculate body: A study with Golgi and Nauta methods in cat. *Journal of Anatomy, 99,* 611–634.

Morest, D.K. & Oliver, D.L. (1984). The neuronal architecture of the inferior colliculus in the cat: Defining the functional anatomy of the auditory midbrain. *Journal of Comparative Neurology, 222,* 209–236.

Moulin, A., Collet, L., & Duclaux, R. (1993). Contralateral auditory stimulation alters acoustic distortion products in humans. *Hearing Research, 65,* 193–210.

Mountain, D.C. & Hubbard, A.E. (1989). Rapid force production in the cochlea. *Hearing Research, 42,* 195–202.

Mountcastle, V.B. (1962). *Interhemispheric Relations and Cerebral Dominance.* Baltimore: Johns Hopkins Press.

Muchnik, C., Ari-Even Roth, D., Othman-Jebara, R., Putter-Katz, H., Shabtai, E.L., & Hildesheimer, M. (2004). Reduced medial olivocochlear bundle system function in children with auditory processing disorders. *Audiology and Neuro-otology, 9,* 107–114.

Mummery, C., Ashburner, J., Scott, S., & Wise, R. (1999). Functional neuroimaging of speech perception in six normal and two aphasic subjects. *Journal of the Acoustical Society of America, 106,* 449–457.

Murugasu, E. & Russell, I.J. (1996). The effect of efferent stimulation on basilar membrane displacement in the basal turn of the guinea pig cochlea. *Journal of Neuroscience, 16,* 325–332.

Musiek, F.E. (1986a). Neuroanatomy, neurophysiology, and central auditory assessment. II. The cerebrum. *Ear and Hearing, 7,* 283–294.

Musiek, F.E. (1986b). Neuroanatomy, neurophysiology, and central auditory assessment. III. Corpus callosum and efferent pathways. *Ear and Hearing, 7,* 349–358.

Musiek, F.E. (1991a). Auditory evoked responses in site-of-lesion lesion assessment. In: W.F. Rintelmann (Ed.), *Hearing Assessment* (2nd ed.) (pp. 383–428). Boston: Allyn & Bacon.

Musiek, F.E. (1991b). Evidence of central vestibulo-auditory dysfunction in atypical Cogan's syndrome: A case report. *American Journal of Otology, 12,* 76.

Musiek, F.E. & Baran, J.A. (1986). Neuroanatomy, neurophysiology and central auditory assessment. I. The brainstem. *Ear and Hearing, 7,* 207–219.

Musiek, F.E., Baran, J.A., & Pinheiro, M.L. (1990). Duration pattern recognition in normal subjects and patients with cerebral and cochlear lesions. *Audiology, 29,* 304–313.

Musiek, F.E., Baran, J.A., & Pinheiro, M.L. (1992). P300 results in patients with lesions of the auditory areas of the cerebrum. *Journal of the American Academy of Audiology, 3,* 5–15.

Musiek, F.E., Baran, J.A., & Pinheiro, M.L. (1994). *Neuroaudiology, Case Studies.* San Diego: Singular Publishing Group.

Musiek, F.E., Charette, L., Kelly, T., Lee, W.W., & Musiek, E. (1999). Hit and false positive rates for the middle latency response in patients with central nervous system involvement. *Journal of the American Academy of Audiology, 10,* 124–132.

Musiek, F.E., Charette, L., Morse, D., & Baran, J.A. (2004). Central deafness associated with a midbrain lesion. *Journal of the American Academy of Audiology, 15,* 133–151.

Musiek, F.E., Geurkink, N.A., & Spiegel, P. (1987). Audiologic and other clinical findings in a case of basilar artery aneurysm. *Archives of Otolaryngology-Head and Neck Surgery, 113,* 772–776.

Musiek, F.E. & Gollegly, K.M. (1988). Maturational considerations in the neuroauditory evaluation of children. In: F.H. Bess (Ed.), *Hearing Impairment in Children* (pp. 231–250). Parkton, MD: York Press.

Musiek, F.E, Gollegly, K.M., & Baran, J.A. (1984a). Myelination of the corpus callosum in learning disabled children: Theoretical and clinical implications. *Seminars in Hearing, 5,* 231–241.

Musiek, F.E., Gollegly, K.M., Kibbe, K.S., & Verkest, S.B. (1988). Current concepts on the use of ABR and auditory psychophysical tests in the evaluation of brainstem lesions. *American Journal of Otology, 9,* 25–33.

Musiek, F.E. & Hoffman, D.W. (1990). An introduction to the functional neurochemistry of the auditory system. *Ear and Hearing, 11,* 395–402.

Musiek, F.E. & Kibbe, K. (1986). Auditory brainstem response wave IV-V abnormalities from the ear opposite large cerebellopontine lesions. *American Journal of Otolaryngology, 7,* 253–257.

Musiek, F.E., Kibbe K., & Baran J.A. (1984b). Neuroaudiological results from split-brain patients. *Seminars in Hearing, 5,* 219–229.

Musiek, F.E. & Lee, W.W. (1999). Auditory middle and late potentials. In: F.E. Musiek & W.F. Rintelmann (Eds.), *Contemporary Perspectives in Hearing Assessment* (pp. 243–271). Boston: Allyn & Bacon.

Musiek, F.E., McCormick, C.A., & Hurley, R.M. (1996). Hit and false alarm rates of selected ABR indices in differentiating cochlear disorders from acoustic tumors. *American Journal of Audiology, 5,* 90–96.

Musiek, F.E. & Pinheiro, M.L. (1985). Dichotic speech tests in the detection of central auditory dysfunction. In: M.L. Pinheiro & F.E. Musiek (Eds.), *Assessment of Central Auditory Dysfunction: Foundations and Clinical Correlates* (pp. 201–218). Baltimore: Williams & Wilkins.

Musiek, F.E. & Pinheiro, M.L. (1987). Frequency patterns in cochlear, brainstem, and cerebral lesions. *Audiology, 26,* 79–88.

Musiek, F.E., Pinheiro, M.L., & Wilson, D.H. (1980). Auditory pattern perception in "split-brain" patients. *Archives of Otolaryngology, 106,* 610–612.

Musiek, F.E. & Reeves, A.G. (1990). Asymmetries of the auditory areas of the cerebrum. *Journal of the American Academy of Audiology, 1,* 240–245.

Musiek, F.E., Reeves, A.G., & Baran, J.A. (1985). Release from central auditory competition in the split-brain patient. *Neurology, 35,* 983–987.

Naatanen, R., Paavilainen, P., Tiitinen, H., Jiang, D., & Alho, K. (1993). Attention and mismatched negativity. *Psychophysiology, 30,* 436–450.

Nakamura, H., Takada, S., Shimabuku, R., Matsuo, M., Matsuo, T., & Negishi, H. (1985). Auditory nerve and brainstem responses in newborn infants with hyperbilirubinemia. *Pediatrics, 75,* 703–708.

Nauta, W.J.H. & Feirtag, M. (1986). *Fundamental Neuroanatomy.* New York: W.H. Freeman & Co.

Neely, S.T. & Kim, D.O. (1983). An active cochlear model showing sharp tuning and high sensitivity. *Hearing Research, 9,* 123–130.

Neely, S.T., Norton, S.J., Gorga, M.P., & Jesteadt, W. (1988). Latency of auditory brainstem responses and otoacoustic emissions using tone-burst stimuli. *Journal of the Acoustical Society of America, 83,* 652–656.

Neff, W. (1961). Neural mechanisms of auditory discrimination. In: W.A. Rosenblith (Ed.), *Sensory Communication* (pp. 259–278). Cambridge, MA: MIT Press.

Nehlig, A. & Vert, P. (1997). Cerebral metabolic consequences of neonatal pathologies in the immature rat. *Acta Paediatric Japonica, 39* (Suppl. 1), S26–S32.

Netter, F.H. (1958). *The Ciba Collection of Medical Illustrations.* Vol. 1. *Nervous System.* Summit, NJ: Ciba Pharmaceutical Products.

Ngan, E.M. & May, B.J. (2001). Relationship between the auditory brainstem response and auditory nerve thresholds in cats with hearing loss. *Hearing Research, 156,* 44–52.

Nguyen, B.H., Javel, E., & Levine, S.C. (1999). Physiological identification of the VIIIth nerve set divisions: Direct recordings of bipolar and monopolar electrodes. *American Journal of Otology, 20,* 522–534.

Niparko, J.K. (1999). Activity influences on neuronal connectivity within the auditory pathway. *Laryngoscope, 109,* 1721–1730.

Noffsinger, D., Martinez, C.D., & Schaefer, A.B. (1985). Puretone techniques in the evaluation of central auditory function. In: J. Katz (Ed.), *Handbook of Clinical Audiology* (3rd ed.)(pp. 337–354). Baltimore: Williams and Wilkins.

Norton, S.J., Mott, J.B., & Champlin, C.A. (1989). Behavior of spontaneous otoacoustic emissions following intense ipsilateral acoustic stimulation. *Hearing Research, 38,* 243–258.

Norton, S.J. & Neely, S.T. (1987). Tone-burst-evoked otoacoustic emissions from normal-hearing subjects. *Journal of the Acoustical Society of America, 81,* 1860–1872.

Nuttall, A.L. & Ren, T. (1995). Electromotile hearing: Evidence from basilar membrane motion and otoacoustic emissions. *Hearing Research, 92,* 170–177.

Obert, A.D. & Cranford, J.L. (1990). Effects of neocortical lesions on the P300 component of the auditory-evoked response. *American Journal of Otology, 11,* 447–453.

Oghalai, J.S., Patel, A.A., Nakagawa, T., & Brownell, W.E. (1998). Fluorescence-imaged microdeformation of the outer hair cell lateral wall. *Journal of Neuroscience, 18,* 48–58.

Ohl, F.W., Wetzel, W., Wagner, T., Rech, A., & Scheich, H. (1999). Bilateral ablation of auditory cortex in Mongolian gerbil affects discrimination of frequency modulated tones but not pure tones. *Learning and Memory, 6,* 347–362.

O'Leary, D.S., Andreasen, N.C., Hurtig, R.R., Hichwa, R.D., Watkins, G.L., Ponto, L., Rogers, M., & Kirchner, P.T.

(1996). Positron emission tomography study of binaurally and dichotically presented stimuli: The effects of level of language and directed attention. *Brain and Language, 53,* 20–39.

Oliver, D., He, D.Z., Klocker, N., Ludwig, J., Schulte, U., Waldegger, S., Ruppersberg, J.P., Dallos, P., & Fakler, B. (2001). Intracellular anions as the voltage sensor of prestin, the outer hair cell motor protein. *Science, 292,* 2340–2343.

Oliver, D.L. & Morest, D.K. (1984). The central nucleus of the inferior colliculus in the cat. *Journal of Comparative Neurology, 222,* 237–264.

Oliver, D.L. & Schneiderman, A. (1991). The anatomy of the inferior colliculus: A cellular basis for integration of monoaural and binaural information. In: R.A. Altschuler, R.P. Bobbin, B.M. Clopton, & D.W. Hoffman (Eds.), *Neurobiology of Hearing: The Central Auditory System* (pp. 195–222). New York: Raven Press.

Olsen, W.O., Bauch, C.D., & Harner, S.G. (1983). Application of Silman and Gelfand (1981) 90th percentile levels for acoustic reflex thresholds. *Journal of Speech and Hearing Disorders, 48,* 330–332.

Olsen, W.O., Noffsinger, D., & Kurdziel, S. (1975). Speech discrimination in quiet and in white noise by patients who have peripheral and central lesions. *Acta Otolaryngologica, 80,* 375–382.

Oonishi, S. & Katsuki, Y. (1965). Functional organization in integrative mechanism of the auditory cortex of the cat. *Japanese Journal of Physiology, 15,* 342–365.

Orchik, D.J., Ge, N.N., & Shea, J.J. (1998). Action potential latency shift by rarefaction and condensation clicks in Meniere's disease. *Journal of the American Academy of Audiology, 9,* 121–126.

Osborne, M.P., Comis, S.D., & Pickles, J.O. (1988). Further observations on the fine structure of tip links between stereocilia of the guines pig cochlea. *Hearing Research, 35,* 99–108.

Osen, K.K. (1969). Cytoarchitecture of the cochlear nucleus in the cat. *Journal of Comparative Neurology, 136,* 453–484.

Ostapoff, E.M., Morest, D.K., & Parham, K. (1999). Spatial organization of the reciprocal connections between the cat dorsal and anteroventral cochlear nuclei. *Hearing Research, 130,* 75–93.

Ozdamar, O. & Dallos, P. (1976). Input-output functions of cochlear whole-nerve action potentials: Interpretation in terms of one population of neurons. *Journal of the Acoustical Society of America, 59,* 143–147.

Ozesmi, C., Ascioglu, M., Suer, C., Golgeli, A., Dolu, N., & Sahin, O. (2002). Evaluation of auditory evoked potentials from the inferior colliculus in rat. *International Journal of Neuroscience, 112,* 1001–1009.

Palmer, A.R. & Evans, E.F. (1982). Intensity coding in the auditory periphery of the cat: Responses of cochlear nerve and cochlear nucleus neurons to signals in the presence of band-stop masking noise. *Hearing Research, 7,* 305–323.

Palmer, A.R., Jiang, D., & McAlpine, D. (2000). Neural responses in the inferior colliculus to binaural masking level differences created by inverting the noise in one ear. *Journal of Neurophysiology, 84,* 844–852.

Palmer, A.R. & Russell, I.J. (1986). Phase-locking in the cochlear nerve of the guinea-pig and its relation to the receptor potential of inner hair-cells. *Hearing Research, 24,* 1–15.

Pandya, D.N. (1995). Anatomy of the auditory cortex. *Revue Neurologique, 151,* 486–494.

Pandya, D.N. & Rosene, D.L. (1985). Some observations on trajectories and topography of commissural fibers. In: A.G. Reeves (Ed.), *Epilepsy and the Corpus Callosum* (pp. 21–35). New York: Plenum Press.

Parent, A. (1996). *Carpenter's Human Neuroanatomy* (9th ed.). Baltimore: Williams & Wilkins.

Parham, K. & Willott, J.F. (1990). Effects of inferior colliculus lesions on the acoustic startle response. *Behavioral Neuroscience, 104*, 831–840.

Parham, K., Zhao, H.B., Ye, Y., & Kim, D.O. (1998). Responses of anteroventral cochlear nucleus neurons of the unanesthetized decerebrate cat to click pairs as simulated echoes. *Hearing Research, 125*, 131–146.

Peiffer, A.M., Rosen, G.D., & Fitch, R.H. (2002). Rapid auditory processing and MGN morphology in microgyric rats reared in varied acoustic environments. *Developmental Brain Research, 138*, 187–193.

Penhune, V.B., Zatorre, R.J., MacDonald, J.D., & Evans, A.C. (1996). Interhemispheric anatomical differences in human primary auditory cortex: Probabilistic mapping and volume measurement from magnetic resonance scans. *Cerebral Cortex, 6*, 661–672.

Penner, M.J., Glotzbach, L., & Huang, T. (1993). Spontaneous otoacoustic emissions: Measurement and data. *Hearing Research, 68*, 229–237.

Perkins, W.H. & Kent, R.D. (1986). *Functional Anatomy of Speech, Language, and Hearing: A Primer.* Austin: Pro-Ed.

Perlman, H. & Case, T. (1939). Latent period of the crossed stapedius reflex in man. *Annals of Otology, Rhinology, and Laryngology, 48*, 663–675.

Perlman, M., Fainmesser, P., Sohmer, H., Tamari, A., Wax, Y., & Pevsmer, B. (1983). Auditory nerve-brainstem evoked responses in hyperbilirubinemic. *Pediatrics, 72*, 658–664.

Pfeiffer, R.R. (1966). Classification of response patterns of spike discharges for units in the cochlear nucleus: Tone burst stimulation. *Experimental Brain Research, 1*, 220–235.

Pfingst, B.E. & O'Connor, T.A. (1981). Characteristics of neurons in auditory cortex of monkeys performing a simple auditory task. *Journal of Physiology, 45*, 16–34.

Phillips, D.P. (1987). Stimulus intensity and loudness recruitment: Neural correlates. *Journal of the Acoustical Society of America, 82*, 1–12.

Phillips, D.P. (1989). The neural coding of simple and complex sounds in the auditory cortex. In: J.S. Lund (Ed.), *Sensory Processing in the Mammalian Brain: Neural Substrates and Experimental Strategies* (pp. 172–207). New York: Oxford University Press.

Phillips, D.P. (1990). Neural representation of sound amplitude in the auditory cortex: Effects of noise masking. *Behavioral Brain Research, 37*, 197–214.

Phillips, D.P. & Hall, S.E. (1987). Responses of single neurons in cat auditory cortex to time-varying stimuli: Linear amplitude modulations. *Experimental Brain Research, 67*, 479–492.

Phillips, D.P. & Hall, S.E. (1990). Response timing constraints on the cortical representation of sound time structure. *Journal of the Acoustical Society of America, 88*, 1403–1411.

Phillips, D.P., Judge, P.W., & Kelly, J.B. (1988). Primary auditory cortex in the ferret (Mustela putorius): Neural response properties and topographic organization. *Brain Research, 443*, 281–294.

Phillips, D.P., Orman, S.S., Musicant, A.D., & Wilson, G.G. (1985). Neurons in the cat's primary auditory cortex distinguished by their responses to tones and wide-spectrum noise. *Hearing Research, 18*, 73–86.

Phillips, D.P., Reale, R.A., & Brugge, J.F. (1991). Stimulus processing in the auditory cortex. In: R.A. Altschuler, R.P. Bobbin, B.M. Clopton, & D.W. Hoffman (Eds.), *Neurobiology of Hearing: The Central Auditory System* (pp. 335–366). New York: Raven Press.

Phillips, D.P., Semple, M.N., Calford, M.B., & Kitzes, L.M. (1994). Level dependent representation of stimulus frequency in the cat's primary auditory cortex. *Experimental Brain Research, 102*, 210–226.

Pickles, J.M. (1988a). Retropharyngeal abscess complicating a neck wound (a case report). *Journal of Laryngology and Otology, 102*, 552–553.

Pickles, J.O. (1988b). *Introduction to the Physiology of Hearing* (2nd ed.). London: Academic Press.

Pickles, J.O. & Comis, S.D. (1973). Role of the centrifugal pathways to cochlear nucleus in detection of signals in noise. *Journal of Neurophysiology, 29*, 1131–1137.

Pickles, J.O., Comis, S.D., & Osborne, M.P. (1984). Cross-links between stereocilia in the guinea pig organ of Corti, and their possible relation to sensory transduction. *Hearing Research, 15*, 103–112.

Pickles, J.O. & Corey, D.P. (1992). Mechanoelectrical transduction by hair cells. *Trends in Neurosciences, 15*, 254–259.

Pinheiro, M.L. & Musiek, F.E. (1985). Sequencing and temporal ordering in the auditory system. In: M.L. Pinheiro & F.E. Musiek (Eds.), *Assessment of Central Auditory Dysfunction: Foundations and Clinical Correlates* (pp. 219–238). Baltimore: Williams & Wilkins.

Pinheiro, M.L. & Ptacek, P.H. (1971). Reversals in the perception of noise and tone patterns. *Journal of the Acoustical Society of America, 49*, 1778–1783.

Pinheiro, M.L. & Tobin, H. (1969). Interaural intensity difference for intracranial lateralization. *Journal of the Acoustical Society of America, 46*, 1482–1487.

Polich, J. (1989). Frequency, intensity, and duration as determinants of P300 from auditory stimuli. *Journal of Clinical Neurophysiology, 6*, 277–286.

Pollmann, S., Maertens, M., von Cramon, D.Y., Lepsien, J., & Hugdahl, K. (2002). Dichotic listening in patients with splenial and nonsplenial callosal lesions. *Neuropsychology, 16*, 56–64.

Polyak, S.L., McHugh, G., & Judd, D.K. (1946). *The Human Ear* (pp. 8–86). Elmsford, NY: Sonatone Corporation.

Poon, P. & Chiu, T. (1997). Single cell responses to AM tones of different envelopes at the auditory midbrain. In: J. Syka (Ed.), *Acoustical Signal Processing in the Auditory System* (pp. 236–252). New York: Plenum Press.

Popelar, J. & Syka, J. (1982). Response properties of neurons in the inferior colliculus of the guinea-pig. *Acta Neurobiologiae Experimentalis, 42*, 299–310.

Popelka, G. (1981). The acoustic reflex in normal and pathological ears. In: G. Popelka (Ed.), *Hearing Assessment with the Acoustic Reflex* (pp. 5–21). New York: Grune and Stratton.

Portmann, M., Sterkers, J., Charachon, R., & Chouard, C. (1975). *The Internal Auditory Meatus: Anatomy, Pathology and Surgery.* New York: Churchill Livingstone.

Powers, N.L., Salvi, R.J., Wang, J., Spongr, V., & Qiu, C.X. (1995). Elevation of auditory thresholds by spontaneous cochlear oscillations. *Nature, 375*, 585–587.

Prasher, D., Ryan, S., & Luxon, L. (1994). Contralateral suppression of transiently evoked otoacoustic emission and neurootology. *British Journal of Audiology, 28,* 247–254.

Pratt, H., Polyakov, A., Aharonson, V., Korczyn, A.D., Tadmor, R., Fullerton, B., Levine, R.A., & Furst, M. (1998). Effects of localized pontine lesions on auditory brainstem evoked potentials and binaural processing in humans. *Electroencephalography and Clinical Neurophysiology, 108,* 511–520.

Preis, S., Jancke, L., Schmitz-Hillebrecht, J., & Steinmetz, H. (1999). Child age and planum temporale asymmetry. *Brain and Cognition, 40,* 441–452.

Preyer, S., Hemmert, W., Zenner, H.P., & Gummer, A.W. (1995). Abolition of the receptive potential response of isolated mammalian outer hair cells by hair-bundle treatment with elastase: A test of tip-link hypothesis. *Hearing Research, 89,* 187–193.

Prieve, B.A., Gorga, M.P., Schmidt, A., Neely, S., Peters, J., Schultes, L., & Jesteadt, W. (1993). Analysis of transient-evoked otoacoustic emissions in normal-hearing and hearing-impaired ears. *Journal of the Acoustical Society of America, 93,* 3308–3319.

Probst, R., Coats, A.C., Martin, G.K., & Lonsbury-Martin, B.L. (1986). Spontaneous, click-, and toneburst-evoked otoacoustic emissions from normal ears. *Hearing Research, 21,* 261–275.

Probst, R., Lonsbury-Martin, B.L., & Martin, G.K. (1991). A review of otoacoustic emissions. *Journal of the Acoustical Society of America, 89,* 2047–2067.

Probst, R., Lonsbury-Martin, B.L., Martin, G.K., & Coats, A.C. (1987). Otoacoustic emissions in ears with hearing loss. *American Journal of Otolaryngology, 8,* 73–81.

Ptito, M. & Boire, D. (2003). Binocular input elimination and the reshaping of callosal connection. In: E. Zaidel & M. Iacoboni (Eds.), *The Parallel Brain: The Cognitive Neuroscience of the Corpus Callosum* (pp. 30–32). Cambridge, MA: MIT Press.

Pujol, J., Vendrell, P., Junque, C., Marti-Vilalta, J.L., & Capdevila, A. (1993). When does human brain development end? Evidence of corpus callosum growth up to adulthood. *Annals of Neurology, 34,* 71–75.

Rakic, P. & Yakovlev, P.I. (1968). Development of the corpus callosum and cavum septi in man. *Journal of Comparative Neurology, 132,* 45–72.

Raphael, Y. & Altschuler, R.A. (2003). Structure and innervation of the cochlea. *Brain Research Bulletin, 60,* 397–422.

Rapin, I. & Gravel, J. (2003). "Auditory neuropathy": Physiologic and pathologic evidence calls for more diagnostic specificity. *International Journal of Pediatric Otorhinolaryngology, 67,* 707–728.

Rao, S.M., Bernardin, L., Leo, G.J., Ellington, L., Ryan, S.B., & Burg, L.S. (1989). Cerebral disconnection in multiple sclerosis. Relationship to atrophy of the corpus callosum. *Archives of Neurology, 46,* 918–920.

Rassmussen, G.L. (1964). Anatomical relationships of the ascending and descending auditory systems. In: W. Fields & B. Alford (Eds.), *Neurological Aspects of Auditory and Vestibular Disorders.* Springfield, IL: Charles C. Thomas Publishers.

Reale, R.A. & Brugge, J.F. (1990). Auditory cortical neurons are sensitive to static and continuously changing interaural phase cues. *Journal of Neurophysiology, 64,* 1247–1260.

Recio, A. & Rhode, W.S. (2000). Representation of vowel stimuli in the ventral cochlear nucleus of chinchilla. *Hearing Research, 146,* 167–184.

Rees, A. & Moller, A.R. (1983). Responses of neurons in the inferior colliculus of the rat to AM and FM tones. *Hearing Research, 10,* 301–330.

Rees, A. & Moller, A.R. (1987). Stimulus properties influencing the responses of inferior colliculus neurons to amplitude-modulated sounds. *Hearing Research, 27,* 129–143.

Rees, A. & Palmer, A.R. (1988). Rate-intensity functions and their modification by broadband noise for neurons in the guinea pig inferior colliculus. *Journal of the Acoustical Society of America, 83,* 1488–1498.

Rees, A. & Sarbaz, A. (1997). The influence of intrinsic oscillations on encoding of amplitude modulation by neurons in the inferior colliculus. In: J. Syka (Ed.), *Acoustical Signal Processing in the Central Auditory System* (pp. 253–261). New York: Plenum Press.

Reeves, A.G. (1989). *Disorders of the Nervous System: A Primer* (2nd ed.). West Lebanon, NH: Imperial Company.

Reiter, E.R. & Liberman, M.C. (1995). Efferent-mediated protection from acoustic overexposure: Relation to slow effects of olivocochlear stimulation. *Journal of Neurophysiology, 73,* 506–514.

Reyes, S., Ding, D., Sun, W., & Salvi, R. (2001). Effect of inner and outer hair cell lesions on electrically evoked otoacoustic emissions. *Hearing Research, 158,* 139–150.

Rhee, C.K., Park, H.M., & Jang, Y.J. (1999). Audiological evaluation of neonates with severe hyperbilirubinemia using transiently evoked otoacoustic emissions and auditory brainstem response. *Laryngoscope, 109,* 2005–2008.

Rhode, W.S. (1971). Observations of the vibration of the basilar membrane in squirrel monkeys using the Mossbauer technique. *Journal of the Acoustical Society of America, 49,* 1218–1231.

Rhode, W.S. (1991). Physiological-morphological properties of the cochlear nucleus. In: R.A. Altschuler, R.P. Bobbin, B.M. Clopton, & D.W. Hoffman (Eds.), *Neurobiology of Hearing: The Central Auditory System* (pp. 47–78). New York: Raven Press.

Rhode, W.S. (1998). Neural encoding of single-format stimuli in the ventral cochlear nucleus of the chinchilla. *Hearing Research, 117,* 39–56.

Rhode, W.S. & Cooper, M. (1996). Non-linear mechanics in the apical turn of the chinchilla cochlea in vivo. *Auditory Neuroscience, 3,* 101–121.

Rhode, W.S. & Smith, P.H. (1986a). Encoding timing and intensity in the ventral cochlear nucleus of the cat. *Journal of Neurophysiology, 56,* 261–286.

Rhode, W.S. & Smith, P.H. (1986b). Physiological studies on neurons in the dorsal cochlear nucleus of the cat. *Journal of Neurophysiology, 56,* 287–307.

Risse, G.L., LeDoux, J., Springer, S.P., Wilson, D.H., & Gazzaniga, M.S. (1978). The anterior commisure in man: Functional variation in a multisensory system, *Neuropsychologia, 16,* 23–31.

Rivier, F. & Clarke, S. (1997). Cytochrome oxidase acetylcholinesterase and NADPH-diaphorase staining in human supratemporal and insular cortex: Evidence of multiple auditory areas. *Neuroimage, 6,* 288–304.

Roberts, M.P., Hanaway, J., & Morest, D.K. (1987). *Atlas of the Human Brain in Section.* Philadelphia: Lea and Febiger.

Roberts, W.M., Howard, J., & Hudspeth, A.J. (1988). Hair cells: Transduction, tuning, and transmission in the inner ear. *Annual Review of Cell Biology, 4,* 63–92.

Robertson, D. (1984). Horseradish peroxidase injection of physiologically characterized afferent and efferent neurones in the guinea pig spiral ganglion. *Hearing Research, 15,* 113–121.

Robertson, D. & Gummer, M. (1985). Physiological and morphological characterization of efferent neurons in the guinea pig cochlea. *Hearing Research, 20,* 63–77.

Robin, D.A., Tranel, D., & Damasio, H. (1990). Auditory perception of temporal and spectral events in patients with focal left and right cerebral lesions. *Brain and Language, 39,* 539–555.

Robinette, M.S. (1992). Clinical observations with transient-evoked otoacoustic emissions with adults. *Seminars in Hearing, 13,* 23–36.

Robinette, M.S. (2003). Clinical observations with evoked otoacoustic emissions at Mayo Clinic. *Journal of the American Academy of Audiology, 14,* 213–224.

Robinette, M.S. & Glattke, T.J. (Eds.). (2002). *Otoacoustic Emissions: Clinical Applications.* New York: Thieme Medical Publishers.

Rockel, A.J. & Jones, E.G. (1973). The neuronal organization of the inferior colliculus of the adult cat. I. The central nucleus. *Journal of Comparative Neurology, 147,* 11–60.

Romand, R. & Avan, P. (1997). Anatomical and functional aspects of the cochlear nucleus. In: G. Ehret & R. Romand (Eds.), *The Central Auditory System* (pp. 97–192). New York: Oxford University Press.

Rose, D.E. (1978). *Audiological Assessment* (2nd ed.). Englewood Cliffs, NJ: Prentice-Hall.

Rose, J.E., Galambos, R., & Hughes, J.R. (1959). Microelectrode studies of the cochlear nucleus in cat. *Bulletin of Johns Hopkins Hospital, 104,* 211–251.

Rouiller, E., de Ribaupierre, Y., & de Ribaupierre, F. (1979). Phase locked responses to low frequency tones in the medial geniculate body. *Hearing Research, 1,* 213–226.

Rouiller, E., de Ribaupierre, Y., Morel, A., & de Ribaupierre, F. (1983). Intensity functions of single unit responses to tones in the medial geniculate body of the cat. *Hearing Research, 11,* 235–247.

Rouiller, E., de Ribaupierre, Y., Toros-Morel, A., & de Ribaupierre, F. (1981). Neural coding of repetitive clicks in the medial geniculate body of the cat. *Hearing Research, 5,* 81–100.

Roullier, E.M. (1997). Functional organization of the auditory pathways. In: G. Ehret & R. Romand (Eds.), *The Central Auditory System* (pp. 3–96). New York: Oxford University Press.

Rozengurt, N., Lopez, I., Chiu, C.S., Kofuji, P., Lester, H.A., & Neusch, C. (2003). Time course of inner ear degeneration and deafness in mice lacking the Kir4.1 potassium channel subunit. *Hearing Research, 177,* 71–80.

Rubens, A.B. (1977). Anatomical asymmetries of the human cerebral cortex. In: S. Harnard, R.W. Dody, L. Goldstein, J. Jaynes, & G. Krauthamer (Eds.), *Lateralization in the Nervous System* (pp. 503–514). New York: Academic Press.

Ruedi L., Furrer, W., Luthy, F., Nager, G., & Tschirren, B. (1952). Further observations concerning the toxic effects of streptomycin and quinine on the auditory organ of guinea pigs. *Laryngoscope, 62,* 333–351.

Ruggero, M.A. (1992). Responses of sound to the basilar membrane of the mammalian cochlea. *Current Opinion in Neurobiology, 2,* 449–456.

Ruggero, M.A., Kramek, B., & Rich, N.C. (1984). Spontaneous otoacoustic emissions in a dog. *Hearing Research, 13,* 293–296.

Ruggero, M.A., Narayan, S.S., Temchin, A.N., & Recio, A. (2000). Mechanical bases of frequency tuning in neuroexcitation at the base of the cochlea: Comparison of basilar membrane vibrations in auditory nerve fiber responses in chinchilla. *Proceedings of the National Academy of Sciences of the United States of America, 97,* 11744–11750.

Ruggero, M.A., Rich, N.C., & Freyman, R. (1983). Spontaneous and impulsively evoked otoacoustic emissions: Indicators of cochlear pathology? *Hearing Research, 10,* 283–300.

Ruggero, M.A., Rich, N.C., Recio, A., Narayan, S.S., & Robles, L. (1997). Basilar-membrane responses to tones at the base of the chinchilla cochlea. *Journal of the Acoustical Society of America, 101,* 2151–2163.

Russchen, F.T. (1982). Amygdalopetal projections in the cat. II. Subcortical afferent connections. A study with retrograde tracing techniques. *Journal of Comparative Neurology, 207,* 157–176.

Russell, I.J., Richardson, G.P., & Cody, A.R. (1986). Mechanosensitivity of mammalian auditory hair cells in vitro. *Nature, 321,* 517–519.

Russell, I.J. & Sellick, P.M. (1977). The tuning of cochlear hair cells. In: E.F. Evans & J.P. Wilson (Eds.), *Psychophysics and Physiology of Hearing* (pp. 71–87). London: Academic Press.

Russell, I.J. & Sellick, P.M. (1978). Intracellular studies of hair cells in the mammalian cochlea. *Journal of Physiology, 284,* 261–290.

Ruth, R., Lambert, P., & Ferraro, J. (1989). Electrocochleography methods and clinical applications. In: F. Musiek (Ed.), *Contemporary Issues in Clinical Audiology* (pp. 1–11). Philadelphia: Decker.

Ryan, A. & Dallos, P. (1975). Effect of absence of cochlear outer hair cells on behavioural auditory threshold. *Nature, 253,* 44–46.

Ryan, A., Dallos, P., & McGee, T. (1979). Psychophysical tuning curves and auditory thresholds after hair cell damage in the chinchilla. *Journal of the Acoustical Society of America, 66,* 370–378.

Ryan, A.F. (2001). Circulation of the inner ear. II. The relationship between metabolism and blood flow in the cochlea. In: A.F. Jahn & J. Santos-Sacchi (Eds.), *Physiology of the Ear* (2nd ed.) (pp. 321–332). San Diego: Singular Publishing Group.

Ryugo, D.K. & Weinberger, N.M. (1976). Corticofugal modulation of the medial geniculate body. *Experimental Neurology, 51,* 377–391.

Sachs, M.B. & Blackburn, C.C. (1991). Processing of complex sounds in the cochlear nucleus. In: R.A. Altschuler, R.P. Bobbin, B.M. Clopton, & D.W. Hoffman (Eds.), *Neurobiology of Hearing: The Central Auditory System* (pp. 79–98). New York: Raven Press.

Sachs, M.B. & Kiang, N.Y.S. (1968). Two-tone inhibition in auditory-nerve fibers. *Journal of the Acoustical Society of America, 43,* 1120–1128.

Sahley, T.L., Chernicky, C.L., Nodar, R.H., & Musiek, F.E. (1995). Dynorphin-like immunoreactivity in chinchilla superior olive and cochlear nucleus. Paper presented at the Annual Meeting of the American Speech-Language-Hearing Association, Orlando, FL.

Sahley, T.L., Kalish, R.B., Musiek, F.E., & Hoffman, D.W. (1991). Effects of opioid drugs on auditory evoked potentials suggest a role of lateral efferent olivocochlear dynorphins in auditory function. *Hearing Research, 55,* 133–142.

Sahley, T.L., Musiek, F.E., & Hoffman, D.W. (1992). Lateral efferents may modulate auditory sensitivity through opioid neuropeptide action. *Abstract from the Association for Research in Otolaryngology,* #25.

Sahley, T.L., Musiek, F.E., & Nodar, R.H. (1996). Naloxone blockade of pentazocine-induced changes in auditory function. *Ear and Hearing, 17,* 341–353.

Sahley, T.L., Nodar, R.H., & Musiek, F.E. (1997). *Efferent Auditory System.* San Diego: Singular Publishing Group.

Saini, V.K. (1964). Vascular pattern of a human tympanic membrane. *Archives of Otolaryngology, 79,* 193–196.

Saint Marie, R.L., Ostapoff, E.M., Morest, D.K., & Wenthold, R.J. (1989). Glycine-immunoreactive projection of the cat lateral superior olive: Possible role in midbrain ear dominance. *Journal of Comparative Neurology, 279,* 382–396.

Saito, K. (1983). Fine structure of the sensory epithelium of guinea-pig organ of Corti: Subsurface cisternae and lamellar bodies in the outer hair cells. *Cell and Tissue Research, 229,* 467–481.

Salamy, A. (1978). Commissural transmission: Maturational changes in humans. *Science, 200,* 1409–1411.

Salvi, R.J., McFadden, S.L., & Wang, J. (2000). Anatomy and physiology of the peripheral auditory system. In: R.J. Roeser, M. Valente, & H. Hosford-Dunn (Eds.), *Audiology Diagnosis* (pp. 19–44). New York: Thieme Medical Publishers.

Sanchez-Longo, L.P. & Forster, F.M. (1958). Clinical significance of impairment of sound localization. *Neurology, 8,* 119–125.

Sando, I. (1965). The anatomical interrelationship of cochlear nerve fibers. *Acta Otolaryngologica, 59,* 417–436.

Santarelli, R. & Arslan, E. (2002). Electrocochleography in auditory neuropathy. *Hearing Research, 170,* 32–47.

Sauerwein, H.C. & Lassonde, M. (1994). Cognitive and sensorimotor functioning in the absence of the corpus callosum: Neuropsychological studies in callosal agenesis and callosotomized patients. *Behavioral Brain Research, 64,* 229–240.

Schaefer, G.B., Thompson, J.N., Bodensteiner, J.B., Hamza, M., Tucker, R.R., Marks, W., Gay, C., & Wilson, D. (1990). Quantitative morphometric analysis of brain growth using magnetic resonance imaging. *Journal of Child Neurology, 5,* 127–130.

Scherg, M., Vajar, J., & Picton, T.W. (1989). A source analysis of the late human auditory-evoked potentials. *Journal of Cognitive Neuroscience, 1,* 336–355.

Schneider, P., Scherg, M., Dosch, H.G., Specht, H.J., Gutschalk, A., & Rupp, A. (2002). Morphology of Heschl's gyrus reflects enhanced activation in the auditory cortex of musicians. *Nature Neuroscience, 5,* 688–694.

Schonweiser, M., von Cramon, D.Y., & Rubsamen, R. (2002). Is it tonotopy after all? *Neuroimage, 17,* 1144–1161.

Schreiner, C.E. & Urbas, J.V. (1986). Representation of amplitude modulation in the auditory cortex of the cat. I. The anterior auditory field (AAF). *Hearing Research, 21,* 227–241.

Schreiner, C.E. & Urbas, J.V. (1988). Representation of amplitude modulation in the auditory cortex of the cat, II. Comparison between cortical fields. *Hearing Research, 32,* 49–63.

Schreiner, C.E., Urbas, J.V., & Mehrgardt, S. (1983). Temporal resolution of amplitude modulation in complex signals in the auditory cortex of the cat. In: R. Klinke & R. Hartman (Eds.), *Hearing: Physiological Basis and Psychophysics* (pp. 169–174). New York: Springer-Verlag.

Schuknecht, H.F. (1974). *Pathology of the Ear.* Cambridge, MA: Harvard University Press.

Schuknecht, H.F. (1975). Pathophysiology of Meniere's disease. *Otolaryngology Clinics of North America, 8,* 507–514.

Schuknecht, H.F. (1993). *Pathology of the Ear.* Philadelphia: Lea & Febiger.

Schuknecht, H.F. & Kirchner, J.C. (1974). Cochlear otosclerosis: Fact or fantasy. *The Laryngoscope, 84,* 766–782.

Schulte, B.A. & Steel, K.P. (1994). Expression of alpha and beta subunit isoforms of Na, K-ATPase in the mouse inner ear and changes with mutations at the Wv or Sld loci. *Hearing Research, 78,* 65–76.

Schwaber, M.K. (1997). Vestibular disorders. In: G.B. Hughes & M.L. Pensak (Eds.), *Clinical Otology* (2nd ed.) (pp. 345–365). New York: Thieme Medical Publishers.

Schwartz, I. (1992). Superior olivary complex in the lateral lemniscal nuclei. In: D.B. Webster, A.N. Popper, & R.R. Fay (Eds.), *The Mammalian Auditory Pathway: Neuroanatomy* (pp. 117–167). New York: Springer-Verlag.

Schwarz, D.W., Tennigkeit, F., & Puil, E., (2000). Metabotropic transmitter actions in auditory thalamus. *Acta Otolaryngologica, 120,* 251–254.

Schweitzer, V.G. (1993). Ototoxicity of chemotherapeutic agents. *Otolaryngology Clinics of North America, 26,* 759–789.

Seggie, J. & Berry, M. (1972). Ontogeny of interhemispheric evoked potentials in the rat: Significance of myelination of the corpus callosum. *Experimental Neurology, 35,* 215–232.

Sellick, P.M., Patuzzi, R., & Johnstone, B.M. (1982). Measurement of basilar membrane motion in the guinea pig using the Mossbauer technique. *Journal of the Acoustical Society of America, 72,* 131–141.

Sellick, P.M. & Russell, I.J. (1978). Intracellular studies of cochlear hair cells: Filling the gap between basilar membrane mechanics and neural excitation. In: R.F. Naunton & C. Fernandez (Eds.), *Evoked Electrical Activity in the Auditory Nervous System* (pp. 113–139). New York: Academic Press.

Selters, W.A. & Brackmann, D.E. (1977). Acoustic tumor detection with brainstem electric response audiometry. *Archives of Otolaryngology, 103,* 181–187.

Seltzer, B. & Pandya, D.N. (1978). Afferent cortical connections and architectonics of the superior temporal sulcus and surrounding cortex in Rhesus monkeys. *Brain Research, 149,* 121–124.

Sha, S.H., Taylor, R., Forge, A., & Schacht, J. (2001). Differential vulnerability of basal and apical hair cells is based on intrinsic susceptibility to free radicals. *Hearing Research, 15,* 1–8.

Shaw, E.A. (1974). The external ear. In: W.D. Keidel & W.D. Neff (Eds.), *Handbook of Sensory Physiology* (Vol. 5) (pp. 450–490). New York: Springer-Verlag.

Shinn, J. (2005). *The auditory steady state response (ASSR) and lesions of the central auditory nervous system (CANS).* Unpublished dosctoral dissertation, University of Connecticut.

Silman, S., Gelfand, S.A., & Silverman, C.A. (1984). Late-onset auditory deprivation: Effects of monaural versus binaural hearing aids. *Journal of the Acoustical Society of America, 76,* 1357–1362.

Silman, S. & Silverman, C. (1991). *Auditory Diagnosis: Principles and Application.* New York: Academic Press.

Slepecky, N. (1996). Cochlear structure. In: P. Dallos, A.N. Popper, & R.R. Fay (Eds.), *The Cochlea* (pp. 44–129). New York: Springer-Verlag.

Slepecky, N. & Chamberlain, S.C. (1982). Distribution and polarity of actin in the sensory hair cells of the chinchilla cochlea. *Cell and Tissue Research, 224,* 15–24.

Smith, C. (1973). Vascular patterns of the membranous labyrinth. In: A. De Lorenzo (Ed.), *Vascular Disorders and Hearing Defects* (pp. 1–22). Baltimore: University Press.

Snow, J. & Suga, F. (1973). Control of cochlear blood flow. In: A. De Lorenzo (Ed.), *Vascular Disorders and Hearing Defects* (pp. 167–184). Baltimore: University Press.

Sokoloff, L., Reivich, M., Kennedy, C., Des Rosiers, M.H., Patlak, C.S., Pettigrew, K.D., Sakurada, O., & Shinohara, M. (1977). The [14C] deoxyglucose method for the measurement of local cerebral glucose utilization: Theory, procedure, and normal values in the conscious and anesthetized albino rat. *Journal of Neurochemistry, 28,* 897–916.

Spangler, K.M., Cant, N.B., Henkel, C.K., Farley, G.R., & Warr, W.B. (1987). The superior olivary complex to the cochlear nucleus of the cat. *Journal of Comparative Neurology, 259,* 452–465.

Spangler, K.M. & Warr, W.B. (1991). The descending auditory system. In: R.A. Altschuler, R.P. Bobbin, B.M. Clopton, & D.W. Hoffman (Eds.), *Neurobiology of Hearing: The Central Auditory System* (pp. 27–46). New York: Raven Press.

Spicer, S.S. & Schulte, B.A. (1996). The fine structure of spiral ligament cells relates to ion return to the stria and varies with place-frequency. *Hearing Research, 100,* 80–100.

Spirou, G.A., May, B.J., Wright, D.D., & Ryugo, D.K. (1993). Frequency organization of the cat dorsal cochlear nucleus. *Journal of Comparative Neurology, 329,* 36–52.

Spoendlin, H. (1967). Innervation of the organ of Corti. *Journal of Laryngology and Otology, 81,* 717–738.

Spoendlin, H. (1969). Innervation patterns in the organ of Corti of the cat. *Acta Otolaryngologica, 67,* 239–244.

Spoendlin, H. (1972). Innervation densities of the cochlea. *Acta Otolaryngologica, 73,* 235–248.

Spoendlin, H. & Gacek, R. (1983). Electromicroscopic study of the afferent and efferent innervation of the organ of Corti. *Annals of Otology, 72,* 660–686.

Spoendlin, H. & Schrott, A. (1989). Analysis of the human auditory nerve. *Hearing Research, 43,* 25–38.

Springer, S.P. & Deutsch, G. (1978). *Left Brain, Right Brain.* San Francisco: W.H. Freeman & Co.

Springer, S.P. & Gazzaniga, M.S. (1975). Dichotic testing of partial and complete split brain subjects. *Neuropsychologia, 13,* 341–346.

Starr, A., Picton, T.W., & Kim, R. (2001). Pathophysiology of auditory neuropathy. In: Y. Sininger & A. Starr (Eds.), *Auditory Neuropathy: A New Perspective on Hearing Disorders* (pp. 67–82). San Diego: Singular Publishing Group.

Starr, A., Picton, T.W., Sininger, Y.S., Hood, L.J., & Berlin, C.I. (1996). Auditory neuropathy. *Brain, 119,* 741–753.

Starr, A., Sininger, Y., Nguyen, T., Michalewski, H.J., Oba, S., & Abdala, C. (2001). Cochlear receptor (microphonic and summating potentials, otoacoustic emissions) and auditory pathway (auditory brain stem potentials) activity in auditory neuropathy. *Ear and Hearing, 22,* 91–99.

Starr, A., Sininger, Y., & Pratt, H. (2000). The varieties of auditory neuropathies. *Journal of Basic and Clinical Physiology and Pharmacology, 11,* 215–230.

Starr, A. & Wernick, J.S. (1968). Olivocochlear bundle stimulation: Effect on spontaneous and tone-evoked activities of single units in cat cochlear nucleus. *Journal of Neurophysiology, 31,* 549–564.

Stavroulaki, P., Apostolopoulos, N., Dinopoulou, D., Vossinakis, I., Tsakanikos, M., & Douniadakis, D. (1999). Otoacoustic emissions: An approach for monitoring aminoglycoside induced ototoxicity in children. *International Journal of Pediatric Otorhinolaryngology, 50,* 177–184.

Steel, K.P. (1983). The tectorial membrane of mammals. *Hearing Research, 9,* 327–359.

Steel, K.P. & Barkway, C. (1989). Another role for melanocytes: Their importance for normal stria vascularis development in the mammalian inner ear. *Development, 107,* 453–463.

Steinmetz, H., Rademacher, J., Huang, Y.X., Hefter, H., Zilles, K., Thron, A., & Freund, H.J. (1989). Cerebral asymmetry: MR planimetry of the human planum temporale. *Journal of Computer Assisted Tomography, 13,* 996–1005.

Steinschneider, M., Arezzo, J., & Vaughan, H.G. (1982). Speech evoked activity in the auditory radiation and cortex of the awake monkey. *Brain Research, 252,* 353–365.

Steinschneider, M., Kurtzberg, D., & Vaughan, H. (1992). Event-related potentials in developmental neural psychology. In; I. Lapin & S. Segalowitz (Eds.), *Handbook of Neural Psychology.* Vol. 6. *Child Neuropsychology* (pp. 239–299). Amsterdam: Elsevier.

Stepien, I., Stepien, L., & Lubinska, E. (1990). Function of dog's auditory cortex in tests involving auditory location cues and directional instrumental response. *Acta Neurobiologiae Experimentalis, 50,* 1–12.

Stiebler, I. & Ehret, G. (1985). Inferior colliculus of the house mouse. I. A quantitative study of tonotopical organization, frequency representation, and tone threshold distribution. *Journal of Comparative Neurology, 238,* 65–76.

Streitfeld, B.D. (1980). The fiber connections of the temporal lobe with emphasis on Rhesus monkey. *International Journal of Neuroscience, 11,* 51–71.

Sudakov, K., MacLean, P.D., Reeves, A., & Marino, R. (1971). Unit study of exteroceptive inputs to claustrocortex in awake, sitting, squirrel monkeys. *Comparative Brain Research, 18,* 19–34.

Sugishita, M., Otomo, K., Yamazaki, K., Shimizu, H., Yoshioka, M., & Shinohara, A. (1995). Dichotic listening in patients with partial section of the corpus callosum. *Brain, 118,* 417–427.

Swadlow, H. (1986). The corpus callosum as a model system of mammalian cerebral axons: A comparison of results from primate and rabbit. In: A.G. Reeves (Ed.), *Epilepsy and the Corpus Callosum* (pp. 55–71). New York: Plenum Press.

Syka, J., Rybalko, N., Mazelova, J., & Druga, R. (2002). Gap detection in the rat before and after auditory cortex ablation. *Hearing Research, 172,* 151–159.

Takeda, S., Hirashima Y., Ikeda H., Yamamoto H., Sugino M., & Endo, S. (2003). Determination of indices of the corpus callosum associated with normal aging in Japanese individuals. *Neuroradiology, 45,* 513–518.

Tallal, P., Miller, S.L., Bedi, G., Byma, G., Wang, X., Nagarajan, S.S., Schreiner, C., Jenkins, W.M., & Merzenich, M.M. (1996). Language comprehension in language-learning impaired children improved with acoustically modified speech. *Science, 271,* 81–84.

Talmadge, C.L., Long, G.R., Murphy, W.J., & Tubis, A. (1993). New off-line method for detecting spontaneous otoacoustic emissions in human subjects. *Hearing Research, 71,* 170–182.

Talwar, S.K., Musial, P.G., & Gerstein, G.L. (2001). Role of mammalian auditory cortex in the perception of elementary sound properties. *Journal of Neurophysiology, 85*, 2350–2358.

Tanriover, N., Kawashima, M., Rhoton, A.L., Ulm, A.J., & Mericle, R.A. (2003). Microsurgical anatomy of the early branches of the middle cerebral artery: Morphometric analysis and classification with angiographic correlation. *Journal of Neurosurgery, 98*, 1277–1290.

Tasaki, I., Davis, H., & Eldredge, D. (1954). Exploration of cochlear potentials with a microelectrode. *Journal of the Acoustical Society of America, 26*, 765–773.

Terr, L.I. & Edgerton, B.J. (1985). Three dimensional reconstruction of the cochlear nuclear complex in humans. *Archives of Otolaryngology, 111*, 495–501.

Thai-Van, H., Bounaix, M.J., & Fraysse, B. (2001). Meniere's disease: Pathophysiology and treatment. *Drugs, 61*, 1089–1102.

Thompson, M.E. & Abel, S.M. (1992a). Indices of hearing in patients with central auditory pathologies. I. Detection and discrimination. *Scandinavian Audiology, 35* (Suppl.) 3–15.

Thompson, M.E. & Abel, S.M. (1992b). Indices of hearing in patients with central auditory pathology. II. Choice response times. *Scandinavian Audiology, 35*, (Suppl.) 17–22.

Thompson, P., Narr, K., Blanton, R., & Toga, A. (2003). Mapping structural alterations of the corpus callosum during brain development and degeneration. In: E. Zaidel & M. Iacoboni (Eds.), *The Parallel Brain: The Cognitive Neuroscience of the Corpus Callosum* (pp. 93–130). Cambridge, MA: MIT Press.

Thornton, A.R., Mendel, M.I., & Anderson, C.V. (1977). Effects of stimulus frequency and intensity on the middle latency components of the averaged auditory electroencephalic response. *Journal of Speech and Hearing Research, 20*, 81–94.

Tobias, J.M. & Zerlin, S. (1959). Lateralization threshold as a function of stimulus duration. *Journal of the Acoustical Society of America, 31*, 1591–1594.

Tonndorf, J. (1957). The mechanism of hearing loss in early cases of endolymphatic hydrops. *Annals of Otology, Rhinology, and Laryngology, 66*, 766–784.

Tonndorf, J. (1960). Response of cochlear models to aperiodic signals and to random noises, *Journal of the Acoustical Society of America, 32*, 1344–1355.

Tonndorf, J. & Khanna, S.M. (1968). Submicroscopic displacement amplitudes of the tympanic membrane (cat) measured by laser interferometer. *Journal of the Acoustical Society of America, 44*, 1546–1554.

Tonnquist-Uhlen, I. (1996). Topography of auditory evoked cortical potentials in children with severe language impairment. *Scandinavian Audiology, 44* (Suppl.) 1–40.

Trautwein, P., Hofstetter, P., Wang, J., Salvi, R., & Nostrant, A. (1996). Selective inner hair cell loss does not alter distortion product otoacoustic emissions. *Hearing Research, 96*, 71–82.

Tsuchitani, C. (1977). Functional organization of lateral cell groups of cat superior olivary complex. *Journal of Neurophysiology, 40*, 296–318.

Tsuzuku, T. (1993). 40-Hz steady state response in awake cats after bilateral chronic lesions in auditory cortices or inferior colliculi. *Auris Nasus Larynx, 20*, 263–274.

Ture, U., Yasargil, D.C., Al-Mefty, O., & Yasargil, M.G. (1999). Topographic anatomy of the insular region. *Journal of Neurosurgery, 90*, 720–733.

Van Wagenen, W.P. & Herren, R.Y. (1940). Surgical division of commissural pathways in the corpus callosum. Relation to spread of an epilcptic attack. *Archives of Neurology and Psychiatry, 44*, 740–759.

Velasco, M., Velasco, F., Almanza, X., & Coats, A.C. (1982). Subcortical correlates of the auditory brain stem potentials in man: Bipolar EEG and multiple unit activity and electrical stimulation. *Electroencephalography and Clinical Neurophysiology, 53*, 133–142.

Villa, A.E. (1990). Physiological differentiation within the auditory part of the thalamic reticular nucleus of the cat. *Brain Research Reviews, 15*, 25–40.

von Bekesy, G. (1936). Zur physic des mittelohres und uber das horen bei fehlerhaftem trommelfell, *Akustik, Zeitshrift, 1*, 13–23.

von Bekesy, G. (1941). Uber die messung der schwingungsamplitude der gehorknochelchen mittels einer kapizitvien sonde, *Akustik, Zeitschrift, 6*, 1–16.

von Bekesy, G. (1947). The variation of phase along the basilar membrane with sinusoidal vibrations. *Journal of the Acoustical Society of America, 19*, 452–460.

von Bekesy, G. (1953). Description of some mechanical properties of the organ of Corti. *Journal of the Acoustical Society of America, 25*, 770–785.

von Bekesy, G. (1960). *Experiments in Hearing*. New York: McGraw Hill.

von Bekesy, G. (1970). Traveling waves as frequency analyzers of the cochlea. *Nature, 225*, 1207–1209.

Wada, J.A., Clarke, R., & Hamm, A. (1975). Cerebral asymmetry in humans. Cortical speech zones in 100 adults and 100 infant brains. *Archives of Neurology, 32*, 239–246.

Wada, S.I. & Starr, A. (1983). Generation of the auditory brainstem responses (ABRs). III. Effects of lesions of the superior olive, lateral lemniscus, and inferior colliculus on the ABR in guinea pig. *Electroencephalography and Clinical Neurophysiology, 56*, 352–366.

Waddington, M. (1974). *Atlas of Cerebral Angiography with Anatomic Correlation*. Boston: Little, Brown and Company.

Waddington, M. (1984). *Atlas of Human Intracranial Anatomy*. Rutland VT: Academy Books.

Walton, J.P., Frisina, R.D., Ison, J.R., & O'Neill, W.E. (1997). Neural correlates of behavioral gap detection in the inferior colliculus of young CBA mouse. *Journal of Comparative Physiology, 181*, 161–176.

Walton, J.P., Frisina, R.D., & O'Neill, W.E. (1998) Age-related alteration in processing of sound features in the auditory midbrain of the CBA mouse. *Journal of Neuroscience, 18*, 2764–2776.

Wang, J., Powers, N.L., Hofstetter, P., Trautwein, P., Ding, D., & Salvi, R. (1997). Effect of selective inner hair cell loss on auditory nerve fiber threshold, tuning, spontaneous and driven discharge rate. *Hearing Research, 107*, 67–82.

Wangemann, P. (2002a). K+ cycling and the endocochlear potential. *Hearing Research, 165*, 1–9.

Wangemann, P. (2002b). K(+) cycling and its regulation in the cochlea and the vestibular labyrinth. *Audiology and Neurootology, 7*, 199–205.

Wangemann, P. & Schacht, J. (1996). Homoestatic mechanisms in the cochlea. In: P. Dallos, A.N. Popper, & R.R. Fay (Eds.), *The Cochlea* (pp. 130–185). New York: Springer-Verlag.

Warr, W.B. (1980). Efferent components of the auditory system. *Annals of Otorhinolaryngology, 89(Suppl.),* 114–120.

Warr, W.B. (1992). Organization of olivocochlear efferent systems in mammals. In: D.B. Webster, A.N. Popper, & R.R. Fay (Eds.), *The Mammalian Auditory Pathway: Neuroanatomy* (pp. 410–448). New York: Springer-Verlag.

Warr, W.B., Guinan, J.J., & White, J.S. (1986). Organization of the efferent fibers: The lateral and medial olivocochlear systems. In: R.A. Altschuler, R.P. Bobbin, & D.W. Hoffman (Eds.), *Neurobiology of Hearing: The Cochlea* (pp. 333–348). New York: Raven Press.

Watanabe, T., Yanagisawa, K., Kanzaki, J., & Katsuki, Y. (1966). Cortical efferent flow influencing unit responses of medial geniculate body to sound stimulation. *Experimental Brain Research, 2,* 302–317.

Webster, M. & Webster, D.B. (1981). Spiral ganglion neuron loss following organ of Corti loss: A quantitative study. *Brain Research, 212,* 17–30.

Weider, D.J. (1992). Treatment and management of perilymphatic fistula: A New Hampshire experience. *The American Journal of Otology, 13,* 158–166.

Wenthold, R. (1991). Neurotransmitters of brainstem auditory nuclei. In: R.A. Altschuler, R.P. Bobbin, B.M. Clopton, & D.W. Hoffman (Eds.), *Neurobiology of Hearing: The Central Auditory System* (pp. 121–140). New York: Raven Press.

Wenthold, R.J. (1978). Glutamic acid and aspartic acid in subdivisions of the cochlear nucleus after auditory nerve lesion. *Brain Research, 143,* 544–548.

Wenthold, R., Hunter, C., & Petralia, R. (1993). Excitatory amino acid in the rat cochlear nucleus. In: M. Merchan, J. Juiz, D. Godfrey, & E. Mugnaina (Eds.), *The Mammalian Cochlear Nuclei: Organization and Function* (pp. 179–194). New York: Plenum Press.

Wester, K., Irvine, D.R., & Hugdahl, K. (2001). Auditory laterality and attentional deficits after thalamic haemorrhage. *Journal of Neurology, 248,* 676–683.

Wever, E.G. & Bray, C.W. (1930). Action currents in the auditory nerve in response to acoustical stimulation. *Proceedings of the National Academy of Sciences of the United States of America, 16,* 344–350.

Whitehead, M.L., McCoy, M.J., Lonsbury-Martin, B.L., & Martin, G.K. (1995). Dependence of distortion-product otoacoustic emissions on primary levels in normal and impaired ears. I. Effects of decreasing L2 below L1. *Journal of the Acoustical Society of America, 97,* 2346–2358.

Whiteside, S.P. & Cowell, P.E. (2001). Comment on delayed left-ear accuracy in dichotic listening. *Perceptual and Motor Skills, 92,* 548–550.

Whitfield, I.C. & Evans, E.F. (1965). Responses of auditory cortical neurons to stimuli of changing frequency. *Journal of Neurophysiology, 28,* 655–672.

Wiederhold, M.L. & Kiang, N.Y.S. (1970). Effect of electrical stimulation of the crossed olivocochlear bundle on single auditory-nerve fibers in the cat. *Journal of the Acoustical Society of America, 4,* 950–965.

Wiener, F.M. & Ross, D.A. (1946). Pressure distribution in the auditory canal in a progressive sound field. *Journal of the Acoustical Society of America, 18,* 401–408.

Wilkinson, I. (1988). *Central Neurology.* Boston: Blackwell Scientific Publications.

Williams, E.A., Brookes, G.B., & Prasher, D.K. (1994). Effects of olivocochlear bundle section on otoacoustic emissions in humans: Efferent effects in comparison with control subjects. *Acta Otolaryngologica, 114,* 121–129.

Wilson, R.H. & McBride, L.M. (1978). Threshold and growth of the acoustic reflex. *Journal of the Acoustical Society of America, 63,* 147–154.

Wilson, RH. & Margolis, R.H. (1999). Acoustic-reflex measurements. In: F.E. Musiek & W.F. Rintelmann (Eds.), *Contemporary Perspectives in Hearing Assessment* (pp. 131–166). Boston: Allyn & Bacon.

Winer, J.A. (1984a). The non-pyramidal cells in layer III of cat primary auditory cortex (AI). *Journal of Comparative Neurology, 229,* 512–530.

Winer, J.A. (1984b). Anatomy of layer IV in cat primary auditory cortex (AI). *Journal of Comparative Neurology, 224,* 535–567.

Winer J.A. (1984c). The pyramidal neurons in layer III of the cat primary cortex (AI). *Journal of Comparative Neurology, 229,* 476–496.

Winer, J.A. (1985). Structure of layer II in cat primary auditory cortex (AI). *Journal of Comparative Neurology, 238,* 10–37.

Winer, J.A. (1992). The functional architecture of the medial geniculate body in primary auditory cortex. In: D.B. Webster, A.N. Popper, & R.R. Fay (Eds.), *The Mammalian Auditory Pathway: Neuroanatomy* (pp. 222–409). New York: Springer-Verlag.

Winer, J.A. & Morest, D.K. (1983). The neuronal architecture of the dorsal division of the medial geniculate body of the cat: A study with the rapid Golgi method. *Journal of Comparative Neurology, 221,* 1–30.

Winslow, R.L. & Sachs, M.B. (1987). Effects of electric stimulation of the crossed olivocochlear bundle on auditory nerve response to tones in noise. *Journal of Neurophysiology, 57,* 1002–1021.

Winslow, R.L. & Sachs, M.B. (1988). Single-tone intensity discrimination based on auditory-nerve rate responses in backgrounds of quiet, noise, and with stimulation of the crossed olivocochlear bundle. *Hearing Research, 35,* 165–189.

Wit, H.P., Feijen, R.A., & Albers, F.W. (2003). Cochlear aqueduct flow resistance is not constant during evoked inner ear pressure change in the guinea pig. *Hearing Research, 175,* 190–199.

Withnell, R.H., Yates, G.K., & Kirk, D.L. (2000). Changes to low-frequency components of the TEOAE following acoustic trauma to the base of the cochlea. *Hearing Research, 139,* 1–12.

Wlodyka, J. (1978). Studies on cochlear aqueduct patency. *Annals of Otology, Rhinology, and Laryngology, 87,* 22–28.

Wollberg, Z. & Newman, J.D. (1972). Auditory cortex of squirrel monkey: Response patterns of single cells to species-specific vocalizations. *Science, 175,* 212–214.

Woolsey, C. (1960). Organization of cortical auditory system: A revealing synthesis. In: G.L. Rasmussen & W.F. Windle (Eds.), *Neural Mechanisms of the Auditory and Vestibular Systems* (pp. 125–185). Springfield, IL: Charles C. Thomas Publishers.

Woolsey, C. (1964). Electrophysiological studies on thalamocortical relations in the auditory system. In: A. Abrams, H.H. Gamer, & J.E.D. Toman (Eds.), *Unfinished Tasks in the Behavioral Sciences* (pp. 45–57). Baltimore: Williams and Wilkins.

Wright, A. (1981) Scanning electron microscopy of the human cochlea: The organ of Corti. *Archives of Otorhinolaryngology, 230*, 11–19.

Wright, A. (1984). Dimensions of the cochlea stereocilia in man and guinea pig. *Hearing Research, 13*, 89–98.

Xue, S., Mountain, D.C., & Hubbard, A.E. (1995a). Acoustic enhancement of electrically evoked otoacoustic emissions reflects basilar membrane tuning: A model. *Hearing Research, 91*, 93–100.

Xue, S., Mountain, D.C., & Hubbard, A.E. (1995b). Electrically evoked basilar membrane motion. *Journal of the Acoustical Society of America, 97*, 3030–3041.

Yakovlev, P.I. & LeCours, A. (1967). *Regional Development of the Brain.* Oxford, England: Blackwell.

Yaniv, D., Schafe, G.E., LeDoux, J.E., & Richter-Levin, G. (2001). A gradient of plasticity in the amygdala revealed by cortical and subcortical stimulation, in vivo. *Neuroscience, 106*, 613–620.

Yeomens, J.S. & Franklind, P.W. (1995). The acoustic startle reflex: Neurons and connections. *Brain Research Review, 21*, 301–314.

Yirmiya, R. & Hocherman, S. (1987). Auditory- and movement-related neural activity interact in the pulvinar of the behaving Rhesus monkey. *Brain Research, 402*, 93–102.

Yost, W.A. (2000). *Fundamentals of Hearing: An Introduction* (4th ed.). San Diego: Academic Press.

Yvert, B., Fischer, C., Guenot, M., Krolak-Salmon, P., Isnard, J., & Pernier, K. (2002). Simultaneous intracerebral EEG recordings of early auditory thalamic and cortical activity in human. *European Journal of Neuroscience, 16*, 1146–1150.

Zappia, J.J. & Altschuler, R.A. (1989). Evaluation of the effect of ototopical neomycin on spiral ganglion cell density in the guinea pig. *Hearing Research, 40*, 29–37.

Zappoli, R. (2003). Permanent or transitory effects on neurocognitive components of the CNV induced by brain dysfunctions, lesions and ablations in humans. *International Journal of Psychophysiology, 48*, 189–220.

Zappoli, R., Zappoli, F., Picchiecchio, A., Chiaramonti, R., Grazia Ameodo, M., Zappoli Thyrion, G.D., & Zerauschek, V. (2002). Frontal and parieto-temporal cortical ablations and diaschisis-like effects on auditory neurocognitive potentials evocable from apparently intact ipsilateral association areas in humans: Five case reports. *International Journal of Psychophysiology, 44*, 117–142.

Zatorre, R.J. (1988). Pitch perception of complex tones in human temporal-lobe function. *Journal of the Acoustical Society of America, 84*, 566–572.

Zatorre, R.J., Evans, A.C., Meyer, E., & Gjedde, A. (1992). Lateralization of phonetic and pitch discrimination in speech processing. *Science, 256*, 846–849.

Zatorre, R.J. & Penhune, V.B. (2001). Spatial localization after excision of human auditory cortex. *Journal of Neuroscience, 21*, 6321–6328.

Zemlin, W.R. (1998). *Speech and Hearing Science: Anatomy and Physiology* (4th ed.). Boston: Allyn & Bacon.

Zhao, S.R. & Wei, B.L. (1989). Origin of the auditory middle latency response Pa in guinea pig. *Sheng Li Xue Bao, 41*, 308–312.

Zheng, J., Shen, W., He, D.Z., Long, K.B., Madison, L.D., & Dallos, P. (2000). Prestin is the motor protein of cochlear outer hair cells. *Nature, 405*, 149–155.

Zheng, X.Y., Ding, D.L., McFadden, S.L., & Henderson, D. (1997). Evidence that inner hair cells are the major source of cochlear summating potentials. *Hearing Research, 113*, 76–88.

Zrull, M.C. & Coleman, J.R. (1996). Effects of tectal grafts on sound detection deficits induced by inferior colliculus lesions in hooded rats. *Cell Transplantation, 5*, 293–304.

Zwislocki, J.J. (2002). *Auditory Sound Transmission: An Autobiographical Perspective.* Philadelphia: Lawrence Erlbaum Associates.

Zwislocki, J.J. & Sokolich, W.G. (1973). Velocity and displacement responses in auditory nerve fibers. *Science, 182*, 64–66.

Index